Mental Disorder

Mental Disorder

Publisher: iConcept Press Ltd.
Cover design: Pineapple Design Ltd.
Interior design: iConcept Press Ltd.
Typesetting and copy editing: iConcept Press Ltd. and Pineapple Design Ltd.

ISBN: 978-1-922227-96-6

Printed in the United States of America

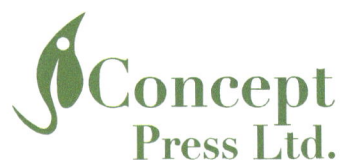

iConcept
Press Ltd.

www.iconceptpress.com

Contents

Preface

Mental disorder is a psychological pattern or anomaly, potentially reflected in behaviour, that is generally associated with distress or disability, and which is not considered part of normal development in a person's culture. The recognition and understanding of mental health conditions have changed over time and across cultures and there are still variations in definition, assessment and classification. The causes of mental disorders are varied and in some cases unclear, and theories may incorporate findings from a range of fields. Services are based in psychiatric hospitals or in the community, and assessments are carried out by psychiatrists, clinical psychologists and clinical social workers, using various methods but often relying on observation and questioning. *Mental Disorder* explains the latest research on mental disorders. It serves as an essential start to mastering the science and art of clinical practice.

There are totally 10 chapters in this book. Chapter 1 examines youth suicide ideation from a cross-cultural perspective and to focus specifically on gender differences by examining data from 19 countries and cities. Chapter 2 examines the relationship between the locus of control scale as an indicator of internality-externality and the Kessler 10 scale as an indicator of psychological distress, and analyses the effects of socio-demographic and employment-related factors on this relationship. The results of this study may help improve mental health clinicians' understanding of psychological distress in workplaces, as well as guide mental health promotion, prevention, and screening programs to target relevant factors and populations. Chapter 3 examines the prevalence of mental health issues and future aspirations among service-seeking youth living in the slums of Kampala. Chapter 4 reviews the literature regarding cognitive deficits in children with type 1 diabetes mellitus as well as explores original research investigating prospective memory in this cohort. This study demonstrates the need for additional studies clarifying the relationship between prospective memory and glycemic control.

Chapter 5 discusses HCV (Hepatitis C Virus) among patients with mental disorders. Guidelines and universal strategies are suggested to minimize, prevent and treat HCV among patients with mental patients. Future prospects and new concepts in modeling HCV among these patients have also been highlighted and evaluated in this chapter. Chapter 6 compares a single (pharmacological treatment) versus a multi-element interventions (pharmacological treatment, social skills training, psychoeducation for relatives and family therapy for first episode-psychosis patients and their relatives) know as integrated treatment to determine clinical and functional outcome improvements. It shows that a greater proportion of patients receiving integrated treatment fulfilled the remission criteria and a higher psychosocial functioning improvement when compared to those receiving standard treatment. In addition, a higher number of patients of integrated treatment fulfilled both criteria: symptomatic remission and a better level of psychosocial functioning achieving better functional outcome compared to patients of standard treatment. Chapter 7 describes concept of social anxiety disorder, and presents recent evidence-based treatment algorithm and available further treatment options for them including pharmacotherapy and psychotherapy. Chapter 8 focuses on delayed matching-to-sample procedures that could be useful for identifying problems of short-term memory in people with dementia. The results with use of a titrated delayed matching-to-sample, showed that small titrating steps were more useful than larger titrating steps.

Chapter 9 presents the process of adult hippocampal neurogenesis and its relationship with neurological disorders, as well as reviews its role in relation to disease etiology, pathogenesis and areas of future therapeutic targeting. Chapter 10 provides knowledge, information and clinical skills that are related to examine Psychosis.

Editing and publishing a book is never an easy task. Each chapter in this book has gone through a peer review, a selection and an editing process so as to guarantee its quality. Without the supports and contributions of the authors and reviewers, this book can never be able to complete. We would like to thank all of the authors in this book and all of the reviewers who participated in the reviewing process: Zena Al-Sharbati, Naeem Aslam, Shervin Assari, Tandy Aye, Paul N. Baird, Rajshekhar Bipeta, Stefan Britsch, Suprakash Chaudhury, Sandhya Cherkil, Qu Cui, L. K. Davis, D. T. Hemanth, Mario Herrera-Marschitz, Lucrezia Islam, Michael Kaess, Reza Khadivi, Remigiusz J. Kijak, Soo-In Kim, Honghua Li, Wei Li, Ivan Y. Lourov, Penelope A. E. Main, Ludise Malkova, Marianne Melau, Pedro J. Modrego, Evalill Nilsson, Susana Ochoa, C. M. Pariante, Susie H. Park, Annemie Ploeger, Ravishankar Rajashree, Enisha Sarin, Vishal Saxena, Akihiro Shiina, N. Shuba, R. Smieskova, Mona Srivastava, Paweł Stankiewicz, Ghada R. A. Taha, Mehdi Tehrani-Doost, J. K. Trivedi, Tuulikki Vehko, Wei Wang and Yung-Chieh Yen. We hope that you, the reader, will find this book interesting and useful. Any advices please feel free and are always welcome to tell us.

iConcept Press Ltd
November 2014

Prevalence and Gender Differences in Suicide Ideation of Youth: A Cross-national Comparison of 19 Countries and Cities

Monica H. Swahn
School of Public Health
Georgia State University, USA

Jane B. Palmier
School of Public Health,
Georgia State University, USA

Sarah M. Braunstein
School of Public Health,
Georgia State University, USA

1   Introduction

Every year, almost one million people die from suicide; a "global" mortality rate of 16 per 100,000, or one death every 40 seconds (World Health Organization [WHO], 2011). Suicide is among the three leading causes of death among those aged 15-44 years in some countries; however, these figures do not include suicide attempts which are up to 20 times more frequent than completed suicide (WHO, 2011). Suicide worldwide is estimated to represent 1.8% of the total global burden of disease in 1998 and escalate to 2.4% in countries with market and former socialist economies in 2020 (WHO, 2011).

In the U.S., where much of the suicide research has been conducted, suicide is the 10th leading cause of death (Centers for Disease Control and Prevention [CDC], 2012a). However, suicide deaths are only part of this public health problem. Fortunately, more people survive suicide attempts than actually die. Those who have attempted suicide are often seriously injured and in need of medical care. As such, injuries from suicide attempts are also an issue that needs attention. For example, while over 38,000 people in the U.S. kill themselves, there are also more than 487,700 people with self-inflicted injuries who are also treated in emergency rooms each year (CDC, 2012b). Suicide, by definition, is fatal. Those who attempt suicide and survive may have serious injuries such as broken bones, brain damage, or organ failure depending on the suicide method used. Also, people who survive a suicide attempt often have depression and other mental health concerns following the attempt. Suicide and suicide attempts also affect the health of the community. Family and friends of people who commit suicide and of those who attempt suicide may feel shock, anger, guilt, and depression. In addition, the medical costs and lost wages associated with suicide also take their toll on the community. It is estimated that the medical and lost work costs of suicide and suicide attempts in the U.S. alone are approximately $41.2 billion combined (CDC, 2012b). Suicidal behavior ranges in degree from merely thinking about ending one's life (suicidal ideation), through developing a plan to commit suicide (suicide planning) and obtaining the means to do so, attempting to kill oneself (suicide attempt), to finally carrying out the act (''completed suicide'') (Krug, E.G., Dahlberg, L.L., Mercy, J.A., Zwi, A.B., & Lozano, R., 2002). Suicide ideation is a critically important part of this continuum and is a prevalent problem for youth.

The focus of this chapter is specifically on suicide ideation among youth from a cross-cultural perspective. There is substantial research conducted on suicide ideation in North America and in Europe; however, research from most other countries remain scarce. As such, cross country comparisons have been limited and any regional or cultural variations with respect to suicide ideation among youth have been difficult if not impossible to ascertain. While definitions of suicide ideation may vary slightly, typically it is defined as thinking about suicide or contemplating a suicide attempt. This issue is particularly relevant for youth. There are three specific goals of this chapter: 1. to briefly summarize the literature on gender differences in suicide ideation among youth; 2. to briefly summarize the literature on differences in suicidal ideation among youth between countries; and 3. to examine empirically the prevalence and gender differences among youth across countries.

1.1   Gender Differences in Suicide Ideation among Youth

There is extensive research on suicide ideation among youth in North America and in Europe (Mark *et al.*, 2013; Swahn *et al.*, 2012a; Scocco, de Girolamo, Vilagut & Alonso, 2008) where suicide prevention research has been prioritized and long standing. From this large body of work, it is very clear that in these regions of the world, there are substantial and consistent gender differences with respect to suicide ideation among youth. In fact, globally, girls appear to have higher rates of suicidal ideation and behavior, but lower rates of suicide mortality than boys (Canetto, 2008). There are numerous studies that report a higher rate of suicidal ideation among girls relative to boys (Grunbaum, Kann, Kinchen, Ross, Hawkins, & Lowry, et al., 2004; Krug et al, 2002; Beautrais, 2002; Bakken & Gunter, 2012; Swahn & Bossarte, 2007; Swahn et al., 2012a) even when examined longitudinally (Boeninger, Masyn, Feldman, & Conger, 2010). As a rough estimate, it is typically noted that girls are twice as likely to report suicide ideation as boys (Beautrais, 2002). Although, while these gender differences are typically observed, there are a few studies that report no gender differences in suicide ideation among youth including a recent study of Catalonian high school students in Spain (Kirchner, Ferrer, Forns, & Zanini, 2011). There is also an emerging body of research that is conducted in countries which have traditionally not examined this issue previously. One recent study in Korea for example, found that suicide ideation differed by gender and that the mean level of suicide ideation was higher among girls than boys in their small sample of adolescents (Sook-Park, Schepp, & Jang, 2006). In India, a very small study also reported that suicide ideation was significantly higher among adolescent girls than boys (Upadhayay & Singh, 2006). Another recent study examined suicidal ideation and attempts in an urban Chinese sample of adolescents and observed several sex-differences (Juan, Xiao-Juan, Jia-Ji, Xin-Wang & Liang, 2010). In their study, girls were significantly more like to report suicidal ideation than boys among those who felt sad or hopeless, but boys were more likely to report suicidal attempts than girls among those who did not feel sad or hopeless. Similarly, recent research from Uganda also indicates that suicide ideation is more common among girls and young women, compared to boys and young men, among youth who live in the slums of Kampala (Swahn et al, 2012b).

Research of U.S. adolescents demonstrates particularly strong gender differences with respect to suicide ideation. Data from the Youth Risk Behavior Survey, a bi-annual, nationally representative surveillance system that surveys high school students continuously, between 1991 and 2011 show persistent gender differences in terms of suicide attempts in the past year (see Figure 1).

These gender differences observed in the U.S. and elsewhere have received great interest and have been examined from a number of different perspectives to determine the underlying factors including any potential gender differences in the developmental trends of suicide ideation among youth (Boeninger et al., 2010). The substantial interest in suicide ideation specifically has been fueled in part because this gender –paradox, typically the gender differences are the opposite of those observed for completed suicide. More specifically, boys or men in the U.S. have higher rates of suicide completion than girls or women (CDC, 2012c). Even in aggregate estimates of the global suicide rates, it is clear that males have substantially higher rates than females (see Figure 2). As such, the key explanatory factors for the higher levels of suicide ideation observed among adolescent girls remain unclear.

1.2   Cross-national Comparisons of Suicide Ideation among Youth

Surprisingly, there are relatively few studies that examine and compare the prevalence of suicide ideation among youth across countries. However, there appears to be a renewed interest in this topic with several recent studies contributing to this important area. As an example, a recent study in Europe compared sex, suicidal ideation, smoking, alcohol use, physical fighting, bullying, and communication with parents among three countries, Estonia, Lithuania, and Luxembourg using data from The Health Behavior in School-Aged Children study. Prevalence of suicide ideation was 13.9% in Estonia, 18.3% in Lithuania, and 17.9% in Luxembourg with an overall proportion of suicide ideation of among the three countries as 16.7% (Mark et al., 2013).

Seriously Considered Attempting Suicide

■ Total   ■ Female   ■ Males

Year	1991	1993	1995	1997	1999	2001	2003	2005	2007	2009	2011
■ Total	29	24.1	24.1	20.5	19.3	19	16.9	16.9	14.5	13.8	15.8
■ Female	37.2	29.6	30.4	27.1	24.9	23.6	21.3	21.8	18.7	17.4	19.3
■ Males	20.8	18.8	18.3	15.1	13.7	14.2	12.8	12	10.3	10.5	12.5

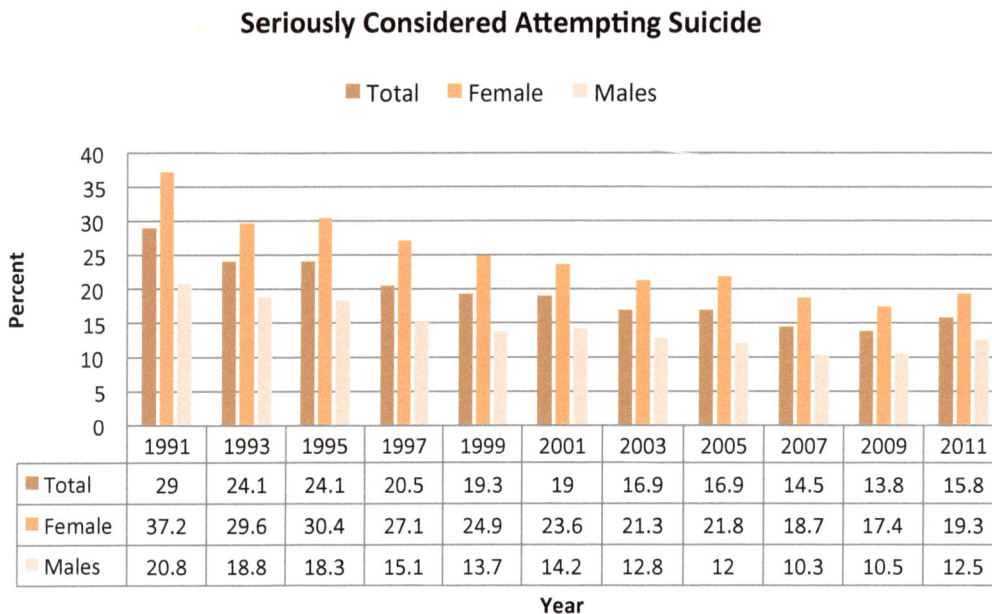

Figure 1: Suicide Ideation defined as seriously considered attempting suicide (12 months prior to survey), from 1991-2011 Youth Risk Behavioral Survey, United States

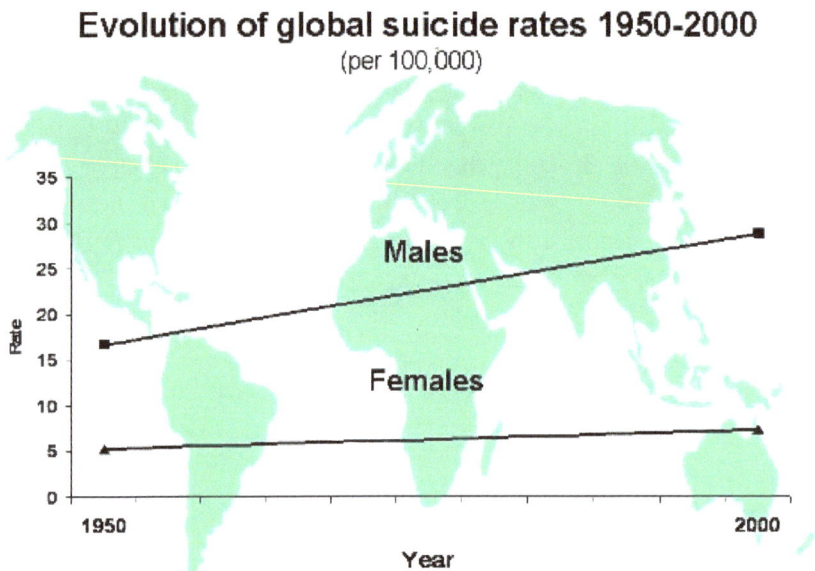

Evolution of global suicide rates 1950-2000
(per 100,000)

Figure 2: "Reproduced, with the permission of the publisher, from *mental health*. Geneva, World Health Organization, 2002 (Evolution 1950-2000 of global suicide rates (per 100,000); http://www.who.int/mental_health/prevention/suicide/evolution/en/index.html, accessed 24 July 2013)".

Similarly, in Asia, a recent study indicates that suicide ideation among urban youth (15-24 years of age) appears higher in Taipei (17.0%), than Shanghai (8.1%) and Hanoi (2.3%) (Blum, Sudhinaraset & Emerson, 2012). Another study of youth (ages 16-34) in rural China demonstrates that about 5.2% report suicidal ideation (Dai *et al.*, 2011). A few previous studies on suicidal behavior among youth in sub-Saharan Africa have been conducted using the Global School-based Student Health Survey (GSHS) (Swahn, Bossarte, Eliman, Gaylor & Jayaraman, 2010a; Rudatsikira, Muula, Siziya & Twa-Twa, 2007a; Rudatsikira, Siziya, & Muula, 2007; Muula, Kazembe, Rudatsikira & Siziya, 2007; Omigbodun *et al.*, 2008). These studies demonstrate substantial differences in the prevalence of suicide ideation ranging from 18.5% to 8.6%. In Zambia the prevalence was 18.5%, in Kenya, 16.4%, in Botswana, 12.7%, and in Uganda, 8.6% (Swahn *et al.*, 2010a) (see Figure 3).

It appears that of all the regions in the world, the levels of suicide ideation appear particularly high in sub-Saharan Africa although this region is among the least represented in the scientific literature (Schlebusch, Burrows, & Vawda, 2009). There is a clear need for epidemiologic data on suicide and suicidal behaviors in Africa and other underserved regions.

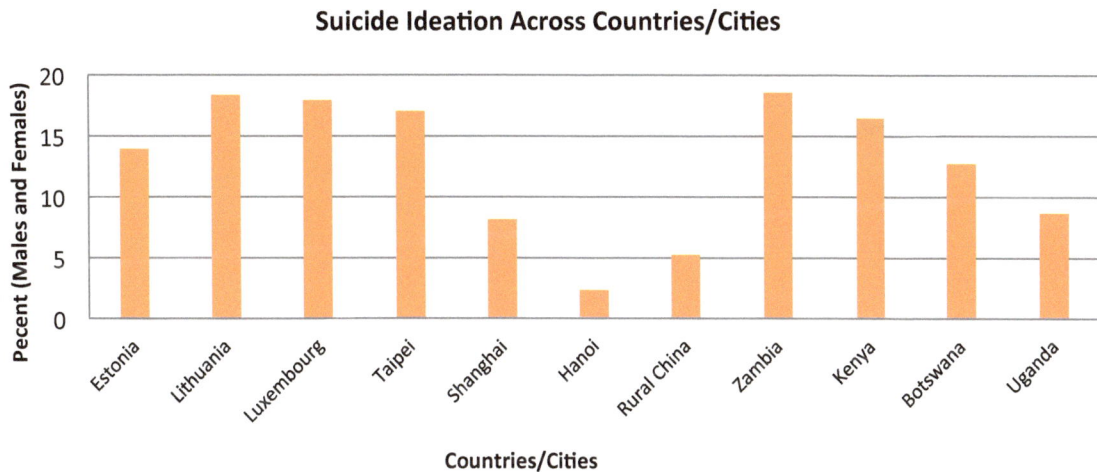

Figure 3: Prevalence of Suicide Ideation in Countries and Cities from prior studies (Mark *et al.*, 2013; Blum *et al.*, 2012; Dai *et al.*, 2011; Swahn *et al.*, 2010a).

1.3 Data Collection to Address Need for Cross-national Comparisons of Youth Health Behaviors

In an effort to obtain more information on youth health and behavior around the world (primarily South America, Africa and Asia), the World Health Organization and the Centers for Disease Control and Prevention created the Global School-based Student Health Survey (GSHS), which has been implemented in over 40 countries (CDC, 2009a; WHO, 2009a). The GSHS datasets will be used in this study to gain an understanding of suicidal ideation among students across 19 countries and cities. This information can be used to provide an overview of suicide ideation among youth across countries and cultures by highlighting similarities and differences. As mentioned previously, data on suicide ideation or suicide behavior are scarce across some regions of the world and have been largely absent in discussion of prevention and intervention strategies aimed at youth. As such, these basic descriptive data analyses fill a void in the current literature by demonstrating the basic self-reported levels of suicide ideation by youth. Moreover, analyses presented separately for boys and girls are prioritized so that analyses and discussion of potential gender differences can be initiated regarding any cross-national patterns and findings and also to guide strategies for prevention and intervention efforts for school-attending youth.

2   Methods

The current study is based on data from the Global School-based Student Health Survey (GSHS) (CDC, 2009a; WHO, 2009a). The GSHS was developed and supported by the World Health Organization in collaboration with the United Nations Children's Fund, the United Nations Educational, Scientific, and Cultural Organization, the Joint United Nations Programme on HIV/AIDS, and with technical assistance from the Centers for Disease Control and Prevention. The goal of the GSHS is to provide data on health behaviors and relevant risk and protective factors among students across all regions served by the United Nations. Country specific questionnaires, fact sheets, public-use data files, documentation and reports are publicly available from the Centers for Disease Control and Prevention and the World Health Organization and have been described in more detail elsewhere (WHO, 2009b). Briefly, the GSHS is comprised of a self-report questionnaire, administered primarily to students aged 13 to 16 years-old. The survey uses a standardized scientific sample selection process, common school-based methodology, and a combination of core questionnaire modules, core-expanded questions, and country-specific questions.

This study conducted secondary analyses of the publicly available data files for 19 countries (see Figure 4). The 17 countries were selected because a complete nationally-representative data file was publicly available at the time of the initiation of our analyses. Additionally, two cities (i.e., Dar Es Salam in Tanzania and Beijing in China) were also included to provide a more balanced representation of regions where limited data were included. All selected countries and cities used a two-stage cluster sample design. The first stage selected schools with probability proportional to enrollment size and the second stage randomly selected classrooms in participating schools. All students in selected classrooms were eligible to participate in the survey.

As a means of comparison, this study also included information from the biannual, nationally representative Youth Risk Behavior Survey (YRBS) of high school students in the United States (CDC, 2013). To maintain comparability with data from the GSHS, this study analyzed data from the 2009 YRBS (N=16,410). U.S. high school students voluntarily completed the anonymous, self-administered questionnaire in school following local parental permission procedures. All 9th through 12th grade students in public, Catholic, or other private schools in the 50 states and District of Columbia were included in the sampling frame (CDC, 2009b).

The details of the sample and survey details including the year of data collection, sample size, response rates and sex distribution are presented in Table 1. More specifically, all surveys were conducted between 2003 and 2009. Also, the sample sizes ranged from 1,212 (Guyana) to 15,790 in the United Arab Emirates. The U.S. sample was 16,410. School response rates were generally good. U.S. had the lowest school response rate (82%). All other countries exceeded 92% response rate. Similarly, student response rates were also generally good and all countries exceeding 75%. Combining the school response and student response rate yielded the participation rate which ranged from a low of 69% in Uganda to the highest of 99% in China (Beijing). Lastly, the distribution of boys and girls were nearly split in half with no country exceeding a 5% differential.

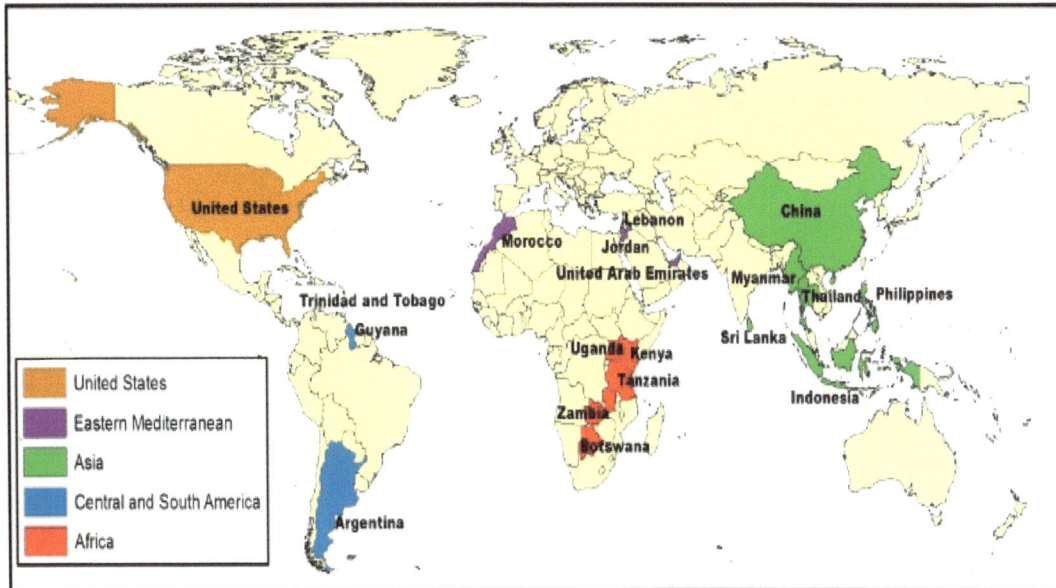

Figure 4: Map of Regions and Countries where the Global School Based Student Health Surveys were conducted and that were included in the current analysis.

Analyses of these complex multistage surveys were conducted with the SAS 9.2 and SUDAAN 10 statistical software packages to accommodate the sampling design and to produce weighted estimates. Approval to conduct these analyses was obtained from the Georgia State University Institutional Review Board.

The prevalence of suicide ideation was assessed by one survey question which asked students to report if they had seriously considered attempting suicide in last 12 months. For ease of analyses and presentation, we dichotomized this measure to indicate any versus no suicide ideation in the past year. The wording of the question in the GSHS and YRBS was equivalent. Bivariate regression analyses were conducted to determine gender differences in the prevalence of suicide ideation across the selected countries, with girls used as the reference group.

3 Results

The prevalence of suicide ideation in the past year across the countries and cities examined varied from 1.15% in Myanmar to 31.47% in Zambia (Table 2). For boys the prevalence of suicide ideation varied from 1.14% to 31.43% and for girls it varied from 1.16% to 31.51% (Table 2).

Gender differences were also examined. In most countries, there were no statistically significant differences with respect to suicide ideation. However, in seven countries, statistically significant differences were observed between boys and girls in that boys were significantly <u>less</u> likely than girls to report suicide ideation. These differences were noted in the following countries: Argentina (OR=0.66; 95% CI:0.46-0.93), Guyana (OR=0.64; 95% CI:0.45-0.89), Trinidad/Tobago (OR=0.60; 95% CI:0.45-0.82), Lebanon (OR=0.80; 95% CI:0.68-0.94), Morocco (OR=0.74; 95% CI:0.56-0.98), Uganda (OR=0.73; 95% CI:0.59-0.92) and the U.S. (OR=0.55; 95% CI:0.48-0.64).

Country	Year	Total Sample	Type of Representation	School Response Rate	Student Response Rate	Participation Rate	Boys Wtd. %	Girls Wtd. %
AFRICA								
Botswana	2005	2,197	National	100%	95%	95%	45.0%	55.0%
Kenya	2003	3,691	National	96%	87%	84%	48.7%	51.3%
Uganda	2003	3,215	National	90%	76%	69%	51.2%	48.8%
Tanzania	2006	2,176	Dar Es Salaam	100%	87%	87%	47.9%	52.1%
Zambia	2004	2,257	National	94%	75%	70%	48.9%	51.1%
CENTRAL AND SOUTH AMERICA								
Argentina	2007	1,980	National	94%	82%	77%	48.0%	52.0%
Guyana	2004	1,212	National	100%	80%	80%	49.0%	51.0%
Trinidad and Tobago	2007	2,969	National	100%	78%	78%	49.8%	50.2%
ASIA								
Indonesia	2007	3,116	National	98%	95%	93%	49.9%	50.1%
Myanmar	2007	2,806	National	100%	95%	95%	50.8%	49.2%
Sri Lanka	2008	2,611	National	100%	89%	89%	50.0%	50.0%
Thailand	2008	2,767	National	100%	93%	93%	48.5%	51.5%
China	2003	2,348	Beijing	100%	99%	99%	50.5%	49.5%
Philippines	2003	7,338	National	99%	85%	84%	43.2%	56.8%
EASTERN MEDITERRANEAN								
Jordan	2004	2,457	National	100%	95%	95%	50.3%	49.7%
Lebanon	2005	5,115	National	92%	96%	88%	47.7%	52.3%
Morocco	2006	2,670	National	100%	84%	84%	54.7%	45.3%
United Arab Emirates	2005	15,790	National	97%	91%	89%	50.0%	50.0%
UNITED STATES								
US	2009	16,410	National	81%	88%	71%	47.8%	52.2%

Table 1: Survey Details and Sample Characteristics of the Global School Based Student Health Surveys included in the analyses.

The distribution of the mean prevalence suicide ideation across the regions is presented in Figure 5. The highest mean prevalence of suicide ideation was noted in the African region (22.63%) followed by the Central and Southern American Region (17.74%), the Eastern Mediterranean (14.56%), the U.S. (13.78%) and Asia (9.32%). With the U.S. excluded, one-way ANOVA determined that the prevalence of suicide varies significantly by region (F (3, 14) = 5.450, p <.05), however, post hoc testing revealed that Africa and Asia were the only regions that were significantly different.

Country	Prevalence of Suicide Ideation %			Bivariate Logistic Regression Analysis of the Association between Gender and Suicide Ideation	
	AFRICA				
	Overall	Boys	Girls	OR*	OR (95% CI)
Botswana	22.89	21.70	23.97	0.88	0.67 – 1.16
Kenya	27.90	27.52	28.26	0.96	0.74 – 1.26
Uganda	19.60	17.24	22.11	**0.73**	**0.59 – 0.92**
Tanzania	11.31	11.64	11.04	1.06	0.82 – 1.38
Zambia*	31.47	31.43	31.51	1.00	0.76 – 1.30
	CENTRAL AND SOUTH AMERICA				
Argentina	17.00	13.96	19.78	**0.66**	**0.46 – 0.93**
Guyana	18.37	14.91	21.63	**0.64**	**0.45 – 0.89**
Trinidad and Tobago	17.86	14.15	21.47	**0.60**	**0.45 – 0.82**
	ASIA				
Indonesia	4.23	3.52	4.94	0.70	0.49 – 1.00
Myanmar*	1.15	1.14	1.16	0.98	0.57 – 1.69
Sri Lanka	10.32	11.39	9.26	1.26	0.89 – 1.79
Thailand	8.78	9.94	7.72	1.32	0.87 – 1.99
China	14.26	13.35	15.18	0.86	0.70 – 1.06
Philippines	17.16	18.44	16.20	1.17	0.98 – 1.39
	EASTERN MEDITERRANEAN				
Jordan	15.38	13.48	17.25	0.75	0.52 – 1.07
Lebanon	16.06	14.49	17.49	**0.80**	**0.68 – 0.94**
Morocco	13.86	12.19	15.83	**0.74**	**0.56 – 0.98**
United Arab Emirates	12.92	13.38	12.47	1.08	0.91 – 1.30
	UNITED STATES				
US	13.78	10.47	17.41	**0.55**	**0.48 – 0.64**

*Note females are the reference group.

Table 2: Prevalence and Gender Difference in Suicide Ideation across 19 Countries and 2 Cities.

4   Discussion

This study examines cross-national population-based data to report on the prevalence of suicide ideation across countries and regions of the world. Our study shows that suicide ideation varies dramatically across regions and that while it is a rare experience in some parts of the world, it is relatively common in other places. Most noteworthy, the African region overall had the highest mean prevalence of suicide ideation. Statistically speaking, when excluding the United States, the only significant difference was observed between Africa and Asia. This is very troubling given the limited resources and attention to mental health concerns in the African region (Schlebusch *et al.*, 2009).

As has been discussed in recent research (Swahn *et al.*, 2012b), suicidal behavior in Africa was thought to be rare in the past.

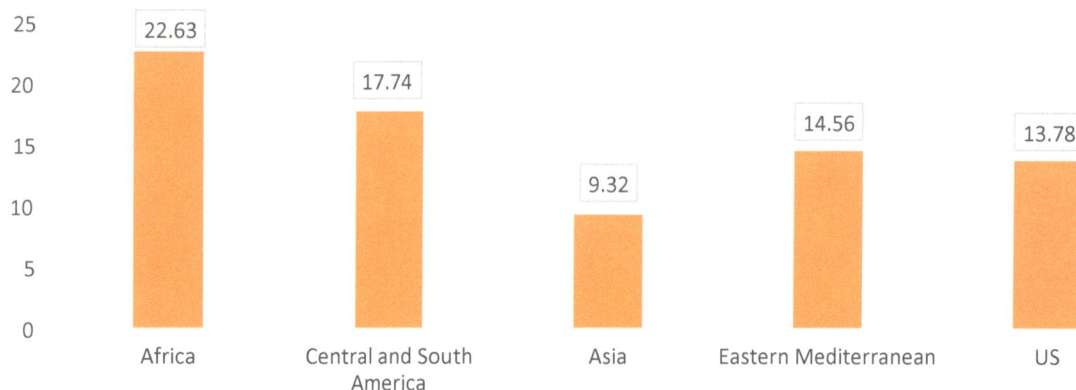

Figure 5: Mean Prevalence of Suicide by Region and for the US.

However, new findings suggest that suicidal behaviors represent a substantial public health burden (Ovuga, Boardman & Wassermann, 2005; Bertolote & Fleischmann, 2009) which is confirmed by our comparisons. Findings from previous research of youth in Nigeria, South Africa, Zambia, and Uganda (Swahn *et al.*, 2010a; Rudatsikira *et al.*, 2007a; Rudatsikira *et al.*, 2007b; Muula *et al.*, 2007; Omigbodun *et al.*, 2008) indicate that suicidal behavior is relatively common, but also varies across countries (Swahn *et al* 2010a) within the African continent.

While this study cannot possibly begin to explain the high levels of suicidal ideation among youth in sub-Saharan Africa, it is reasonable to speculate that mental health concerns among youth may have been exacerbated by the severe psychosocial stress and other adverse health outcomes associated with the high prevalence of HIV/AIDS in Africa (Krug *et al.*, 2002) as well as scarce food supply in some settings (Swahn, Bossarte, Eliman, Gaylor & Walingo, 2010b; FAO agriculture fact sheet) and other distressing circumstances (Swahn *et al.*, 2012b). In addition, the stigma, discrimination, isolation, lack of support from family and friends, loss of parents or family members from HIV/AIDS further increases the risk of suicidal behavior (Schlebusch *et al.*, 2009). However, these factors need to be considered in future research of the underlying factors that may contribute to suicide ideation among youth from a psychosocial perspective.

Moreover, the dramatic variation in the prevalence of suicide ideation across countries and regions indicate that cultural norms and practices may play an important role in the expression of suicide ideation and that they may either buffer against or contribute to the occurrence of suicidal thoughts (Wasserman, 2009). Future research should seek to determine those sociocultural factors that may affect youth reporting of suicide ideation to provide a greater understanding of the associated risk factors. How religion and differential cultural factors serve as contributing and buffering factors for suicide risk is very important for prevention and intervention (Orbach & Iohan-Barak, 2009).

Finally, in contrast to popular convention about gender differences with respect to suicide ideation in which girls are expected to report higher levels of suicide ideation than boys, our study found that true in only 7 of the 19 countries and cities examined. Our findings suggest that when examined from a global perspective, boys and girls are more alike in terms of suicidal ideation. This is a surprising finding and warrants additional consideration and research.

4.1   Limitations

Interpretation of the findings in this report is subject to several limitations. First, all participants were school-attending youth and, as such, the findings may not reflect the experiences of youth who have dropped out of school or may not be able to attend school. Findings from a U.S. study indicate that school attendance may be a protective factor for reporting suicide ideation for both male and female students, thereby indicating a potential for underreporting of suicidal ideation and behaviors among school-attending youth (Blum, Ireland & Blum, 2003; Borowsky, Ireland & Resnick, 2001).

Moreover, the status of school attendance as a financial privilege in some countries may further impact these results. Second, reports of suicide ideation (and suicidal behavior) may be considered a socially undesirable behavior, for religious and other reasons, thus potentially affecting the validity of self-report data. Third, comparisons across regions may be biased by the countries and cities selected for inclusion, as well as the year for which data was collected. Lastly, the analyses and comparisons do not consider other demographic characteristics, or societal level factors that may be relevant to suicide ideation. Despite these limitations, the findings of this study maintain important implications for providing relatively recent and descriptive data on the prevalence and gender differences in suicide ideation among youth, an understudied topic from a global health context.

4.2   Conclusions

Given the variability in the prevalence of suicidal ideation across countries and regions in this study, future research should examine the risk factors for suicidal ideation and also for suicidal behavior including suicide attempt from an international and comparative perspective in order to inform prevention strategies that may have broader global relevance. As noted earlier, it appears that of all the regions in the world, the mental health concerns of youth in sub-Saharan Africa appear to be among the least represented in the scientific literature. Accordingly, there is a growing and urgent need to focus on effective research and preventive efforts, with greater collaboration among African and non-African researchers being pivotal to this process. Major investment is needed, for both research and for preventive efforts. While short-term efforts contribute to an understanding of why suicide occurs and what can be done to prevent it, longitudinal research studies are necessary to fully understand the role of biological, psychosocial and environmental factors in suicide. There is also a great need for rigorous and long-term evaluations of interventions.

Research examining trends within countries and regions are also needed to determine the factors that may reduce or exacerbate risk. Considerable gaps in research regarding the correlates and risk factors of suicide ideation and attempt also remain for several parts of the world. This study, which employed cross-sectional analyses of relatively recent population-based surveillance data to understand the current prevalence and context of suicide ideation, provides insight for addressing these gaps. Furthermore, this study may also lead to discussions about designing interventions that target suicide ideation that may be a component of a broader mental health prevention effort or school wellness programs. Interventions that combine an understanding of cultural and gender variations of suicidal behaviors, while focusing attention on the underlying factors, will likely have the greatest opportunities for impact.

4.3   Implications and Recommendations

The prevalence of suicidal ideation varied dramatically across the countries examined. Moreover, gender differences were only observed in 7 of the 19 countries and cities examined, challenging the commonly held belief that girls across the world are more likely to report suicide ideation. More cross-national research is needed on this understudied topic to better understand the context of suicidal ideation and behavior to inform strategies and prevention efforts.

Future research is also needed to better determine strategies for providing additional services and treatment to youths in schools, but also to those who may be difficult to reach and who are not attending schools (Swahn *et al.*, 2012b). This is particularly important given the acute shortage of psychiatrists, psychologists, nurses, and social workers in Africa (Saxena, Thornicroft, Kapp & Whiteford, 2007). Moreover, future projection indicates that suicides will increase substantially by the year 2030 (WHO, 2008). As such, it is of critical importance, as has been suggested in prior research and reports, to strengthen the infrastructure of mental health services and to add capacity, perhaps by incorporating mental health into primary care (WHO, 2008) and increasing the scope and training of lay workers (Ovuga, Boardman & Wassermann, 2007). Similarly, as this study examined youth attending school, these settings would be highly suitable for screenings and also potentially brief interventions as relatively cost-effective approaches to reach as many youth as possible in need. With such strategies we may be better able to address the needs of youth and reduce their risk of suicide ideation.

References

Bakken, N., & Gunter, W. (2012). Self-cutting and suicidal ideation among adolescents: Gender difference in the causes and correlates of self-injury. Deviant Behavior, 33(5), 339–356.

Beautrais, A. L. (2002). Gender issues in youth suicidal behavior. Emergency Medicine, 14(1), 35.

Bertolote, J. M., & Fleischmann, A. (2009). A global perspective on the magnitude of suicide mortality. In D. Wasserman & C. Wasserman (Eds.), Oxford Textbook of Suicidology and Suicide Prevention (pp. 92–98). Oxford University Press. Retrieved from http://oxfordmedicine.com/view/10.1093/med/9780198570059.001.0001/med-9780198570059-chapter-14

Blum J., Ireland, M., & Blum, R.W. (2003). Gender differences in juvenile violence: A report from Add Health. Journal of Adolescent Health, 32(3), 234–240.

Blum, R., Sudhinaraset, M., & Emerson, M. R. (2012). Youth at risk: Suicidal thoughts and attempts in Vietnam, China, and Taiwan. Journal of Adolescent Health, 50(3, Supplement), S37–S44. doi:10.1016/j.jadohealth.2011.12.006

Boeninger, D. K., Masyn, K. E., Feldman, B. J., & Conger, R. D. (2010). Sex Differences in Developmental Trends of Suicide Ideation, Plans, and Attempts among European American Adolescents. Suicide and Life Threatening Behavior, 40(5), 451–464.

Borowsky, I.W., Ireland, M., & Resnick, M.D. (2001). Adolescent suicide attempts: Risk and protectors Pediatrics, 107, 485–495.

Canetto, S. (2008). Women and suicidal behavior: A cultural analysis. American Journal of Orthopsychiatry, 78(2), 259-266.

Center for Disease Control. (2012b) Fact Sheet: Understanding Suicide. Retrieved from: http://www.cdc.gov/violenceprevention/pdf/suicide_factsheet_2012-a.pdf

Centers for Disease Control and Prevention. (2012a). Suicide facts at a glance. Retrieved from www.cdc.gov/violenceprevention/pdf/Suicide-DataSheet-a.pdf

Centers for Disease Control and Prevention. (2012c) Injury prevention and control. Retrieved from http://www.cdc.gov/violenceprevention/pub/youth_suicide.html

Centers for Disease Control and Prevention. Global School-based Student Health Survey (GSHS) [Online]. 2009a. Available from: http://www.cdc.gov/gshs/

Centers for Disease Control and Prevention. Youth Risk Behavior Surveillance System (YRBSS): Youth Online [Online]. 2013. Available from: http://www.cdc.gov/HealthyYouth/yrbs/index.htm

Centers for Disease Control and Prevention. Youth Risk Behavior Surveillance System (YRBSS): Youth Online [Online]. 2009b. Available from: http://apps.nccd.cdc.gov/youthonline/App/Default.aspx

Dai, J., Chiu, H. F. K., Conner, K. R., Chan, S. S. M., Hou, Z. J., Yu, X., & Caine, E. D. (2011). Suicidal ideation and attempts among rural Chinese aged 16–34 years — Socio-demographic correlates in the context of a transforming China. Journal of Affective Disorders, 130(3), 438–446. doi:10.1016/j.jad.2010.10.042

Food and Agriculture Organization. The state of food insecurity in the World 2011. Available online: http://www.fao.org/docrep/014/i2330e/i2330e00.htm (Retrieved on 11 October 2011).

Grunbaum, J. A., Kann, L., Kinchen, S., Ross, J., Hawkins, J., Lowry, R., et al. (2004). Youth risk behavior surveillance— United States, 2003. MMWR, 53(SS02), 1-96.

Juan, W., Xiao-Juan, D., Jia-Ji, W., Xin-Wang, W. & Liang, Xu (2010). The associations between health risk behaviors and suicidal ideations and attempts in an urban Chinese sample of adolescents. Journal of Affective Disorders, 126, 180-187.

Kirchner, T., Ferrer, L., Forns, M., & Zanini, D. (2011). Self-harm behavior and suicidal ideation among high school students. Gender differences and relationship with coping strategies. Actas Españolas De Psiquiatría, 39(4), 226–235.

Krug, E.G., Dahlberg, L.L., Mercy, J.A., Zwi, A.B., & Lozano, R (2002). World report on violence and health. World Health Organization. Geneval: Author. Retrieved from http://whqlibdoc.who.int/publications/2002/9241545615_eng.pdf

Mark, L., Samm, A., Tooding, L.-M., Sisask, M., Aasvee, K., Zaborskis, A., Värnik, A. (2013). Suicidal ideation, risk factors, and communication with parents: An HBSC study on school children in Estonia, Lithuania, and Luxembourg. Crisis: The Journal of Crisis Intervention and Suicide Prevention, 34(1), 3–12. doi:10.1027/0227-5910/a000153.

Muula, A.S., Kazembe, L.N., Rudatsikira, E., & Siziya, S. (2007). Suicidal ideation and associated factors among in-school adolescents in Zambia. Tanzania Health Res Bull, 9(3):202-06.

Omigbodun, O., Dogra, N., Esan, O., & Adedokun, B. (2008). Prevalence and correlates of suicidal behavior among adolescents in Southwest Nigeria. Int J Soc Psychiatry, 54(1), 34-46.

Orbach, I., & Iohan-Barak, M. (2009). Psychopathology and risk factors for suicide in the young. In D. Wasserman & C. Wasserman (Eds.), Oxford Textbook of Suicidology and Suicide Prevention (pp. 634–642). Oxford University Press. Retrieved from http://m.oxfordmedicine.com/mobile/view/10.1093/med/9780198570059.001.0001/med-9780198570059-chapter-87

Ovuga, E., Boardman, J. & Wassermann, D. (2007). Integrating mental health into primary health care: Local initiatives from Uganda. World Psychiatry, 6, 60–61.

Ovuga, E., Boardman, J., & Wassermann, D. (2005). Prevalence of suicide ideation in two districts of Uganda. Arch Suicide Res 9(4), 321-322

Rudatsikira, E., Muula, A.S. Siziya, S. & Twa-Twa, J. (2007a). Suicidal ideation and associated factors among school-going adolescents in rural Uganda. BMC Psychiatry, 7, 67.

Rudatsikira, E., Siziya, S., Muula, A.S. (2007b). Suicidal ideation and associated factors among school-going adolescents in Harare, Zimbabwe. Journal of Psychiatry in Africa, 17(1), 93-98.

Saxena, S., Thornicroft, G., Knapp, M. & Whiteford, H. (2007). Resources for mental health: Scarcity, inequity and inefficiency. Lancet, 370, 878–889.

Schlebusch, L., Burrows S. & Vawda, N. Suicide prevention and religious traditions on the African continent. In D. Wasserman and C. Wasserman (Eds.) Suicidology and suicide prevention: A global perspective (pp. 63-69) Oxford England: Oxford University Press, 2009.

Scocco, P., de Girolamo, G., Vilagut, G., & Alonso, J. (2008). Prevalence of suicide ideation, plans, and at tempts and related risk factors in Italy: Results from the European Study on the Epidemiology of Mental Disorders-World Mental Health study. Comprehensive Psychiatry, 49(1), 13–21. doi:10.1016/j.comppsych.2007.08.004

Sook-Park, H., Schepp, K. G., & Jang, E. H. (2006). Predictors of suicidal ideation among high school students by gender in South Korea. Journal of School Health, 76(5), 181–188. doi:10.1111/j.1746-1561.2006.00092.x

Swahn, M. H., & Bossarte, R. M. (2007). Gender, early alcohol use, and suicide ideation and attempts: Findings from the 2005 youth risk behavior survey. The Journal of Adolescent Health: Official Publication of the Society for Adolescent Medicine, 41(2), 175–181. doi:10.1016/j.jadohealth.2007.03.003

Swahn, M. H., Bossarte, R. M., Choquet, M., Hassler, C., Falissard, B., & Chau, N. (2012a). Early substance use initiation and suicide ideation and attempts among students in France and the United States. International Journal of Public Health, 57(1), 95–105. doi:10.1007/s00038-011-0255-7.

Swahn, M.H., Bossarte, R.M., Eliman, D.M., Gaylor E. & Jayaraman, S. (2010a.) Prevalence and correlates of suicidal ideation and physical fighting: a comparison of students in Botswana, Kenya, Uganda, Zambia and the Unites States. Int Public Health Journal, 2(2), 195-206.

Swahn, M.H., Bossarte, R.M., Eliman, D.M., Gaylor E., & Walingo, M.K. (2010b). Associations between hunger and emotional and behavioral problems: a comparison of students in Botswana, Kenya, Uganda, Zambia and the Unites States. Int Public Health Journal, 2(2), 185-194.

Swahn, M.H., Palmier, J.B., Kasirye, R.. & Yao, H. (2012b). Correlates of suicide ideation and attempt among young living in the slums of Kampala. Int. J. Environ. Res. Public Health, 9, 596-609.

Upadhayay, B. K., & Singh, R. (2006). Suicide ideation and psychopathology among adolescents. Europe's Journal of Psychology, 2(3).

Wasserman, C. Suicide: Considering religion and culture. In D. Wasserman and C. Wasserman (Eds.) Suicidology and suicide prevention: A global perspective (pp.3-6) Oxford England: Oxford University Press, 2009.

World Health Organization (2011). Suicide prevention (SUPRE). Retrieved from http://www.who.int/mental_health/prevention/suicide/suicideprevent/en/)

World Health Organization. Global School-based Student Health Survey (GSHS) [Online]. 2009a. Available from: http://www.who.int/chp/gshs/en/

World Health Organization. Global School-based Student Health Survey (GSHS) purpose and methodology [Online]. 2009b. Available from: http://www.who.int/chp/gshs/methodology/en/index.html

World Health Organization. World Health Statistics; 2008. Available online: http://www.who.int/whosis/whostat/2008/en/index.html (Retrieved on 23 October 2011).

Figures/graphs

Centers for Disease Control and Prevention (CDC). 1991-2011 High School Youth Risk Behavior Survey Data. Available at http://apps.nccd.cdc.gov/youthonline. Retrieved on July 29, 2013.

World Health Organization. (2002). [Evolution of global suicide rates 1950-2000]. Mental Health Global Charts. Retrieved from http://www.who.int/mental_health/prevention/suicide/evolution/en/index.html

Effects of Job Satisfaction and Locus of Control on Psychological Distress in Japanese Employees

Masahito Fushimi

Akita Prefectural Mental Health and Welfare Center, Japan
Akita Occupational Health Promotion Center, Japan

1 Introduction

Japan has one of the highest suicide rates among developed countries, and mental health problems are blamed for the majority of reported suicides. Thus, issues related to mental health are of significant concern for the country (Fushimi et al., 2005; Fushimi et al., 2010; Fushimi et al., 2012). Occupational safety and health programs typically invite employees to complete a voluntary health assessment questionnaire consisting of brief self-report health scales at the workplace. The Kessler 10 (K10) is a brief, validated scale that assesses psychological distress and effectively predicts mental disorders (Fushimi, 2012; Fushimi et al., 2010; Fushimi et al., 2012; Kessler et al., 2003). In this study, the K10 scale was employed to assess the psychological distress of employees.

It is important to employ proactive health screening to identify stressful situations and the stress management skills of employees. Several previous studies on stress have explored the relationship between stressors and psychological distress, and some of these studies have assessed moderating factors such as locus of control (LOC) (Fushimi, 2011; Fushimi; 2012; Newton & Keenan, 1990; Parkes, 1985; Rotter, 1966). LOC refers to beliefs concerning personal control, represented by the continuum from internality to externality. "Internals" believe that "reinforcements are contingent upon their own behavior, capacities, or attributes." In contrast, "externals" believe that "reinforcements are not under their personal control, but rather are under the control of powerful others, luck, chance, fate, etc." (Rotter, 1966). Therefore, LOC may be related to the long-term coping pattern of individuals. An individual's response to perceived stress (i.e., coping behavior) is crucial to understanding the processes related to occupational stress; however, not all coping occurs during stressful incidents or episodes. Therefore, it is important to study the long-term pattern of coping behavior (i.e., coping style) because psychological distress builds up over months or years, rather than as a mere response to a single stressful incident. Consequently, this study does not focus on individual stressful incidents, but rather on LOC, which is thought to be related to the long-term coping pattern of individuals (Fushimi, 2011; Fushimi, 2012).

2 Materials and Methods

The research design of this study was cross-sectional sampling, and information presented in this report was collected as part of the Akita Occupational Health Promotion Center's Study for Mental Health (Fushimi, 2011; Fushimi, 2012; Fushimi et al., 2010; Fushimi et al., 2012). The participants in this study were recruited as follows: Employers were selected through random systematic sampling, and their employees were invited to complete a self-administered questionnaire during a one-month survey period (September – October 2007). In all, 15 employers from public and private sector firms in Akita prefecture, Japan, agreed to participate in the study. The questionnaires were distributed to the participants using paper-based methods. The demographic information collected during this study included gender, age (29 years or younger, 30 to 39 years, 40 to 49 years, and 50 years and older), and the highest level of education obtained (compulsory or senior high school, tertiary education, and graduate degree or higher). The questionnaire survey also elicited information about the employees' jobs (full-time work, managerial class, job category, and average number of working hours per day). Participants were asked to select their job category from the following: clerical or administrative support, sales- or service-related, professional or technical support, and other. In addition, the questionnaire assessed employment satisfaction (accomplishment, personal growth, salary, evaluations, and workplace human relations) on a

4-point scale ("satisfied," "somewhat satisfied," "somewhat disappointed," and "disappointed"). Participation in the survey was voluntary and confidential. The Japan Labour Health and Welfare Organization, which was represented by occupational health promotion centers in each administrative division of the firms, approved the study protocol.

The K10 scale was used to assess psychological distress over the past 30 days. The psychological dimensions explored in K10 make it sensitive and specific to mental disorders, such as affective and anxiety disorders (Fushimi, 2012; Fushimi et al., 2010; Fushimi et al., 2012; Kessler et al., 2003). Each of the 10 items on the K10 scale is rated on a 5-point scale ranging from 1 ("none of the time") to 5 ("all of the time"). The total score can range from 10 to 50. Previous studies using the K10 indicate that scores between 30 and 50 represent very high psychological distress, scores between 22 and 29 indicate high psychological distress, scores between 16 and 21 indicate moderate psychological distress, and scores between 10 and 15 represent low psychological distress (Avery et al., 2004; Baillie, 2005; Fushimi, 2012). The present study was divided into two categories of psychological distress: (1) high or very high psychological distress (22 – 50), defined as "serious psychological distress"; and (2) moderate or low distress (10 – 21), defined as "no serious psychological distress."

The LOC scale was used to measure the internality-externality trait of the participants. Kambara and his colleagues (Kambara et al., 2001; Sasaki & Kanachi, 2005) developed an alternative to the original LOC scale developed by Rotter (1966). This alternative Japanese version of the LOC scale has 18 items (9 items each for internality and externality). Each item is evaluated using a 4-point rating scale, indicating the level of agreement or disagreement with each item. Therefore, the sum of the response scores can range from 18 to 72, with higher scores indicating internality. In the previous study quoted here, internal consistency reliability was estimated at 0.78, and the test-retest reliability was 0.76 (Kambara et al., 2001; Sasaki & Kanachi, 2005). Further information about this scale can be found in Kambara et al. (2001).

Statistical analyses were performed using SPSS version 11.0J for Windows (SPSS, Tokyo, Japan). Statistical differences in each category were measured using binomial multivariate logistic regression. Three binomial logistic regression analyses with K10 scores as the dependent variable (less than 22 or 22 and higher) were performed. Gender was included as an independent variable in one regression. The remaining two logistic regressions were conducted on separate data sets for males and females.

3   Results

Of the 2,145 employees, 1,873 responded to the questionnaire (response rate: 87.3%); however, the number of questionnaires with satisfactory responses, excluding those with insufficient data, was 1,512 (70.5%), which included 624 males and 888 females (Fushimi, 2012). Mean scores and standard deviations from the K10 scale were 20.23 ± 8.04 (19.52 ± 8.19 for males and 20.74 ± 7.90 for females). The prevalence of serious psychological distress was 37.2% (33.7% for males and 39.6% for females).

Figure 1 shows the distribution of scores for the K10 scale according to the low (10 – 15), moderate (16 – 21), high (22 – 29) and very high (30 – 50) psychological distress groups (Fushimi, 2012). Figure 2 shows the percentage of each employment satisfaction category: "satisfied," "somewhat satisfied," "somewhat disappointed," and "disappointed." Table 1 presents the adjusted odds ratio (OR) from the binomial logistic regression for serious psychological distress by socio-demographic status, employment related variables, and internality-externality (LOC scale). There were no significant effects

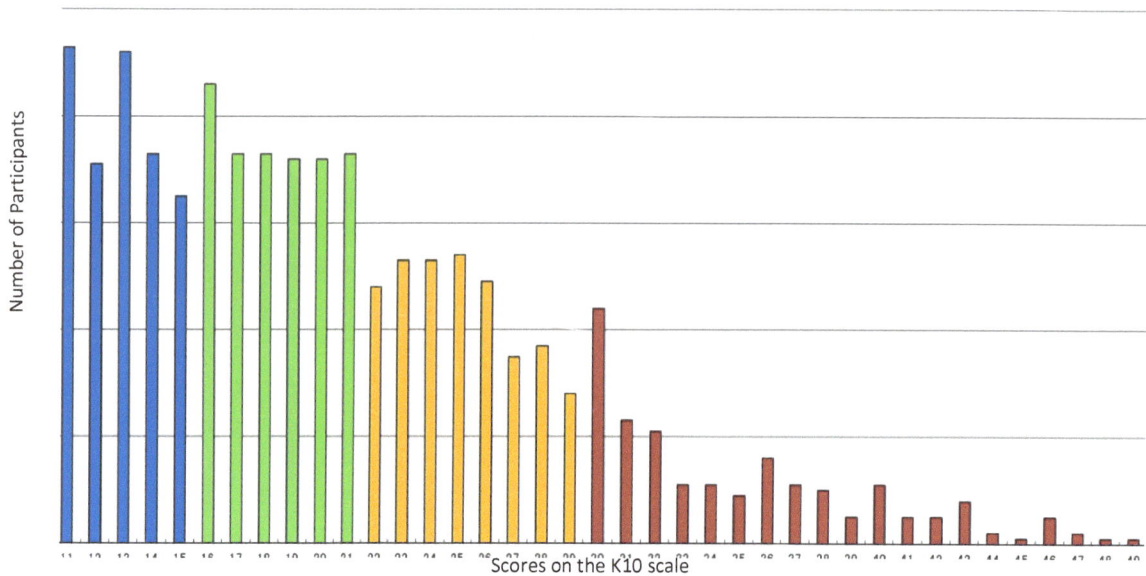

Figure 1: Distribution of scores from the K10 scale by low (10 – 15), moderate (16 – 21), high (22 – 29) and very high (30 – 50) psychological distress groups (Fushimi, 2012). The present study was divided into two categories of psychological distress: high or very high psychological distress, defined as "serious psychological distress"; and moderate or low distress, defined as "no serious psychological distress."

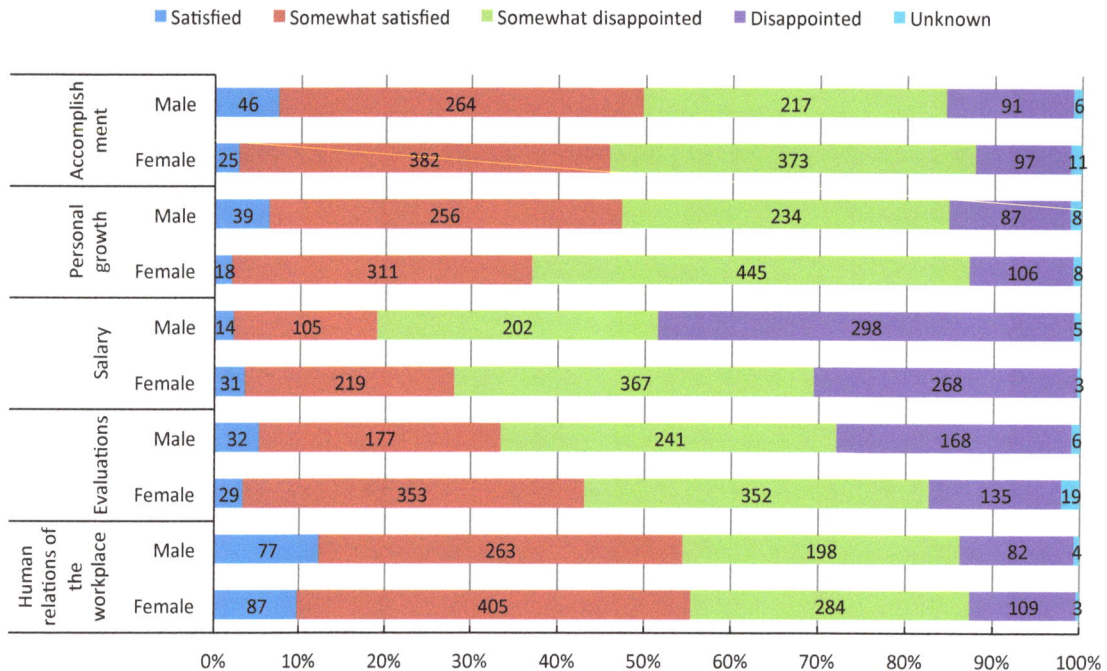

Figure 2: Level of employment satisfaction related to accomplishment, personal growth, salary, evaluations, and workplace human relations.

	Total			Male			Female		
	OR	95% CI	p-value	OR	95% CI	p-value	OR	95% CI	p-value
Gender									
Male	0.9	0.6 – 1.2	0.34						
Female		Ref.							
Age									
≤ 29	1.9	1.3 – 2.9	< 0.005	1.2	0.7 – 2.3	0.51	2.0	1.2 – 3.4	<0.01
30 – 39	1.9	1.3 – 2.7	< 0.005	2.4	1.4 – 4.2	<0.005	1.5	0.9 – 2.4	0.11
40 – 49	1.4	1.0 – 2.0	0.07	1.7	1.0 – 2.9	0.05	1.1	0.7 – 1.7	0.77
≥ 50		Ref.			Ref.				
Education									
Compulsory / senior high school	1.1	0.6 – 1.9	0.74	1.2	0.6 – 2.5	0.60	1.0	0.4 – 2.3	0.92
Some tertiary education	1.3	0.8 – 2.3	0.28	1.1	0.5 – 2.3	0.90	1.5	0.7 – 3.4	0.34
Graduate degree or higher		Ref.			Ref.			Ref.	
Job Category									
Clerical / administrative	0.8	0.5 – 1.3	0.44	0.9	0.5 – 1.7	0.79	0.8	0.4 – 1.6	0.55
Sales / service	1.4	0.9 – 2.1	0.17	1.2	0.6 – 2.1	0.66	1.7	0.8 – 3.4	0.14
Professional / technical	1.2	0.9 – 1.8	0.23	1.4	0.8 – 2.3	0.18	1.2	0.7 – 2.0	0.57
Others (on-site workers, etc.)		Ref.			Ref.			Ref.	
Employment status									
Full-time work	0.7	0.5 – 1.1	0.18	0.8	0.4 – 1.7	0.64	0.7	0.4 – 1.2	0.15
No full-time work		Ref.			Ref.				
Employee type									
Managerial class	1.3	0.8 – 1.9	0.25	1.0	0.6 – 1.8	0.93	1.4	0.7 – 2.9	0.31
No managerial class		Ref.			Ref.			Ref.	
Working hours per day									
8 hours or less	0.8	0.6 – 1.0	0.07	0.9	0.6 – 1.3	0.50	0.8	0.6 – 1.1	0.16
More than 8 hours		Ref.			Ref.			Ref.	
Level of Satisfaction related to the employment - Accomplishment									
Satisfied	1.1	0.5 – 2.5	0.88	0.5	0.1 – 2.0	0.35	2.1	0.6 – 7.4	0.26
Somewhat satisfied	0.8	0.5 – 1.3	0.41	1.0	0.5 – 2.1	0.99	0.6	0.3 – 1.3	0.19
Somewhat disappointed	0.8	0.5 – 1.2	0.28	1.2	0.6 – 2.5	0.57	0.5	0.3 – 1.0	0.05
Disappointed		Ref.			Ref.			Ref.	
Level of Satisfaction related to the employment - Personal growth									
Satisfied	0.4	0.2 – 1.0	0.05	0.6	0.2 – 2.2	0.43	0.2	0.0 – 1.0	0.05

	OR	95% CI	p	OR	95% CI	p	OR	95% CI	p
Somewhat satisfied	0.5	0.3 – 0.9	0.01	0.5	0.2 – 1.0	0.06	0.6	0.3 – 1.1	0.09
Somewhat disappointed	0.7	0.5 – 1.1	0.10	0.4	0.2 – 0.9	0.02	0.9	0.5 – 1.6	0.65
Disappointed		Ref.			Ref.			Ref.	
Level of Satisfaction related to the employment – Salary									
Satisfied	1.5	0.6 – 3.6	0.35	5.3	1.1 – 25.2	0.04	0.9	0.3 – 2.7	0.80
Somewhat satisfied	1.1	0.8 – 1.6	0.64	1.7	0.9 – 3.3	0.09	0.9	0.5 – 1.4	0.59
Somewhat disappointed	0.9	0.7 – 1.3	0.59	1.3	0.8 – 2.2	0.26	0.8	0.5 – 1.1	0.16
Disappointed		Ref.			Ref.			Ref.	
Level of Satisfaction related to the employment – Evaluations									
Satisfied	0.7	0.3 – 1.5	0.36	0.6	0.2 – 1.9	0.38	0.8	0.2 – 2.7	0.74
Somewhat satisfied	0.6	0.4 – 1.0	0.04	0.5	0.2 – 0.9	0.02	0.9	0.5 – 1.6	0.61
Somewhat disappointed	1.1	0.7 – 1.5	0.75	0.8	0.5 – 1.4	0.48	1.4	0.8 – 2.3	0.27
Disappointed		Ref.			Ref.			Ref.	
Level of Satisfaction related to the employment – Human relations of the workplace									
Satisfied	0.4	0.2 – 0.7	<0.005	0.5	0.2 – 1.1	0.08	0.3	0.2 – 0.7	<0.005
Somewhat satisfied	0.3	0.2 – 0.5	<0.001	0.3	0.2 – 0.6	<0.005	0.3	0.2 – 0.5	<0.001
Somewhat disappointed	0.5	0.7 – 1.5	<0.005	0.6	0.3 – 1.2	0.14	0.4	0.2 – 0.7	<0.005
Disappointed		Ref.			Ref.			Ref.	
LOC scale (Internality – Externality)									
≤ 44	3.6	2.6 – 4.8	<0.001	3.2	2.0 – 5.1	<0.001	3.9	2.6 – 6.0	<0.001
45 – 49	2.2	1.6 – 3.0	<0.001	1.4	0.9 – 2.3	0.17	2.8	1.9 – 4.2	<0.001
≥ 50		Ref.			Ref.			Ref.	

Table 1: Effects of socio-demographic and employment factors on psychological distress. Total K10 score can range between 10 and 50, and scores of 22 or higher indicate serious psychological distress. LOC: locus of control; OR: odds ratio; CI: confidence interval; Ref: reference group to which all other categorical variables are compared.

of gender, education, job category, employment status, employee type, and hours worked per day on the prevalence of serious psychological distress. The prevalence of psychological distress varied significantly and substantially by age. Controlling for other variables, employees in the age group 50 years and older had the lowest OR for serious psychological distress. The prevalence of psychological distress varied significantly by the level of satisfaction with employment in terms of the quality of workplace relationships. Controlling for other variables, employees who selected "disappointed" in response to the item assessing the quality of relationships have a significantly increased OR for serious psychological distress. The prevalence of psychological distress also varied significantly by internality-externality. Controlling for other variables, a high score on the LOC scale (50 and above) was significantly associated with a decreased OR of serious psychological distress.

4   Discussion

In the present study, 37.2% of the employees exhibited serious psychological distress. Another study conducted in Australia estimated the risk of serious (*i.e.*, high or very high) levels of psychological distress on the K10 psychological distress scale among the general population to be 10.6%, and among the sub-group of employed individuals to be 8.4% (Avery *et al.*, 2004; Fushimi, 2012). The 37.2% prevalence rate of serious psychological distress among employees noted in this study is clearly much higher than the prevalence rate estimated among the general population of Australia (Avery *et al.*, 2004; Fushimi, 2012). The prevalence rates of high scorers on the K10 noted among employees in this study are also much higher than the findings of previous studies for workers in Japan and other countries. Certain assumptions can be made based on these findings. First, Japan's suicide rate increased considerably during the 1990s, which might have been the result of drastic social changes, such as the national economic crisis and the termination of the lifetime employment practice at many major companies (Fushimi *et al.*, 2005). Therefore, the reason for higher scores on the psychological distress scale was partly explained by rapid changes in job opportunities or the work environment. Second, I suggest that a culturally different response style to questions relating to emotion has caused higher scores on psychological distress scale. Japanese are reluctant to express their affect positively when compared to American populations (Cho *et al.*, 1998; Iwata *et al.*, 1989; 1998). Further studies are required to clarify this point.

In this study, age was a demographic variable that was significantly associated with psychological distress. This result approximates the trend discovered in another study in Australia, which found that younger age groups were at a relatively higher risk of psychological distress than older age groups (Avery *et al.*, 2004). Other previous studies reveal that depression is most commonly reported among younger respondents, particularly females (Comstock & Helsing, 1976; Craig & van Natta, 1979; Husaini *et al.*, 1980; Madianos *et al.*, 1988; Narrow *et al.*, 1990; Radloff, 1977). The results of the present study support these findings. The level of education has not been significantly associated with psychological distress. It is widely accepted that the prevalence of mental health problems increases with lower levels of educational attainment (Andrews *et al.*, 2001; Bijl *et al.*, 1998; Fushimi *et al.*, 2012; Pratt *et al.*, 2007; Stewart *et al.*, 2003). However, the results of previous studies are inconsistent in terms of the relationship between psychological distress and the level of educational attainment. For example, although the highest prevalence rates of psychological distress were noted among employees with the lowest level of formal education in certain studies, others have noted significantly high levels of psychological distress among employees with a postgraduate degree (Hilton *et al.*, 2008). In this study, employment category was not found to be significantly associated with the prevalence rates of serious psychological distress. Other studies have reported that the highest prevalence of psychological distress was observed among females in operator and/or laborer roles and among males in clerical and/or administrative roles (Hilton *et al.*, 2008; Kessler & Frank, 1997). Moreover, on average, across males and females, the highest prevalence rates for psychological distress were observed among individuals in sales-related positions; on the other hand, the lowest rates were observed among executives or senior managers (Hilton *et al.*, 2008; Kessler & Frank, 1997). In brief, there is no consistent evidence of the relationship between job category and psychological distress in the literature, perhaps due to the complexity of this relationship (Fushimi *et al.*, 2012). The number of hours worked per day was not significantly associated with psychological distress. Generally, high work demand is known to be associated with a decline in mental well-being (D'Souza *et al.*, 2006; Niedhammer *et al.*, 1998; Stansfeld *et al.*, 1999). Pressure to work overtime is associated with poor mental health. Increased working hours may also produce a negative work-to-family spillover, which is associated with an increased risk of depression. A proportion of employees with high psychological distress possibly work longer to complete all the tasks necessary to maintain their employment (Hilton *et al.*, 2008).

In the previous studies, lower income, heavier workload, less personal control, and lower satisfaction on the Social Support Questionnaire in combination with longer working hours were risk factors for mental distress. Therefore, careful monitoring of mental health is necessary (Sugiura-Ogasawara *et al.*, 2012). In contrast, psychological distress increases the OR for workplace accidents or failures, and decreases the OR for workplace successes (Hilton & Whiteford, 2010). The present results are consistent with these previous findings. Regarding the level of employment satisfaction, salary was associated with the lowest level of satisfaction, whereas work relationships were associated with the highest level of satisfaction for both males and females (Figure 1). However, only the variable "workplace relationships" was significantly associated with psychological distress by the binomial multivariate logistic regression (Table 1). According to the results of a nationwide survey on health conditions among workers in Japan published by the Ministry of Heath, Labour and Welfare, respondents indicated that "issues related to personal relationships in the workplace," "issues related to quality of work," and "issues related to amount of work" accounted for a majority of the anxiety and stress related to work and professional life. The survey, conducted every five years, consistently indicates that "issues related to personal relationships in the workplace" is the top response to this question regarding the source of workplace stress. The current study supports these results. It is clear that human relations are important in devising and implementing mental health care measures in the workplace.

The LOC was hypothesized to moderate stressor-strain relations because it appears as the factor most likely to affect the coping styles of individuals. Comparatively little research has been conducted on how coping styles interact with psychological distress in an applied setting, although factors related to coping styles (such as the LOC) have a lengthy tradition of research (Fushimi, 2011; Fushimi, 2012). Therefore, it is worthwhile to consider the effects that socio-demographic and occupational factors may have on these variables. Generally, on observing the correlations between the LOC and the K10 scales, a pattern of findings emerged—the correlations were all negative, indicating that as the LOC score increased (greater internality), the K10 score decreased (less psychological distress). The results of the present study are in accordance with those observed in earlier research on psychological distress from job-related stressors, such as job demands (Fushimi, 2011; Fushimi, 2012; Jackson & Schuler, 1985; Keenan & McBain, 1979). For instance, externals are more likely to report greater psychological distress than others. In contrast, internals are likely to report less psychological distress, even when the number of stressors is relatively larger (Fushimi, 2011; Fushimi, 2012; Rotter, 1966; 1975).

A limitation of this study was cross-sectional sampling, which made it difficult to infer causality. The data sample was selected at random; however, the decision to participate in the project and respond to the survey was left entirely to the employers and employees. Consequently, the current paper presents results based on a realistic approach. In particular, self-selection biases in the current data are representative of those inherent in any employee health assessment survey, unlike large epidemiological surveys based on general population probability samples (Fushimi, 2011; Fushimi, 2012; Fushimi et al., 2010; Fushimi et al., 2012). The assessment of individual personality traits regarding internality-externality (LOC scale) is another limitation of this study, since it was based on a single questionnaire measurement. As noted previously, one reason for studying long-term coping styles is that not all coping behaviors occur in stressful incidents or episodes; psychological distress builds up over months or years rather than being the response to a single stressful incident. One approach to investigating the long-term patterns of coping styles is to measure the coping behavior repeatedly. However, in this type of research design, the response obtained may in part be an artifact of the method utilized by repeatedly focusing the participants' attention on how they cope in the long term (Newton & Keenan, 1990). An alternative to this approach, which reduces the occurrence of such problems, is to examine the long-term patterns of coping styles (Fushimi, 2011; Fushimi, 2012; Newton & Keenan, 1990).

5   Conclusion

Comparatively little research has been conducted on the interaction between internality-externality and psychological distress. This study examined the relationship between the LOC scale as an indicator of the internality-externality and the K10 scale as an indicator of psychological distress, and analyzed the effects of socio-demographic and employment-related factors on this relationship in a cross-sectional design. As part of the Akita Occupational Health Promotion Center's Study for Mental Health, employees from the Akita prefecture in Japan were invited to complete self-administered questionnaires, that included questions on: their socio-demographic status; employment-related variables (including level of employment satisfaction); and psychological distress. A value of 22 or higher on the K10 scale was defined as serious psychological distress. The data from 1,512 employees (males: 624; females: 888) revealed that 37.2% (males: 33.7%; females: 39.6%) had serious psychological distress. Binomial multivariate logistic regression analyses with the identified factors of socio-demographic level and occupation found a high risk for serious psychological distress in younger age groups and a high risk for participants who had low LOC scale scores (i.e., a trend of the greater the internality, the lesser the psychological distress). A low risk was observed for participants who reported satisfaction in their workplace relationships. Among the job-related satisfactory factors, workplace relationships were an important factor in determining psychological distress.

The results of this study may help improve mental health clinicians' understanding of psychological distress. Moreover, the risk factors identified in this study will guide mental health promotion, prevention, and screening programs to target relevant factors and populations.

Acknowledgements

The author would like to thank Tetsuo Shimizu, Katsuyuki Murata, Yasutsugu Kudo, Masayuki Seki, Seiji Saito, and the staff of the Akita Occupational Health Promotion Center for their valuable comments and suggestions.

References

Andrews, G., Henderson, S., & Hall, W. (2001). Prevalence, comorbidity, disability and service utilisation. Overview of the Australian National Mental Health Survey. British Journal of Psychiatry, 178, 145–153.

Avery, J., Dal Grande, E., Taylor, A., & Gill, T. (2004). Which South Australians experience psychological distress?: Kessler psychological distress 10-item scale July 2002-June 2004, South Australian Monitoring and Surveillance System (SAMSS). South Australian Department of Health Population Research and Outcome Studies Unit.

Baillie, A. J. (2005). Predictive gender and education bias in Kessler's psychological distress Scale (K10). Social Psychiatry and Psychiatric Epidemiology, 40, 743–748.

Bijl, R. V., Ravelli, A., & van Zessen, G. (1998). Prevalence of psychiatric disorder in the general population: results of The Netherlands Mental Health Survey and Incidence Study (NEMESIS). Social Psychiatry and Psychiatric Epidemiology, 33, 587–595.

Cho, M. J., Nam, J. J., & Suh, G. H. (1998). Prevalence of symptoms of depression in a nationwide sample of Korean adults. Psychiatry Research, 81, 341–352.

Comstock, G. W. & Helsing, K. J. (1976). Symptoms of depression in two communities. Psychological Medicine, 6, 551–563.

Craig, T. J. & Van Natta, P. A. (1979). Influence of demographic characteristics on two measures of depressive symptoms: the relation of prevalence and persistence of symptoms with sex, age, education, and marital status. Archives of General Psychiatry, 36, 149–154.

D'Souza, R. M., Strazdins, L., Broom, D. H., Rodgers, B., & Berry, H. L. (2006). Work demands, job insecurity and sickness absence from work. How productive is the new, flexible labour force? Australian and New Zealand Journal of Public Health, 30, 205–212.

Fushimi, M. (2011). The relationship between individual personality traits (internality-externality) and psychological distress in employees in Japan. Depression Research and Treatment, 2011:731307.

Fushimi, M. (2012). Relationships among the Kessler 10 Psychological Distress Scale, Socio-Demographic Status, Employment-Related Variables, and Internality-Externality in Japanese Employees. In Psychological Distress: Symptoms, Causes and Coping, Ohayashi, H. & Yamada, S. (eds.), pp. 83-102, Nova Science Publishers.

Fushimi, M., Sugawara, J., & Shimizu, T. (2005). Suicide patterns and characteristics in Akita, Japan. Psychiatry and Clinical Neurosciences, 59, 296–302.

Fushimi, M., Shimizu, T., Saito, S., Kudo, Y., Seki, M., & Murata, K. (2010). Prevalence of and risk factors for psychological distress among employees in Japan. Public Health, 124, 713–715.

Fushimi, M., Saito, S., Shimizu, T., Kudo, Y., Seki, M., & Murata, K. (2012). Prevalence of psychological distress, as measured by the Kessler 6 (K6), and related factors in Japanese employees. Community Mental Health Journal, 48, 328–335.

Hilton, M. F., Whiteford, H. A., Sheridan, J. S., Cleary, C. M., Chant, D. C., Wang, P. S., & Kessler, R. C. (2008). The prevalence of psychological distress in employees and associated occupational risk factors. Journal of Occupational and Environmental Medicine, 50, 746–757.

Hilton, M. F. & Whiteford, H. A. (2010). Associations between psychological distress, workplace accidents, workplace failures and workplace successes. *International Archives of Occupational and Environmental Health, 83, 923–933.*

Husaini, B. A., Neff, J. A., Harrington, J. B., Houghs, M. D., & Stone, R. H. (1980). Depression in rural communities: validating the CES-D scale. *Journal of Community Psychology, 8, 20–27.*

Iwata, N., Okuyama, Y., Kawakami, Y., & Saito, K. (1989). Prevalence of depressive symptoms in a Japanese occupational setting: a preliminary study. *American Journal of Public Health, 79, 1486-1489.*

Iwata, N., Umesue, M., Egashira, K., Hiro, H., Mizoue, T., Mishima, N., et al. (1998). Can positive affect items be used to assess depressive disorders in the Japanese population? *Psychological Medicine, 28, 153-158.*

Jackson, S. E. & Schuler, R. S. (1985). A meta-analysis and conceptual critique of research on role ambiguity and role conflict in work settings. *Organizational Behavior and Human Decision Processes, 36, 16–78.*

Kambara, M., Higuchi, K., & Shimizu, N. (2001). Locus of control scale. In Hori, H. & Yamamoto, Y. (eds.), *Book of psychometric scales Vol. 1*, pp. 180–184, Saiensu-sha, Tokyo, Japan, (in Japanese).

Keenan, A. & McBain, G. D. M. (1979). Effects of type A behaviour, intolerance of ambiguity, and locus of control on the relationship between role stress and work-related outcomes. *Journal of Occupational Psychology, 52, 277–285.*

Kessler, R. C. & Frank, R. G. (1997). The impact of psychiatric disorders on work loss days. *Psychological Medicine, 27, 861–873.*

Kessler, R. C., Barker, P. R., Colpe, L. J., Epstein, J. F., Gfroerer, J. C., Hiripi, E., Howes, M. J., Normand, S. L., Manderscheid, R. W., Walters, E. E., & Zaslavsky, A. M. (2003). Screening for serious mental illness in the general population. *Archives of General Psychiatry, 60, 184–189.*

Madianos, M. G., Tomaras, V., Kapsali, A., Vaidakis, N., Vlachonicolis, J., & Stefanis, C. N. (1988). Psychiatric case identification in two Athenian communities: estimation of the probable prevalence. *Acta Psychiatrica Scandinavica, 78, 24–31.*

Narrow, W. E., Rae, D. S., Moscicki, E. K., Locke, B. Z., & Regier, D. A. (1990). Depression among Cuban Americans: the Hispanic Health and Nutrition Examination Survey. *Social Psychiatry and Psychiatric Epidemiology, 25, 260–268.*

Newton, T. J. & Keenan, A. (1990). The moderating effect of the type A behavior pattern and locus of control upon the relationship between change in job demands and change in psychological strain. *Human Relations, 43, 1229–1255.*

Niedhammer, I., Goldberg, M., Leclerc, A., Bugel, I., & David, S. (1998). Psychosocial factors at work and subsequent depressive symptoms in the Gazel cohort. *Scandinavian Journal of Work, Environment & Health, 24, 197–205.*

Parkes, K. R. (1985). Stressful episodes reported by first-year student nurses: a descriptive account. *Social Science & Medicine, 20, 945–953.*

Pratt, L. A., Dey, A. N., & Cohen, A. J. (2007). Characteristics of adults with serious psychological distress as measured by the K6 scale: United States, 2001-04. *Advance Data, 30, 1–18.*

Radloff, L. S. (1977). The CES-D scale: a report of depression scale for research in the general population. *Applied Psychological Measurement, 1, 385–401.*

Rotter, J. B. (1966). Generalized expectancies for internal versus external control of reinforcement. *Psychological Monographs, 80, 1–28.*

Rotter, J. B. (1975). Some problems and misconceptions related to the construct of internal versus external control of reinforcement. *Journal of Consulting and Clinical Psychology, 43, 56–67.*

Sasaki, H. & Kanachi, M. (2005). The effects of trial repetition and individual characteristics on decision making under uncertainty. *Journal of Psychology, 139, 233–246.*

Stansfeld, S. A., Fuhrer, R., Shipley, M. J., & Marmot, M. G. (1999). Work characteristics predict psychiatric disorder: prospective results from the Whitehall II study. *Occupational and Environmental Medicine, 56, 302–307.*

Stewart, W. F., Ricci, J. A., Chee, E., Hahn, S. R., & Morganstein, D. (2003). Cost of lost productive work time among US workers with depression. *Journal of the American Medical Association, 289, 3135–3144.*

Sugiura-Ogasawara, M., Suzuki, S., Kitazawa, M., Kuwae, C., Sawa, R., Shimizu, Y., Takeshita, T., & Yoshimura, Y. (2012). Career satisfaction level, mental distress, and gender differences in working conditions among Japanese obstetricians and gynecologists. Journal of Obstetrics and Gynaecology Research, 38, 550–558.

Mental Health Disparities among Youth Living in the Slums of Kampala

Monica H. Swahn
School of Public Health
Georgia State University, USA

Jane B. Palmier
School of Public Health,
Georgia State University, USA

Rogers Kasirye
UYDEL Link
Kampala, Uganda

Nina K. Babihuga
School of Public Health
Georgia State University, USA

1   Introduction

The World Health Organization (WHO) defines mental health as a state of well-being in which every individual realizes his or her own potential, can cope with the normal stresses of life, can work productively and fruitfully, and is able to make a contribution to her or his community and not just the absence of mental disorder (World Health Organization, 2007). Mental illness on the other hand is defined as "collectively all diagnosable mental disorders" or "health conditions that are characterized by alterations in thinking, mood, or behavior (or some combination thereof) associated with distress and/or impaired functioning" (U.S. Department of Health and Human Services, 1999).The Centers for Disease Control and Prevention (CDC) highlights that whereas efforts have been made to screen, diagnose and treat people with mental illness, there has been little effort devoted to protect the mental health of people free from mental illness. Research and efforts to protect the mental health of these people should focus on the realms of social, emotional and psychological well-being which comprise the social determinants of mental health and whose support should be put in place (Centers for Disease Control and Prevention, 2011).

The socio-ecological model which takes into account the multifaceted interaction between individual, relationship, community, and societal factors, helps us to understand the risk factors or determinants of mental health (Centers for Disease Control and Prevention, 2013). They include, but are not limited to the following factors; access to drugs and alcohol, displacement, isolation and alienation, lack of education, transport, housing, neighborhood disorganization, peer rejection, poor social circumstances, poor nutrition, poverty, social disadvantage, urbanization, unemployment, violence and delinquency (WHO, 2004). These are not only individual risk factors that include the capability to manage one's thought process, emotions, or relations with others, but also; social, cultural, economic, political and environmental factors including national policies, social protection, living standards, working conditions, and community social support systems (WHO, 2013).

According to the WHO, 450 million people suffer from mental disorders worldwide with many more having mental problems (WHO, 2010). The WHO Global Burden of Disease Survey estimates that depression and anxiety disorders, including stress-related mental health conditions will become the second-ranked cause of disease burden by the year 2020, accounting for 5.7% of Disability Adjusted Life Years (DALYs), just behind ischemic heart disease (WHO, 2004). Mental health issues, including suicide are estimated to cause approximately 1.2 million deaths and 10-20 times more attempted suicides than that by the year 2020, making this a global public health problem that needs further attention (WHO, 2004).

The higher rates of disproportionate mortality among people with mental disorders are a sound basis for the need for extensive research and support systems for these people. 40%-60% of people with major depression have a greater chance of dying prematurely when compared to the general population because of the increased risk from other opportunistic illness that they acquire such as; cancers, cardiovascular diseases, diabetes and suicide (WHO, 2013). While research has found that certain life stressors are necessary to elicit a sense of competition and survival for people, a high level of adverse experiences especially in childhood is a known risk factor for ill mental health (WHO, 2013).

1.1   Mental Health in Africa

Despite renewed interest in the topic, every year, almost one million people die from suicide (WHO, 2011). Suicide is a particular concern among youth 15 to 19 years of age as it is the fourth leading cause of death globally in this age group (Wasserman, Cheng, & Jiang, 2005). Additionally, suicide attempt and ideation are also of concern since they are much more common than completed suicides (WHO, 2011). Unfortunately, research on mental health issues and suicidal behavior specifically, is relatively scarce in sub-Saharan Africa (Ovuga, Boardman, & Wassermann, 2005; Bertolote & Fleischmann, 2009; Swahn, Palmier, Kasirye, & Yao, 2012). The limited progress for mental health research in this region stems primarily from the presence of other critical public health issues and because of political and economic instability (Schlebusch, Burrows, & Vawda, 2009).

Advancement has also been limited because of the previously commonly held belief that depressive symptoms and suicidal ideation and behavior in Africa were rare; more recent research, however, indicate quite the contrary and that suicidal behaviors represent a real public health burden (Ovuga *et al.*, 2005; Bertolote & Fleischmann, 2009). Research across countries indicates that suicidal behavior is common but also underscore that patterns vary by countries (Ovuga, *et al.*, 2005; Omigbodun, Dogra, Esan, & Adedokun, 2008; Joe, Stein, Seedat, Herman, & Williams, 2008; Muula, Kazembe, Rudatsikira, & Siziya, 2007; Hjelmeland *et al.*, 2008). Research based on school-attending youth show that self-reported suicidal ideation ranges between 19.6% in Uganda, 23.1% in Botswana, 27.9% in Kenya, and 31.9% in Zambia (Swahn, Bossarte, Eliman, Gaylor, & Jayaraman, 2010). While not empirically examined, it is assumed that the relatively high levels of suicidal ideation and behavior among youth in sub-Saharan Africa may have been exacerbated by the severe psychosocial stress and other adverse health outcomes associated with the high prevalence of HIV/AIDS in Africa (Krug, Dahlberg, Mercy, Zwi & Lozano, 2002) as well as scarce food supply (Food and Agriculture Organization of the United Nations, 2011) and other distressing circumstances.

The increasing gap between the need for treatment and its provision all over the world is a clear indicator that health systems have not yet adequately responded to the burden of mental health disorders. There is a bigger burden in low and middle income countries with an estimated 76%-85% of people with mental disorders having no treatment. Less than US$2 per person is spent annually on mental health globally and less than US$0.25 per person in low income countries with only 36% of people living in low income countries covered by mental health legislation compared with 92% in high-income countries (WHO, 2013).

1.2   Mental Health in Uganda

Many countries in sub-Saharan Africa do not have appropriate mental health legislation. Uganda in particular has an outdated mental health act which was enacted in 1964 although a new mental health bill has been drafted and are awaiting parliamentary approval since 2010. The new bill addresses community mental health, an urgent need of communities throughout the country (Mental Disability Advocacy Center, 2011).

Although statistics on mental health in the country are very limited, the Uganda Bureau of Statistics report of 2006 revealed that 58% of all households with disabled people had at least one person with a mental disorder, common depression (20%), manic depression (3%), anxiety (4%), Epilepsy (3%) and Schizophrenia (1%); and these account for 20-30% of all hospital outpatient attendance. At least one in five people (approximately 23%) with mental health problems has "suicidal tendencies" and nearly one in four (18%) engage in substance abuse. All in all, an estimated 35% of Ugandans (approximately 9,574,915 people) suffer from some form of psychiatric (mental) disorders; at least 15% of which require treatment. However, these numbers leave out many who are outside the primary care system due to reasons like poverty and lack of appropriate health systems (Chronic Poverty Research Centre, 2007).

1.3   Mental Health of Youth living in the Slums

The United Nations which defines a slum household as a group of individuals living under the same roof in an urban area who lack durable housing, sufficient living space, easy access to safe water, access to adequate sanitation or security of tenure highlights that sub-Saharan Africa's slums are the most deprived (UN-HABITAT, 2005). It is clear that youth who live on the streets and in the slums of sub-Saharan Africa face much of the burden related to poverty, lack of family support as well as infectious and chronic diseases (Mufune, 2000; Chigunta, 2002). However, to date, there is a dearth of research on the specific mental health needs of these vulnerable youth and their strategies for coping and trying to survive in such a challenging environment (Swahn *et al.*, 2012a). Additionally, it is not clear what the specific disparities may be for these youth compared to their peers who may face fewer disadvantages.

Given the dearth of research of the scope of mental health needs and concerns among youth who live on the streets and in the slums in sub-Saharan Africa, this book chapter examines the prevalence of mental health issues and future aspirations among service-seeking youth living in the slums of Kampala. In particular, we focus on nine indicators including; feeling lonely, feeling so worried that they have not been able to sleep, feeling hopeful about the future, feeling so worried that they have wanted to use drugs and/or alcohol in order to feel better, thought they would never have enough money, thought they would die early (as defined by dying before the age of thirty), thought they would be unhappy, thought bad things would happen to them, and thought they would have a nice family when got older.

This book chapter also compares these service-seeking youth living in the slums of Kampala to urban and nationally representative school-attending youth from Uganda on the mental health indicators of; sadness, loneliness, having no friends, worrying, and suicide ideation. The purpose of this research project is to obtain quantitative data to examine the potential mental health disparities across these population groups in order to inform the identification and implementation of prevention and intervention strategies among vulnerable service-seeking youth.

2   Methods

The current study is based on three cross-sectional surveys: the Global School-based Student Health Survey (GSHS: National); conducted in 2003, of nationally representative students across Uganda, the Global School-based Student Health Survey (GSHS: Urban); conducted in 2003, of nationally representative students in Urban areas in Uganda, and the Kampala Youth Survey of service-seeking youth in Kampala. The GSHS surveys were developed and supported by the WHO with technical support from the CDC (CDC, 2012). The goal of the GSHS is to provide data on health behavior and relevant risk and protective factors among students across regions served by the United Nations. Country-specific questionnaires, fact sheet, public-use data files, documentation, and reports are publicly available from CDC and WHO (CDC, 2012).

The Kampala Youth Survey, conducted in 2011, was implemented to quantify and describe high-risk behaviors and exposures in a convenience sample of urban service-seeking youth living on the streets or in the slums. These youth were between the ages of 14 and 24 and were participating in a Uganda Youth Development Link (UYDEL); drop-in center for disadvantaged street youth (UYDEL, 2012). The methods of this survey have been described elsewhere (Swahn *et al.*, 2012a; Swahn *et al.*, 2012b; Swahn, Palmier, & Kasirye, 2013). Brief face-to-face surveys lasting about 30 minutes, were administered by social workers/peer educators employed by UYDEL across 8 drop-in centers to youth ages 14-24. Participating youth received snacks and transportation for completing the survey. Surveys were administered in

English or Luganda, to the extent possible, in private settings and rooms, to ensure privacy of survey questions and responses.

Each social worker/peer educator received training on the study methodology, each of the survey questions and its translation into Luganda (local language) if needed, and recruited potential participants among attendants at their specific drop-in Center. Recruitment took place using word-of-mouth, and each attendant was eligible for participation if they were between 14 and 24 years of age. No exclusion criteria were applied beyond the age range. Participants were informed about the study and read (or were read) the consent forms to indicate their willingness to take the survey. The consent process required that emancipated street youth 14 to 17 years of age provide their own consent for participating in the survey. Because youth 14 to 17 years of age who "cater for their own livelihood" are considered emancipated in Uganda, parental permission/consent had been waived. The same consenting process was followed for youth 18 to 24 years of age.

Over the ten-day survey period, 507 youth were approached for participating in the survey. Among these youth, 46 declined and 461 agreed to participate, yielding a participation rate of 90.9%. Four of the surveys were missing substantial numbers of responses and were therefore excluded, yielding 457 completed surveys for the final analytic sample of youth between the ages of 14 and 24 (31.1% boys and 68.5% girls). The mode for age was 17 years (n=81) and 67% of participants were between ages 16 and 20.

2.1   Measures

The Kampala survey questionnaire was modeled from the Global School-based Student Health Survey (CDC, 2012). For this book chapter, nine specific measures were examined with questions asking about if in the past month: the participants felt lonely, had been so worried that they could not sleep, had been so worried that they wanted alcohol or drugs to feel better, felt hopeful about the future, thought that they would never have enough money, thought that they would die early (defined as dying before the age of thirty), thought they would be unhappy, thought that bad things would happen to them and if they thought that they would have a nice family when they get older.

Additionally, five mental health indicators: sadness, loneliness, having no friends, worrying, and suicide ideation, were then compared between these service-seeking youth living in the slums of Kampala to urban and nationally representative youth from Uganda. These measures were compared between the Kampala Youth Survey and Global Student Health Survey (GSHS). See Table 1 for comparison of questions.

2.2   Analysis

Analyses were conducted to examine the percentage of the participants who experienced any of the nine mental health indicators. Analysis was further broken down to examine the prevalence of responses to the nine mental health indicators; sex and age. A z-test was used to test the significance of difference in proportions. The Kampala statistic was compared to Uganda National and Urban statistic respectively. A z-test is used when the sample size is large or when the population variance is known. In our sample, the smallest cell count was five (5). Therefore, no exact test was needed. Also, to conduct comparative analyses across surveys, the ages of participants were restricted to those between 14 and 17 years of age. GSHS: national; N= 2838, GSHS: Urban; N=1524 and the Kampala Youth Survey; N=192. We present the analyses comparing the three studies first followed by a more in-depth examination of the Kampala Youth Survey specifically.

Measure	Kampala Youth Survey (2011)	GSHS National Survey/ Urban Survey (2003)
Loneliness	In the past month, how often have you felt lonely?	During the past 12 months, how often have you felt lonely?
No Friends	How many close friends do you have?	How many close friends do you have?
Worries	In the past month, how often have you been so worried about something that you could not sleep at night?	During the past 12 months, how often have you been so worried about something that you could not sleep at night?
Sadness	In the past year, did you ever feel so sad or hopeless almost every day for two weeks or more in a row that you stopped doing your usual activities?	During the past 12 months, did you ever feel so sad or hopeless almost every day for two weeks or more in a row that you stopped doing your usual activities?
Suicide Ideation	In the past year, did you ever think of killing yourself?	During the past 12 months, did you ever seriously consider attempting suicide?

Table 1: Description of mental health indicator questions in the Kampala Survey and the GSHS (national/urban).

3   Results

Among the youth in the Kampala Youth Survey, the most frequently reported mental health indicator was loneliness (81.8%) followed by worrying (77.7%) and sadness (75.0%). In the GSHS: National, the two most frequently reported mental health indicators were sadness (43.1%) and suicide ideation (20.1%). In the GSHS: Urban, the two most frequently reported mental health indicators were sadness (43.3%) and suicide ideation (18.5%). Statistical differences were noted across surveys with respect to loneliness, worrying and sadness which were all more prevalent among youth in the Kampala Youth Survey than in either the GSHS: National or the GSHS: Urban. The prevalence of each mental health indicator stratified by sex is presented in Table 2.

The patterns noted overall were also observed for specific gender analyses. Boys and girls in the GSHS National and Urban samples were less likely to report loneliness, worrying (losing sleep) and sadness than were boys and girls in the Kampala Youth Survey.

For the nine mental health indicators, the prevalence for each is presented in Table 3. Analyses for the nine indicators show that 83.3% (N = 373) of the overall respondents said they experienced loneliness, 82.9% (N= 375) of the overall respondents said they were so worried that they have or had lost sleep, 35.2% (N= 159) of the overall respondents said that they were so worried that they wanted to use drugs or alcohol to feel better, 92.9% (N= 419) of the respondents felt hopeful about the future, 70.58% (N= 319) of the respondents thought they would never have enough money, 44.3% (N = 199) of the overall respondents thought they would die early (defined as dying before the age of 30), 66.3% (N=295) of the overall respondents thought they would be unhappy, 77.6% (N=346) of the respondents thought they would have bad things happen to them, and 92.2% (N=413) of the overall respondents thought they would have a nice family when they got older.

The prevalence of the nine mental health indicators broken down by sex is presented in Figure 1. Analyses were computed for responses by sex for the different mental health status indicators. There were no significant differences between boys and girls based on being lonely, having worried, having no money, being unhappy, thinking bad things will happen to them and expecting to have a nice family in the future. However, significant differences were found between boys and girls in their responses to being so worried that they used drugs. Higher number of boys reported that they were worried and used drugs (46.8% boys and 30.1% girls) and this difference was significant with a p-value of 0.0006.

	Kampala Youth Survey (Age 14 - 17) %			GSHS National (Age 14 - 16+) %			GSHS Urban (Age 14 - 16+) %		
	Overall	Boys	Girls	Overall	Boys	Girls	Overall	Boys	Girls
Loneliness	153 (81.8)	61 (87.1)	92 (78.6)	329 (11.9)***	168 (12.1)***	161 (11.7)***	191 (13.0)***	78 (11.0)***	113 (15.0)***
No Friends	16 (8.7)	5 (7.5)	11 (9.3)	281 (10.3)	131 (9.4)	150 (11.3)	155 (10.9)	60 (8.5)	95 (13.1)
Worries	146 (77.7)	57 (82.6)	89 (74.78)	328 (12.1)***	158 (11.3)***	170 (13.0)***	152 (10.3)***	59 (7.8)***	93 (12.7)***
Sadness	141 (75.0)	59 (84.3)	82 (69.5)	1179 (43.1)***	572 (40.6)***	607 (45.7)***	641 (43.3)***	279 (38.5)***	362 (48.0)***
Suicide Ideation	51 (26.8)	14 (19.7)	37 (31.1)	534 (20.1)	249 (17.9)	285 (22.8)	256 (18.5)	109 (16.0)	147 (20.8)

***p < 0.05, All comparisons are made against the Kampala Youth Survey.

Table 2: Prevalence and Comparisons of Mental Health Factors across Three Surveys.

Significant differences were also found between boys and girls based on their responses of expecting to die early. More boys reported thinking that they would die early (52.1% boys and 40.7% girls) and this was a significant difference with a p-value of 0.0241.

The prevalence of the nine mental health indicators broken down by age is presented in Figure 2. Analyses were also computed to assess mental health status indicators by age dichotomized as those under 18 years of age and those 18 years of age and older (<18 and ≥ 18). Respondents did not significantly differ by age group in their responses to being lonely, being hopeful, thinking they will die early, thinking they will have no money, thinking bad things will happen to them, being unhappy or thinking they will have a nice family. There were, however, significant differences based on their age according to the responses for worrying resulting in sleep loss and being so worried that they used drugs. Older youth reported worrying that impacted sleep more often (77.8% < 18 and 86.6% ≥ 18) and this was significant with a p-value of 0.0143 while older youth also reported using drugs more than younger youth because of being so worried (23.7% < 18 and 43.6% ≥ 18) and this was significant with a p-value of 0.0001.

4   Discussion

This book chapter sought to determine whether youth, primarily non-school-attending, living in the slums of Kampala, had greater mental health needs than nationally representative school-attending youth living across Uganda or living in urban areas. In the comparisons, even when restricted to youth living in urban areas specifically, those who live in the slums are at particular disadvantage with respect to sadness, worrying and loneliness indicating that the mental health needs in this vulnerable population are of grave concerns. This is in accordance with previous research among girls and young women living on the streets and in the slums of Kampala (Swahn et al., 2012b).

Indicators of Mental Health Status		
Indicators	**Yes %**	**No %**
Lonely	373 (83.3)	75 (16.7)
Worried No Sleep	375 (82.8)	78 (17.2)
Worried Using Drugs	159 (35.2)	293 (64.8)
Hopeful	419 (92.9)	32 (7.1)
No Money	319 (70.6)	133 (29.4)
Die Early	199 (44.3)	250 (55.7)
Unhappy	295 (66.3)	150 (33.7)
Bad Things	346 (77.6)	100 (22.4)
Nice Family	413 (92.8)	32 (7.2)

Table 3: Nine Mental Health Status Indicators Examined in Kampala Youth Survey (2011).

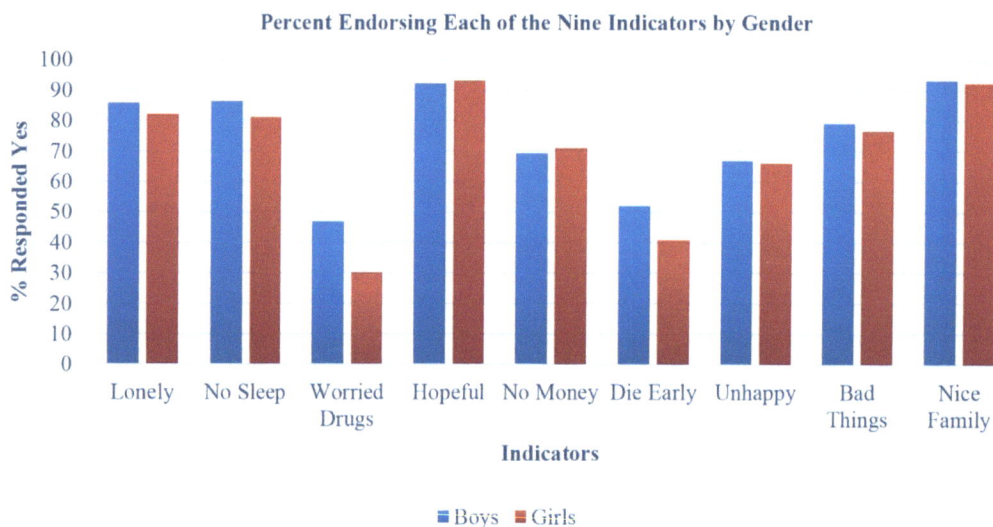

Figure 1: Mental Health Status Indicators Reported by Sex.

This research revealed that there is a high prevalence of youth expecting to be unhappy in the future which is of great concern and highlights the need for interventions to reduce the impact of social disadvantage in their lives through interventions at various levels (Swahn *et al.*, 2012b). These recommendations build on previous research which also proposes that socially-disadvantaged youth have lower levels of collective cognitive and social resources upon which to encourage them to have high hopes for the future (Clinkinbeard & Zohra, 2012; Foster & Spencer, 2011). In the current study we also found no significant differences between boys and girls for the most part with respect to the mental health indicators, a finding that is consistent with previous research examining adolescents' conceptions of the past, the present, and the future which found that females and males reported relatively similar ideas about the past, present, and future (Mello *et al.*, 2009).

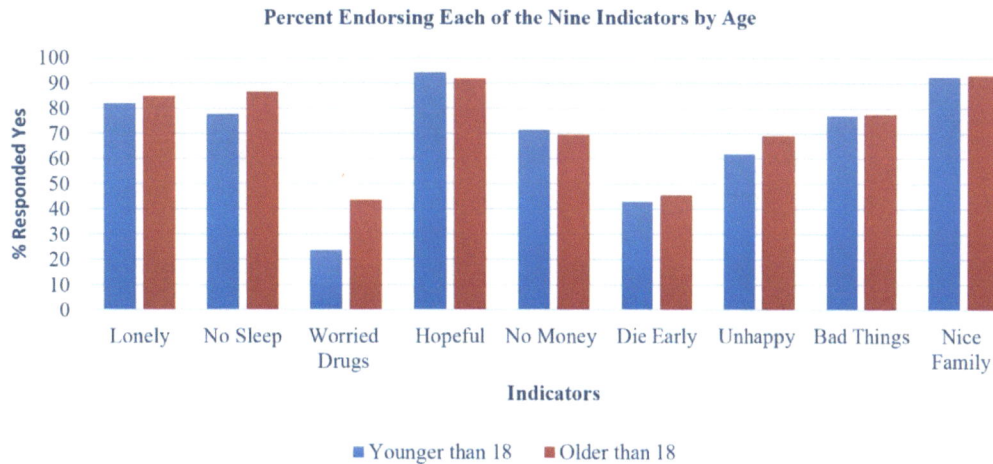

Figure 2: Mental Health Status Indicators by Age.

These findings, while preliminary, demonstrate very high levels of sadness, worry and loneliness among youth living in the slums and reflect great social isolation and despair. As has been suggested previously (Swahn *et al.*, 2012a), while street youth may appear to have higher levels of adaptability and flexibility when faced with adversity than do other youth populations (Ayuku, Devries, Mengech, & Kaplan, 2004), there may still be limits of flexibility that these vulnerable youths can express because of the possible cumulative effect of victimizations (Swahn *et al.*, 2012b) and other adverse health factors that subsequently may be expressed as sadness and isolation as noted in this study. This may be a particular salient issue in the absence of a social network available for support (Swahn *et al.*, 2012a) which is also noted as a disparity among these vulnerable youth.

Given the stark differences with respect to sadness, loneliness and worrying, it was surprising that levels of suicide ideation also did not differ between the groups. However, there may be religious and other contextual and cultural factors that serve to protect these vulnerable youth against suicide ideation even though they have very high levels of sadness and loneliness. Alternatively, it is also highly recognized that the level of stigma and cultural disapproval of suicide may result in under reporting of any suicide-related questions. Additional exploration and research on this topic would be very beneficial in particular for the service provision to these youths. Moreover, the prevalence of reporting sadness varied by sex in the Kampala youth survey indicating that boys had higher levels than girls (84% and 69%, respectively). This observation was not made for either of the GSHS surveys.

4.1   Limitations

The Kampala study is comprised of a relatively small number of participants and included limited measures related to mental health indicators and future aspirations. As such, results of this study should be viewed in the context of several important limitations. Most importantly, the surveys compared herein used very different study methodologies, included questions which were not always worded exactly the same and also did not capture the same time period. The different data collection years could have impacted the findings in multiple and unknown ways. Both surveys also included very brief measures on mental health symptomatology. Moreover, the surveys were also conducted several years apart. These important discrepancies and limitations could have impacted the findings in multiple and unknown ways. Also, the study participants in the Kampala youth survey were not randomly selected, but were youth who self-selected to attend the drop-in centers and to take part of the study. Therefore, the findings may not be representative of street and slum youth in Kampala and may not be generalizable to populations elsewhere. Despite these important limitations, the findings clearly underscore significant mental health disparities among vulnerable urban youth living in the slums compared with urban school-attending youth. However, additional research is needed to replicate these findings and expand comparisons that seek to elucidate the significant and modifiable mental health disparities that may be better addressed in the future to improve the lives and health outcomes of vulnerable youth.

4.2   Further Research

Future research is also needed to better determine strategies for providing additional services and treatment to these youths who may be difficult to reach but who are already service-seeking. Several reports have outlined the dire situation of mental health needs and the acute shortage of psychiatrists, psychologists, nurses, and social workers in Africa (Saxena, Thornicroft, Knapp, & Whiteford, 2007) and in Uganda, more specifically (Swahn et al., 2012a; Ovuga, Boardman, & Wasserman, 2007). However, new strategies have been suggested for the development of child mental health services in low income countries (Omigbodun, 2008) including school based mental health programs (Ibeziako, Omigbodun, & Bella, 2008) that may also be promising for adaptation to be delivered to youth who seek services in drop-in centers. However, these would most ideally involve lay workers but will need to be implemented and evaluated in these informal drop-in centers.

4.3   Implications and Recommendations

The health concerns of street children in Kampala is a particularly pressing issue because they are expected to substantially increase in numbers as Uganda is projected to have the world's highest population growth over the next couple of decades (Swahn et al., 2012a; World watch Institute, 2011). Unfortunately, there is a dearth of information regarding the specific mental health needs and concerns among street youth in sub-Saharan Africa (Ovuga et al., 2005; Bertolote & Fleischmann, 2009; Swahn et al., 2012a; Schlebusch et al., 2009). As such, our findings indicate that there is a significant unmet need among these youths, and given the rapid population growth, these unmet needs will continue to increase and exacerbate the already compromised living situation for these youth. This concern of these youth based on their responses is consistent with findings from a study on self-schemas and possible selves as predictors and outcomes of risky behaviors in adolescents which suggested that the self-concept could be one means through which the behaviors become structuralized into actually enduring parts of the self in the future (Stein, Roeser, & Markus, 1998).

   The findings from these youth are worthy of attention and although challenging to address, they can be met through multisectoral collaborations. This is emphasized in the WHO's mental health action plan 2013-2020 which is a fundamental resource for improving mental health globally. It gives background and insight for nations and communities to improve their mental health outcomes through its major objectives to; strengthen effective leadership and governance for mental health, provide comprehensive, integrated and responsive mental health and social care services in community-based settings, implement strategies for promotion and prevention in mental health and to strengthen information systems, evidence and research for mental health. It lays a foundation for mental health prioritization through six cross cutting principles of Universal health coverage, Human rights, Evidence-based practice, Life course approach, Multi-sectoral approach and Empowerment of persons with mental disorders and psychosocial disabilities (WHO, 2013). This is an exciting advancement for mental health research and priority setting and hopefully these initiatives will reach youth in underserved communities with high need for services, particularly in sub-Saharan Africa.

References

Ayuku, D. O., Devries, M. W., Mengech, H. A., & Kaplan, C. D. (2004). Temperament characteristics of street and non-street children in Eldoret, Kenya. African Health Sciences, 4(1), 24–30.

Bertolote, J. M., & Fleischmann, A. (2009). A global perspective on the magnitude of suicide mortality. In D. Wasserman & C. Wasserman (Eds.), Oxford Textbook of Suicidology and Suicide Prevention: A Global Perspective (pp. 92–98). Oxford Engalnd: Oxford University Press.

Centers for Disease Control and Prevention (CDC). (2011). Mental Health Basics. Retrieved from http://www.cdc.gov/mentalhealth/basics.htm.

Centers for Disease Control and Prevention (CDC). (2013). The social-ecological model: A framework for prevention. Retrieved from http://www.cdc.gov/violenceprevention/overview/social-ecologicalmodel.html.

Centers for Disease Control and Prevention. (2012). Global School-based Student Health Survey (GSHS). Retrieved from http://www.cdc.gov/GSHS/.

Chigunta, F. (2002). The socio-economic situation of youth in Africa: Problems, prospects and options. A Paper Presented at the Youth Employment Summit, Alexandria, Egypt, 1–13.

Chronic Poverty Research Centre (CPRC). (2007). Mental illness and exclusion: Putting mental health on the development agenda in Uganda. Retrieved from http://www.chronicpoverty.org/publications/details/mental-illness-and-exclusion-putting-mental-health-on-the-development-agenda-in-uganda/ss.

Clinkinbeard, S. S., & Zohra, T. (2012). Expectations, fears, and strategies juvenile offender thoughts on a future outside of incarceration. Youth & Society, 44(2), 236–257. doi:10.1177/0044118X11398365.

Food and Agriculture Organization of the United Nations. (2011). The state of food insecurity in the world: how does international price volatility affect domestic economies and food security? Rome: Food and Agriculture Organization of the United Nations. Retrieved from http://www.fao.org/docrep/014/i2330e/i2330e00.htm.

Foster, K. R., & Spencer, D. (2011). At risk of what? Possibilities over probabilities in the study of young lives. Journal of Youth Studies, 14(1), 125–143. doi:10.1080/13676261.2010.506527.

Hjelmeland, H., Knizek, B. L., Kinyanda, E., Musisi, S., Nordvik, H., & Svarva, K. (2008). Suicidal behavior as communication in a cultural context: A comparative study between Uganda and Norway. Crisis: The Journal of Crisis Intervention and Suicide Prevention, 29(3), 137–144. doi:10.1027/0227-5910.29.3.137.

Ibeziako, P. I., Omigbodun, O. O., & Bella, T. T. (2008). Assessment of need for a school-based mental health programme in Nigeria: Perspectives of school administrators. International Review of Psychiatry, 20(3), 271–280. doi:10.1080/09540260802000354.

Joe, S., Stein, D. J., Seedat, S., Herman, A., & Williams, D. R. (2008). Prevalence and correlates of non-fatal suicidal behavior among South Africans. The British Journal of Psychiatry, 192(4), 310–311. doi:10.1192/bjp.bp.107.037697.

Krug, E.G., Dahlberg, L.L., Mercy, J.A., Zwi, A.B., & Lozano, R. (2002). World report on violence and health. Geneva: World Health Organization Retrieved from http://whqlibdoc.who.int/publications/2002/9241545615_eng.pdf.

Mello, Z., Bhadare, D., Fearn, E., Galaviz, M., Hartmann, E., & Worrell, F. (2009). The window, the river, and the novel: Examining adolescents' conceptions of the past, the present, and the future. Adolescence, 44(175), 539–556.

Mental Disability Advocacy Center. (2011). Uganda. Retrieved from http://mdac.info/en/where-we-work/uganda.

Mufune, P. (2000). Street youth in southern Africa. International Social Science Journal, 52(164), 233–243.

Muula, A. S., Kazembe, L. N., & Rudatsikira, E. & S. (2007). Suicidal ideation and associated factors among in-school adolescents in Zambia. Tanzania Health Research Bulletin, 9(3), 202–206.

Omigbodun, O. (2008). Developing child mental health services in resource-poor countries. International Review of Psychiatry, 20(3), 225–235. doi:10.1080/09540260802069276.

Omigbodun, O., Dogra, N., Esan, O., & Adedokun, B. (2008). Prevalence and correlates of suicidal behavior among adolescents in Southwest Nigeria. International Journal of Social Psychiatry, 54(1), 34–46. doi:10.1177/0020764007078360.

Ovuga, E., Boardman, J., & Wasserman, D. (2007). Integrating mental health into primary health care: Local initiatives from Uganda. World Psychiatry: Official Journal of the World Psychiatric Association (WPA), 6(1), 60–61.

Ovuga, E., Boardman, J., & Wassermann, D. (2005). Prevalence of suicide ideation in two districts of Uganda. Archives of Suicide Research: Official Journal of the International Academy for Suicide Research, 9(4), 321–332. doi:10.1080/13811110500182018.

Saxena, S., Thornicroft, G., Knapp, M., & Whiteford, H. (2007). Resources for mental health: scarcity, inequity, and inefficiency. Lancet, 370(9590), 878–889. doi:10.1016/S0140-6736(07)61239-2.

Schlebusch, L., Burrows, S., & Vawda, N. (2009). Suicide prevention and religious traditions on the African continent. In D. Wasserman & C. Wasserman (Eds.), Oxford Textbook of Suicidology and Suicide Prevention (pp. 64–70). Oxford England: Oxford University Press.

Stein, K., Roeser, R., & Markus, H. (1998). Self-Schemas and possible selves as predictors and outcomes of risky behaviors in adolescents. Nursing Research, 47(2), 96–106.

Swahn, M. H., Gressard, L., Palmier, J. B., Kasirye, R., Lynch, C., & Yao, H. (2012b). Serious violence victimization and perpetration among youth living in the slums of Kampala, Uganda. Western Journal of Emergency Medicine, 13(3), 253.

Swahn, M. H., Palmier, J. B., & Kasirye, R. (2013). Alcohol exposures, alcohol marketing, and their associations with problem drinking and drunkenness among youth living in the slums of Kampala, Uganda. ISRN Public Health, 2013, 1–9. doi:10.1155/2013/948675.

Swahn, M. H., Palmier, J. B., Kasirye, R., & Yao, H. (2012a). Correlates of suicide ideation and attempt among youth living in the slums of Kampala. International Journal of Environmental Research and Public Health, 9(12), 596–609. doi:10.3390/ijerph9020596.

Swahn, M.H., Bossarte, R.M., Eliman, D.M., Gaylor E. & Jayaraman, S. (2010). Prevalence and correlates of suicidal ideation and physical fighting: a comparison of students in Botswana, Kenya, Uganda, Zambia and the Unites States. Int Public Health Journal,, 2(2), 195–206.

U.S. Department of Health and Human Services. Mental Health: A Report of the Surgeon General. Rockville, MD: U.S. Department of Health and Human Services, Substance Abuse and Mental Health Services Administration, Center for Mental Health Services, National Institutes of Health, National Institute of Mental Health, 1999.

Uganda Youth Development Link. (2012). Official Website. Retrieved from http://www.uydel.org/.

UN-HABITAT. (2005). Slums: Some definitions. Retrieved from http://ww2.unhabitat.org/mediacentre/documents/sowcr 2006/SOWCR%205.pdf.

Wasserman D., Cheng, Q., & Jiang, G-X. (2005). Global suicide rates among young people aged 15-19. World Psychiatry, 4(2), 114–120.

World Health Organization (WHO). (2007). What is mental health?. Retrieved February 13, 2014, from http://www.who. int/features/qa/62/en/.

World Health Organization, Department of Mental Health and Substance Abuse, & Prevention Research Centre in the Netherlands. (2004). Prevention of mental disorders: effective interventions and policy options summary report. Geneva: World Health Organization. Retrieved from http://www.who.int/mental_health/evidence/en/prevention_of_mental_disorders_sr.pdf

World Health Organization. (2010). Mental health: Strengthening our response fact sheet number 220. Retrieved from http://www.who.int/mediacentre/factsheets/fs220/en/.

World Health Organization. (2011). Suicide prevention (SUPRE). Retrieved from http://www.who.int/mental_health/prevention/suicide/suicideprevent/en/.

World Health Organization. (2013). Mental health action plan 2013-2020. Retrieved from http://apps.who.int/iris/handle/10665/89966.

World watch Institute. (2011). Uganda on track to have world's highest population growth. Retrieved from http://www.worldwatch.org/node/4525

Prospective Memory in Children with Type 1 Diabetes Mellitus

Jennifer Osipoff
Department of Pediatrics, Division of Pediatric Endocrinology
Stony Brook Children's Hospital, USA

Thomas Wilson
Department of Pediatrics, Division of Pediatric Endocrinology
Stony Brook Children's Hospital, USA

Thomas Preston
Neuropsychology Service
Stony Brook University Hospital, USA

1   Background and Significance

Type 1 diabetes mellitus (T1DM) is one of the leading chronic diseases among children and adolescents in the United States. Prospective memory, that is "the cognitive ability of remembering to carry out intended actions [is]… an essential precursor of independent living, as the necessity to prospectively remember is highly prevalent in the organization of one's daily routine and in the challenge of accomplishing occupational and social demands" (Kliegel 2008). For example, one's prospective memory will dictate if a child remembers, without parental prompting, to complete his/her homework afterschool or in the case of a child with T1DM, if he/she remembers to check his/her blood sugar before a meal. To date, our study is the only one that begins to look at the impact of having T1DM on prospective memory (Osipoff *et al.,* 2012). Understanding how T1DM affects one's prospective memory is important clinically for physicians and families in making decisions about insulin regimens. Prospective memory is also an important consideration in one's educational functioning and ability to become self-sufficient as an adult.

A 2002-2003 multicenter study conducted by the Center of Disease Control and Prevention (CDC) and the National Institute of Health (NIH) determined that 15,000 children under the age of 20 are diagnosed with T1DM annually, with an incidence rate of 19 new cases per 100,00 youth (Prevention 2008), constituting a major public health problem. In 2007, an estimated $174 billion dollars was consumed by diabetic care, including $116 billion in direct medical costs and $58 billion in decreased national productivity (Association 2008). The majority of the medical costs were related to inpatient hospital care of diabetics, diabetic medications and supplies, and prescriptions to treat diabetic complications (Association 2008). Discovering ways to enhance compliance with one's diabetic management would help prevent the occurrence of diabetic complications which in turn would decrease the economic burden diabetes care imposes on all of society. If compliance is indeed impaired because of deficits in prospective memory, the development of tools to enhance this neurocognitive component could in turn help individuals with T1DM improve their glycemic control, lower their chances of developing diabetes related co-morbidities, such as retinopathy, nephropathy, neuropathy, and cardiovascular disease, and improve their overall quality of life.

2   Memory and Cognitive Deficits in Children with Type 1 Diabetes Mellitus

The long term medical problems associated with T1DM are well studied and widely recognized. The Diabetes Control and Complications Trial (DCCT) found that adult diabetics who maintained their average hemoglobin A1C at 7% using an intensive insulin regimen had a 60% reduction in the development of microvascular complications compared to diabetics who attained a hemoglobin A1C (HbA1C) of 9% using a standard insulin regimen; macrovascular complications were decreased over 40% in the intensive group (Skyler *et al.,* 2009). The results of the DCCT have served as a foundation for clinical practice, with hemoglobin A1Cs being frequently monitored in diabetic patients.

Though still scarce compared to research involving the aforementioned medical sequelae, a relatively large amount of research involving cognition has been generated in the adult diabetic population. A sub-study of the Action to Control Cardiovascular Risk in Diabetes (ACCORD) trial found that in adult type 2 diabetics, higher HbA1C values were associated with lower cognitive ability (Cukierman-Yaffee 2009). In 2008, Kohl and Seaquist published a review of the literature identifying cognitive dysfunction in patients with type 1 and type 2 diabetes (Kodl and Seaquist 2008). Their work summarized the various deficits documented in earlier studies; problems have been reported in information processing speed, psychomotor efficiency, vocabulary, general intelligence, attention, executive function, academic achievement, mental flexibility, and memory. A meta-analysis of 33 studies investigating cognitive performance in adults with T1DM concluded "A study on the impact of cognitive problems in patients with type 1 diabetes on the day-to-day functioning is still missing" (Brands *et al.*, 2005).

In contrast to the substantial adult research, there is a dearth of information in the pediatric population. Cognitive deficits in children with T1DM did not begin to gain attention until the early 1980s. The impact of T1DM on the developing cognitive and memory skills of pediatric aged patients is largely unexplored and many questions remain in regards to the nature, mechanism, and significance of these impairments. A meta-analysis of cognitive function in children with T1DM conducted in 2008 only found nineteen studies published since 1985 focusing solely on pediatric subjects (Gaudieri *et al.*, 2008). Their review concluded that compared with their healthy peers, children with T1DM have slightly lower overall cognition and score lower on tests of intelligence, psychomotor activity, speed of information processing, attention, executive function, visual motor integration, and academic achievement. Naguib *et. Al.*'s 2008 meta-analysis of neuro-cognitive performance in children with T1DM expanded their review to include studies conducted from 1980-2005 and still only found 24 such studies. Their conclusions echoed those of Gaudeieri *et al.*'s meta-analysis, reporting that children with T1DM had poorer performance on tests of visuospatial ability, motor speed, writing, sustained attention, reading, full intelligence quotient (IQ), performance IQ, and verbal IQ.

The majority of studies involving pediatric T1DM and cognitive functioning have focused on the impact of severe hypoglycemia, defined as an event where a child needs outside assistance to bring up his/her blood sugar, for example the use of glucagon. Such studies have concluded that children with severe episodes of hypoglycemia have more learning difficulties reported by parents (Hannonen *et al.*, 2003), increased need for special education (Hannonen *et al.*, 2003; Rovet *et al.*, 1988), impairments in memory and learning (Hannonen *et al.*, 2003; Rovet and Ehrlich 1999), decreased spatial ability (Hershey *et al.*, 1999; Perantie *et al.*, 2008; Rovet *et al.*, 1988), deficits in executive functioning (Bjorgaas *et al.*, 1997; Hannonen *et al.*, 2003; Rovet and Ehrlich 1999), problems with verbal skills (Hannonen *et al.*, 2003; Hershey 1997; Northam *et al.*, 2001; Rankins *et al.*, 2005; Rovet and Alvarez 1997; Rovet and Ehrlich 1999), poorer verbal short term memory (Hannonen *et al.*, 2003; Naguib *et al.*, 2008), weaker visual and verbal delayed recall (Hershey 1997; Perantie *et al.*, 2008; Rovet and Ehrlich 1999; Strudwick *et al.*, 2005), inferior analytical skills (Perantie *et al.*, 2008), problems with attention (Bjorgaas *et al.*, 1997; Gschwend *et al.*, 1995; Rankins *et al.*, 2005; Rovet and Alvarez 1997; Rovet and Ehrlich 1999; Ryan *et al.*, 1985), and slower motor speeds (Hershey *et al.*, 1999). To date, only one study argued that severe hypoglycemia had no impact on any of the domains of cognitive function (Wysocki *et al.*, 2003). Interestingly, one study concluded that subtle hypoglycemia actually led to an increase in test scores in academic achievement, memory, verbal comprehension and general cognition (Kaufman *et al.*, 1999). Though McCarthy *et al.*, conceded that the aforementioned studies have documented neuropsychological deficits in children with type 1 diabetes, they concluded these findings do not have an appreciable impact on the development of functional academic skills These authors report that although children with type 1 diabetes tend to have more school absences than their age-matched peers, having diabetes did not have a significant impact on school grades and test performance (McCarthy *et al.*, 2002).

Given that severe episodes of hypoglycemia are more likely to occur in young children who lack the skills necessary to recognize and verbalize their symptoms, researchers have begun investigating the cognitive differences in children with diabetes of early onset, generally defined as onset prior to the age of five to seven years, versus those with late onset of disease (Hagen 1990; Kaufman *et al.*, 1999; Rovet *et al* 1988; Ryan *et al.*, 1985, 2006; Schoenle *et al.*, 2002; Strudwick *et al.*, 2005). One study found that children who developed T1DM prior to five years old had deficits in their ability to organize and recall information and more parental reports of inattentiveness and difficulty completing tasks (Hagen 1990). Ryan, Vega and Drash found that compared with non-diabetic controls, children diagnosed with T1DM before the age of five years scored significantly lower in multiple subsets of tests of cognition. The largest differences were seen in general comprehension; vocabulary, digit span and reading; assessment of visuospatial ability, such as block design, embedded figures, and road map; delayed and immediate visual memory; and tests of mental and motor speed using the grooved pegboard and digit symbols (Ryan *et al.*, 1985). Compared with those with later-onset T1DM, this cohort of subjects also scored lower on tests of vocabulary, visuospatial ability, incidental memory, reading, and mental and motor speed. Schoenle *et. al* found that early onset T1DM caused deterioration in performance and verbal IQ, but only in boys who were diagnosed less than six years of age and who had lower capillary blood gases at the time of diagnosis and had higher hemoglobin A1Cs from the time of onset (2012). In contrast, Kaufman *et. al.* found no differences in any form of neurocognitive testing in children with early disease (1999).

To a lesser extent, high blood sugar, hypoglycemic seizures, gender, and socioeconomic status (SES) have been investigated as causal factors of cognitive dysfunction in pediatric T1DM. Conflicting results about the effect of acute hyperglycemia have been published. A 1995 study using insulin-glucose clamping concluded that acute hyperglycemia, defined as a blood sugar> 360 mg/dL, had no effect on cognitive functioning (Gschwend *et al.*, 1995). Davis *et al.*, countered this a year later finding that when blood sugar was acutely raised to between 360-540 mg/dL, eight of twelve children with T1DM had a decrease in their performance IQ (1996). A 2008 study found that more frequent exposure to high blood sugars was associated with lower general intelligence scores (Perantie *et al.*, 2008). One study (Rovet and Ehrlich 1999) followed sixteen children with diabetes diagnosed at a mean age of 4.5 +/- 3 years over a seven year course. Fifty-three per cent of these patients had at least one hypoglycemic seizure. This subgroup of children scored significantly lower on tests of perceptual, fine motor, visuomotor, visual memory, attention, and executive processing compared to the control group of healthy children and to the children with diabetes that did not experience a hypoglycemic seizure. Several studies have found that boys with T1DM have a higher incidence of learning problems compared to girls with T1DM (Fox *et al.*, 2003; Holmes *et al.*, 1992, 1995, 1999). These studies counter the results of an earlier study that concluded that children, particularly girls and those who developed diabetes prior to the age of four years, were at an increased risk of developing difficulties with mathematics, verbal skills, and visuospatial ability (Rovet *et al.*, 1988). Lower SES also has been implicated as an additional risk factor for cognitive incongruities (Holmes 1999).

The aforementioned studies tended to focus on cognitive function as an entity and only subsets of the larger neurocognitive tests looked at the impact of diabetes on developing memory skills. Given the multiple and complex forms of memory, these findings at best can begin to form a foundation upon which other memory studies can be built. Research looking specifically at pediatric T1DM and its effect on memory did not begin to take place until the mid-1990s and to date only a few studies have been published (Hershey *et al.*, 1997, 1999, 2003, 2004; Kovacs *et al.*, 1994; Soutor *et al.*, 2004; Wolters *et al.*, 1996).

Two studies (Kovacs *et al.*, 1994; Wolters *et al.*, 1996) found that compared with their healthy age-matched peers, children with T1DM scored lower on verbal recall tests assessing their short term memory. Wolters noted that children with early onset T1DM scored lower on this measure than those with late onset disease or with healthy controls. Wolters' study also investigated strategies that children used during the short term memory test to enhance their recall. Children who had poorer control of their diabetes, that is a higher HbA1C, used less active rehearsal strategies and subsequently had lower final scores on the short term memory test. However, Kovacs *et al.,* found no association between long term metabolic control and short term memory (1994). A number of studies (Hershey *et al.,* 1997, 1999, 2003, 2004) looked at the effect of severe hypoglycemia on declarative memory, procedural memory and long term-spatial memory. The 1997 study, unlike the aforementioned studies, stratified the children into those who had a history of severe hypoglycemia and those who did not. Children with T1DM who had experienced at least one episode of severe hypoglycemia had significant impairment in delayed verbal recall, whereas the T1DM children without hypoglycemia performed at the same level of the control, non-diabetic sample. Additionally, no intra-group differences were found between the T1DM groups with and without severe hypoglycemia on tests of procedural memory. The remaining three studies (Hershey *et al.,* 1999, 2003, 2004; Skyler *et al* 2009) all supported the hypothesis that severe hypoglycemia negatively impacts long-term spatial memory in patients with TIDM. Albeit limited, the literature clearly suggests that having diabetes does hinder memory skills in children.

Only two publications have looked at the role that memory plays in diabetic management rather than investigating if T1DM impairs different components of memory (Holmes *et al.,* 2006; Soutor *et al.,* 2004). Holme*s et al.,* utilized The Wide Range Assessment of Memory and Learning (WRAML), a test designed to assess immediate and delayed recall of verbal and visual memory. The earlier study, evaluating youth nine to seventeen years old, concluded that rote verbal memory accounted for 5.5% of the variance in the frequency of blood glucose (BG) testing in children 12.5 years and older and quantitative memory accounted for 9.9% of variance in carbohydrate consumption in adolescents 14.8 years and older (Soutor *et al.,* 2004). However, these behaviors did not predict mean HbA1C values over the prior six months. The second paper developed a biopsychosocial model of predictors of diabetes care behavior and metabolic control after studying more than 200 children nine to sixteen years old (Holmes *et al.,* 2006). A significant inverse correlation of modest magnitude was obtained between higher scores on the memory index of the WRAML and lower HbA1C.

The aforementioned studies build a foundation for further research involving memory and T1DM. One important gap in our knowledge is the role of prospective memory, an essential component of executing intended actions at an appropriate time in the future, in children with T1DM. Despite its importance in diabetic care, only one study about prospective memory in diabetic subjects has been published. A novel test of prospective memory was used in adult patients (ages 18-45 years) with T1DM at both euglycemic and hypoglycemic conditions (Warren *et al.,* 2007). Subjects were given a shopping list of 21 tasks to read. These tasks were divided into three categories- "buy" tasks (i.e. buy tennis balls at A and B sports); "do tasks" (i.e. book a table at Smith's restaurant), and "question tasks" (i.e. what is the advertised loan rate at Mercantile Bank). After the subjects looked over the task list, they were shown a video of a pedestrian journey in an urban shopping area. The subjects were to report what task needed to be accomplished as specific shops appeared; they were given points for correctly recalling the task at the appropriate time. The main objective of this study was to determine if acute hypoglycemia impaired the subjects' score on the prospective memory test. Subjects underwent two glucose clamps- one hypoglycemic and one euglycemic. For the hypoglycemic arm of the study, blood glucoses were maintained at 80mg/dL for 40 minutes before being brought down and maintained at 45 mg/dL for the following hour.

For the euglycemic portion, the blood glucose values were stabilized at 80 mg/dL. The authors concluded that prospective memory was significantly impaired under hypoglycemic conditions.

Warren *et al.*'s study began to investigate a relatively unexplored area of diabetes. Although the authors employed an innovative and clinically reproducible approach, this measure of prospective memory cannot simply be replicated in a pediatric population. The themes used in the aforementioned video are not age normed tasks and could therefore artificially impair prospective memory scores in children with T1DM. At the time our study was conducted, there were no gold standards for assessing prospective memory in a pediatric population (Kvavilashvili 2008). The prospective memory test employed in our study, PROMS (see next section), was designed with a pediatric population in mind and the associated tasks are developmentally appropriate, allowing us to investigate prospective memory in a pediatric T1DM population.

To our knowledge, Osipoff *et al.* (2012) was the first study to look into this area and helps advance our knowledge about how T1DM affects children's ability to remember to carry out daily life activities. Prospective memory is particularly important in a diabetic population, as the medical regimen for such patients is rather complex. Along with their academic and personal responsibilities, on a daily basis pediatric T1DM patients must remember to check their blood sugar before meals, snacks, and bedtime, take insulin a minimum of two times per day, count the number of carbohydrates they consume each time they eat, and to remember to adjust insulin doses based on how they are feeling and how much exercise they did that day. Parents and guardians initially play a large role in this intensive care plan, but as children get older and more independent, more and more responsibility is placed upon the diabetic patient. It is not likely a coincidence HbA1C values begin to rise, often at an astronomical rate, during adolescence. Identifying risk factors that impact prospective memory in pediatric T1DM patients will advance the care of such patients. This information will better allow physicians and families to tailor insulin regimens and will be helpful in determining which children need extra guidance in their daily diabetic care. In addition, the results help provide support in advocating for accommodations that these children may need in educational/occupational settings. Optimizing the treatment plan, perhaps through the addition of environmental cues, would not only improve glycemic control, thereby decreasing the risk of developing long term complications from T1DM, but could also improve the child's ability to function in the aforementioned settings.

3   Development of the Prospective Memory Screening Test

Memory can be divided into two main classifications- how long the memory is retained and the temporal direction that the stored information is used for (Lezak *et al.,* 2012). The duration of memory retention is generally divided into three categories: sensory, short term, and long term. Sensory memory is what is perceived after the first 200-500 milliseconds after viewing an item. Short term memory is what can be recalled within several seconds to a few minutes. Short term memory, often described as working memory, connects one's central executive functioning (for example attention) to one's visuospatial abilities and phonological loop. This information gets processed in the frontal cortex where it can be transcribed into long term memory with the assistance of the hippocampus. Long term memory, as its name implies, has the potential to be stored indefinitely. Long term memory is made up of declarative (explicit) and procedural (implicit) memory. Declarative memory requires conscious recall and is further subdivided into semantic memory and episodic memory. Semantic memory allows one to recall abstract knowledge independent of the environmental context. On the contrary, episodic memory is responsible for one's personal memories, such as how he/she felt at a particular point in time. Autobiographical memory and visual memory constitute episodic memory. The other component of long term memory, procedural or implicit memory, does not require any conscious recall and is primarily used in learning motor skills. Retrospective and prospective memory is used to describe the temporality of memory. Retrospective memory, which includes semantic and episodic memory, requires one to recall content from the past. Prospective memory is used to remember future intentions. Prospective memory may be trigged by a time-cue or by environmental-context cues.

The Prospective Memory Screening (PROMS) was originally developed by Sohlberg, Mateer and Geyer (Sohlberg 1985) as a simple, ecologically valid measure of memory for intentions in adult traumatic brain injury (Sohlberg 1989). It has recently been piloted with a pediatric population to determine its potential usefulness with children and adolescents. An initial validation study was conducted with a sample of 167 clinically referred sample of children and adolescents. In this study, the PROMS had seven items, each involving a task to be remembered and carried out at a future time. Three of the items involved event-based prospective memory, in which the examinee was to carry out a task when given a signal by the examiner. Three of the items were time-based, i.e., they required the examinee to carry out some action at a future time on the clock. The seventh and final item required the examinee to remember to mail a postcard to the examiner a day after the examination.

Each event based item of the original PROMS was scored on a 3 point scale, as follows:

- 2 points: Correct action carried out at the correct signal

- 1 point: Incorrect action carried out at the correct signal or Examinee verbalized some knowledge of the need to carry out an action but could not recall the action.

- 0 points: Examinee demonstrates no response at the designated signal.

- Each time based item of the PROMS was scored on a 3 point scale, as follows:

- 3 points: Examinee carried out the correct task at the appropriate time

- 2 points: Examinee carried out the correct task at the incorrect time or Examinee carried out the incorrect task at the correct time or Examinee demonstrated some knowledge, at the correct time that a task needed to be carried out, but could not recall the task

- 1 point: Examinee carried out the incorrect task at the incorrect time

- 0 points: Examinee showed no response

The final, 24 hour task required the examinee to take a postcard from the office and mail it back to the office the following day. Scoring was as follows:

- 3 points: Postcard postmarked on target date

- 2 points: Postmarked within two days of target date

- 1 point: Postcard taken from office and mailed back at any time

- 0 points: Postcard not taken from the office or not received at all

All evaluations involving the PROMS were conducted by a clinical neuropsychologist with over 20 years' professional experience. The age range of the children was 6 through 18 years with a mean age of 11.22 years. There were 54 (72%) boys, and 21 (28 %) girls. Thirty-five (46%) of the subjects had a primary diagnosis of Attention Deficit/Hyperactivity Disorder; 23 (31%) had a primary diagnosis of Learning Disability; and 17 (23%) had mixed neurodevelopmental disorders.

The PROMS was designed to assess prospective memory, and has been well-validated for use with adult populations. An initial validation study to test the psychometric properties has been completed for administration of the PROMS to child and adolescent populations. The scale was tested across several stages, including initial tests for reliability and validity. An exploratory principal-component factor analysis identified 2 factors that accounted for 48% of the total variance (as demonstrated via utilization of the Scree test- see figure 1), with both factors. These two factors were expected, supporting the hypothesis that prospective memory assessment is comprised of event-based and time-based components. Initial tests for reliability were acceptable.

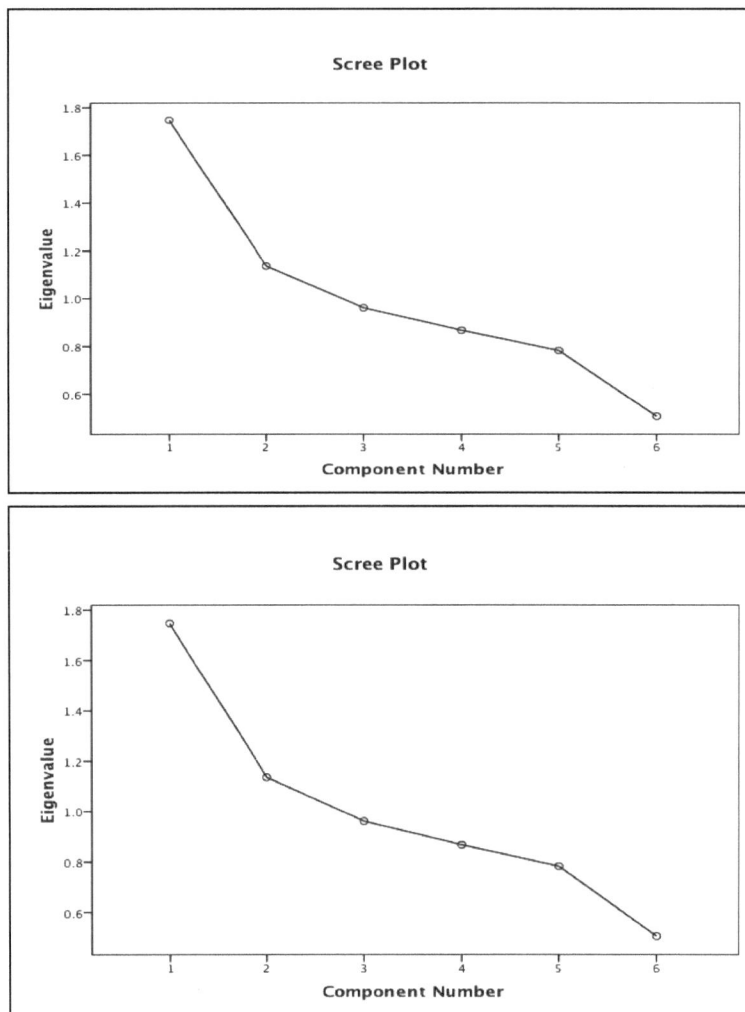

Figure 1: Scree Plot.

The PROMS has been refined in order to make it more sensitive and easier to administer. In its revised form, it has been administered to approximately 50 clinically referred children, and 12 typically developing (non-referred) children, ranging in age from 6-16 years. Preliminary observation of the data indicate that children in the sample with an unequivocal diagnosis of Attention Deficit/Hyperactivity Disorder, with concomitant executive function difficulties, perform significantly more poorly on the PROMS than do typically developing children.

The revised version of the PROMS, as constructed for a broad age range from childhood through adulthood, went through several pilot trials. With respect to test construction and administration, the core problem with any prospective memory measure is the means by which cueing for prospective memory tasks takes place. Prospective memory tasks with event based cues are relatively easy, because the cue is provided by the examiner and execution of the prospective memory task simply involves associative learning between cue and task on the part of the examinee. Time-based tasks are more difficult, because they require the examinee to register and recall a specific time on the clock, associate that time with the prospective memory task, periodically monitor the progression of time on the clock, and wait until the projected time elapses before carrying out the task. It stands to reason that children who are unable to tell time would have great difficulty carrying out these time-based prospective memory tasks, and in the initial phases of revision of the PROMS, they were actually dropped. In the revision and administration process, however, one of the co-investigators on the proposed study (Preston) noted that many typically developing young children who could not yet tell or predict time on the initial screening, or who could do so only partially, nonetheless remembered the target time for the task, monitored the available clock carefully and then carried out the time-based tasks at the appropriate time. After careful consideration, it was decided that the process by which children at all developmental levels learn to tell, predict, and monitor the passage of time is in itself valuable information in relation to prospective memory, and that the PROMS would have far greater psychometric and developmental integrity across a broad age range if all tasks were included for children of all ages.

As it stands now, and as can be seen from the PROMS test form and instructions (see table 1), the examinee is asked at the beginning of the test to read the current time from a digital clock and predict the time 2, 5, 10, and 20 minutes from the current time. Moreover, during the test administration, the examiner carefully but unobtrusively monitors and counts the number of times the examinee checks the available clock. Initial data from the normative developmental study show increasing attention to the clock with age, tapering off in adolescence without significant cost to older children in terms of correct task execution. This mirrors available experimental findings on the "test-wait-test-exit" model of prospective memory (McDaniel 2007).

4 Present Study (Osipoff *et al.*, 2012)

4.1 Methods

One hundred twenty children were recruited during outpatient appointments, hospitalizations, diabetes camp, and via advertising in the local Juvenile Diabetes Research Foundation chapter from July 2009 to November 2010. Eligibility criteria were age six - eighteen years, diagnosed with T1DM for at least three months, and fluency in English. Exclusion criteria were neurologic, psychiatric, or medical disorders known to effect cognition and attendance in special education programs prior to the diagnosis of T1DM.

PROMS Task #	Time (min)	Instructions to Subject	Instructor's Prompt	Subject's Action
1	0	1. When I tap on table, get that book for me (EBT)	Gives first two tasks to carry out	
2		2. In exactly two minutes, write your grade in school (TBT)		
3	2	When I show you a manila folder state your phone number (EBT to occur in 5 minutes)		Writes grade in school
4	7	In exactly 5 minutes, get me that CD (TBT)	Shows manila folder	States phone number
5	12	When I show you a stapler tell me to organize my papers (EBT to occur in 10 minutes)		Gets CD
6	20	In exactly 10 minutes put a penny in the envelope (TBT)	Taps on table	Gets book
7	22	When I show you a green paper, write a problem you are having in school (EBT to occur in 15 minutes)	Shows stapler	Says to organize papers
8	30	In exactly 20 minutes ask me what we are going to do next (TBT)		Puts penny in envelope
	37		Shows green paper	Writes down school problem
	50			Asks what are we doing next?

Table 1: Description of PROMS. A digital clock is placed on the table between the instructor and the child. The instructor ensures that the child is able to determine what time it will be at different time intervals. Then the instructor gives the child the first two tasks to remember to carry out which starts the test. The instructor gives the next task to remember at the predetermined times regardless of whether or not the child has correctly completed the prior tasks. For scoring purposes tasks are divided into event based tasks (EBT) and time based tasks (TBT).

The protocol was approved by the institutional review board and the General Clinical Research Center (GCRC); $40 gift cards were provided for each family to serve as an incentive to participate. Consent and assent were obtained from all parent-child pairs. At the start of the study visit, the child's BG was measured (Accucheck® glucometer) and HbA1C (Siemens DCA Analyzer). Hypoglycemia (random BG < 70 mg/d), if present, was treated prior to testing and ample time was provided for recovery. If the BG was more than 240 mg/dL, urine ketones were checked. No participants had hypoglycemia or moderate or large ketones at the onset of the study.

One GCRC staff member received intensive training from our neuropsychologist (Preston) to administer the PROMS and other cognitive tests. This person had no prior interactions with any of the children and remained blinded to the BG and HbA1C results. If hypoglycemia was suspected during testing, the child's BG was retested and treatment was provided as needed. Only one child experienced low BG during testing.

Prospective memory was assessed using a revised version of the Prospective Memory Screening (Sohlberg 1985, 2009) utilizing a combination of eight event-based prospective memory tasks (EBT) and time-based prospective memory tasks (TBT). The PROMS was conducted concurrently with academic testing in order to provide an index of prospective memory that is both sensitive and ecologically valid (Preston 2011). The 2-subtest version of the Wechsler Abbreviated Scale of Intelligence (WASI) evaluated general intellect (Corporation 1999). Academic skills were measured using the Wechsler Individual Achievement Test – Second Edition (WIAT 2) (Corporation 2002). The California Verbal Learning Test – Children's Version (CVLT C) assessed declarative memory (Delis 1994). Working memory was investigated by the Digit Span subtest of the Wechsler Intelligence Scale for Children – Fourth Edition (WISC 4) (Corporation 2004). At completion, a repeat BG level was obtained.

The accompanying parent answered questions regarding the child's diabetic history and the family's socioeconomic status. The Behavior Rating Inventory of Executive Functions (BRIEF) was also completed to capture parents' observations of their child's capacities across several sub-domains of executive function, including self-regulation, planning/organization, and working memory (Gioia 2000).

4.2 Statistical Analysis

4.2.1 Power Analyses

A projected sample size of 100 participants provided 88% power for detecting significant correlations (e.g., for r = .30), and a two-tailed significance level set at p <0.05. The a priori power analyses for each regression model (IBM SPSS SamplePower 2.0), included seven control variables entered in Step 1 of the equation (chronological age at time of PROMS; age at diabetes diagnosis; parental report of age at first severe episode of hypoglycemia defined as a hypoglycemic seizure, loss of consciousness, or need for glucagon; number of episodes of hypoglycemia; duration of T1DM; gender; socioeconomic status), yielding an R-square of 0 .25. The second step of the regression (entering PROMS score) yielded a unique increment of 0.06 (total R-square for each equation = 0.31), providing a power of 0.80 for the final increment (and 0.95 for all eight variables entered into the regression models) with the given sample size of 100 and alpha set at 0.05. The test was based on Model 2 error, such that variables entered into the regression subsequent to the set of interest served to reduce the error term in the significance test, and therefore were included in the power analysis. This effect was selected as the smallest effect that would be important to detect, in the sense that any smaller effect would not have been of clinical or substantive significance. It was assumed that this effect size was reasonable, in the sense that the effects of this magnitude have been demonstrated by prior research in this field of research (Hershey *et al.,*1999, 2003, 2004; Kovacs *et al* 1992, 1994; Perantie *et al.,* 2008). Thus, the analyses provided adequate power for testing the assumptions underlying the statistical models.

4.2.2 Data Analysis

All variables were examined for accuracy of data entry, missing values, and fit between their distributions and the assumptions of multivariate analysis. The ratio of cases to independent variables appeared satisfactory for each of the regression analyses. The majority of the variables met the assumptions of normality, linearity, and homoscedasticity of residuals, with the exception of HbA1C and number of severe hypoglycemic episodes. Therefore, these two variables were log transformed prior to entry in the regression analyses.

No significant outliers were identified among the residuals. Co-linearity diagnostics performed for each regression analysis determined that the majority of the independent variables appeared sufficiently independent to enter into the regression analyses, with the exception of age, age at diagnosis and duration of illness, and number of episodes of diabetic ketoacidosis and low BG episodes. As a result, age and number of low BG episodes were selected as empirically based variables for the parsimonious regression equations. The levels of association among the background and control, explanatory, and outcome variables were computed with Pearson product moment correlations. Control variables were entered into hierarchical regression analyses at Step 1, followed by the explanatory variable to determine if the explanatory variable contributed additional unique variance to the multivariate models. Hierarchical regression analyses were deemed appropriate, as they provided primarily descriptive and exploratory information related to cognitive and psychosocial factors as predictors of HbA1C values in a reasonably novel study population. Also, this analysis provided the relative contributions of the delineated independent factors to the outcome variables of HbA1c values. All data were analyzed using IBM SPSS for Mac (Version 18.0).

4.3   Results

One hundred child-parent pairs completed the study. Despite agreeing to participate, twenty families ultimately failed to schedule an appointment with the GCRC. Six children were excluded due to medical co-morbidities or special education needs not disclosed prior to participation. Data from 94 participants was analyzed. Demographic and clinical characteristics are shown in table 2.

4.3.1   Associations of Control Variables

No association between total PROMS score and glycemic control was found (see figure 2). Lower HbA1C values were associated with higher (better) scores on the 20 minute EBT on PROMS ($r = -0.2$, $p < 0.05$). Parental concerns about their child's working memory and metacognition as assessed by the BRIEF were related to higher HbA1C ($r = 0.21$, $p < 0.05$ for each). No relationship between PROMS scores and parental ratings of the child's cognition on the BRIEF was found. PROMS scores did not correlate with the child's performance on the standardized cognitive tests, gender, nor BG level at the start of the PROMS.

4.3.2   PROMS as a Predictor of HbA1c Values

A hierarchical regression was performed to determine if the PROMS 20 minute EBT would improve predictions of HbA1c values after controlling for participant age, gender, race, socioeconomic status, IQ, and number of severe hypoglycemic episodes. The equation was significant with all of the independent variables entered ($R^2 = 0.14$, $p < 0.05$). Increased age predicted higher HbA1c. None of the other control variables were significantly associated with HbA1c values when entered in the same block of the regression equation. The addition of the PROMS 20 minute EBT scores predicted additional variance in HbA1c values, with the beta weight indicating that lower PROMS 20 minute EBT scores predicted higher HbA1c values ($\beta = -0.22$, $p < 0.05$). Altogether, 14% (7% adjusted) of HbA1c values were predicted by knowing scores on the independent variable of PROMS 20 minute EBT.

5   Discussion

This study represents the first of its kind investigating prospective memory and glycemic control in children with type 1 diabetes mellitus. While as a whole this was a largely negative study, the association between glycemic control and the PROMS 20 minute EBT warrants further exploration. Deficits in EBT could help explain why children, even those with a long standing T1DM, have difficulty remembering to check BG and take insulin at meal times, as these events require event-based prospective memory. It is not clear why the only significant correlation between HbA1C and PROMS was the 20 minute EBT and

Age (years)	12.5 + 3.4 (range 6.17 -17.95)
Gender (% Female)	49
Ethnicity (% white, not of Hispanic origin)	87.2
Full Scale IQ	106.8 $\pm$ 10.5 (range 79 - 142)
Academic Achievement (%)	
As	53.8
As and Bs	7.7
Bs	28.6
Bs and Cs	5.5
Cs	2.2
Cs and Ds	1.1
As, Bs, and Cs	1.1
Education Level of Mother (%)	
Some High School	1.1
High School Graduate	16
Some College	16
Associate's Degree	13.8
Bachelor's Degree	31.9
Master's Degree	16
Doctorate	3.2
Other	2.1
Education Level of Father (%)	
Some High School	0
High School Graduate	25.5
Some College	19.1
Associate's Degree	8.5
Bachelor's Degree	27.7
Master's Degree	7.4
Doctorate	5.3
Other	6.4
Total household income (%)	
<$25,000	3.2
$25-49,999	7.4
$50-74,999	13.8
$75-99,999	24.5
$100-124,999	23.4
>$125,000	23.4
Didn't answer	4.3
Caregiver completing study questionnaires (% mother)	81.9
Hemoglobin A1C (%)	7.9 + 1.2 (range 5.8 – 14.1)
Type 1 diabetes duration (years)	4.9 + 3.5 (range 0.2 - 12.3)
Age at diagnosis of type 1 diabetes (years)	7.6 + 3.8 (range 0.9 - 14.9)
Blood glucose at start of study (mg/dL)	209.7 + 84.5 (range 87 – 452)
Method of Insulin Delivery	
Multiple daily injections (%)	20
CS II (%)	65.6
History of severe low blood glucose reaction (%)	20.4
History of diabetic ketoacidosis (%)	40.4

Table 2: Demographic Information.

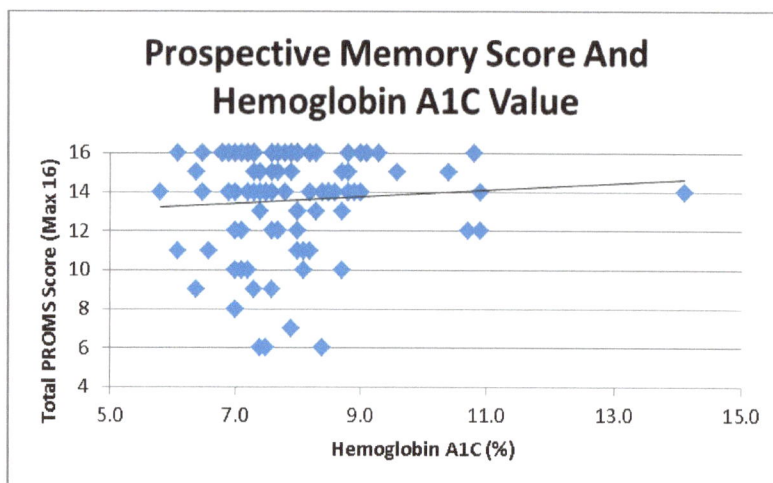

Figure 2: No correlation was found between total PROMS score and A1C

not the shorter EBT. Multiple inputs at the outset of the PROMS and the length of time from request to cue for the task may have contributed to tendency to forget the task. However, this might best mimic expectations outside of the laboratory setting and could impact upon daily diabetic care. Positron emission tomography scans have demonstrated that EBT and TBT activate different areas of the rostral prefrontal cortex (Okuda *et al.,* 2007) and at least one study has shown that deficits in EBT and TBT are not always congruent (Katai *et al.,* 2003).

Our study also found a modest correlation between HbA1C and parental concerns about the children's working memory and metacognition as assessed by the BRIEF. This finding is consistent with that reported by McNally *et al* (2010) who concluded that higher levels of executive functioning (i.e. lower reports of parental concern on the BRIEF) were associated with increased treatment adherence which predicted improved HbA1C levels. The BRIEF parent form is both easy to administer and score. The use of this test in a clinical setting should be considered to help screen for those individuals at increased risk of poor glycemic control.

As stated earlier, most studies involving pediatric T1DM and cognition found that hypoglycemia increased the risk for impairments in executive function (Hannonen *et al.,* 2003; Hershey *et al.,* 1999; Naguib *et al.,* 2008; Perantie *et al.,* 2008; Ryan *et al.,* 1985). Although not one of our primary aims, our study only found a significant correlation between increased hypoglycemic events and increased episodes of diabetic ketoacidosis (r= 0.45, p<0.001). While the relationship between increased episodes of hypoglycemia and lower full-scale IQs trended towards significance (r= -0.185, p= 0.076), more frequent episodes of severe low BG did not impact performance on the PROMS or academic achievement.

Hyperglycemia, gender, and SES have also been investigated as causal factors of cognitive dysfunction in pediatric T1DM. While the mean BG of our participants was approximately 100 mg/dL lower than in either the Davis or the Gschwend studies, no correlations were seen between ambient BG and PROMS scores, performance on digit span testing, or full scale IQ. Studies testing prospective memory under both euglycemic and hyperglycemic conditions in the same child need to be conducted before conclusions regarding the effect of elevated BG on this component of memory can be made. Additionally, our data did not support prior findings (Fox *et al* 2003; Holmes *et al* 1992, 1995, 1999) that boys with T1DM have more cognitive problems as being male did not impact prospective memory or cognitive test scores nor did parents of sons report more concerns on the BRIEF. Although lower SES has also been implicated as an additional risk factor for cognitive incongruities (Holmes 1999) this was not found amongst our children.

There are several limitations of this study. Most important with regard to prospective memory, while there was a positive correlation between one of the prospective memory tasks and HbA1C levels, it was just one of the eight tasks given in the PROMS. There are several possible reasons for this. First, the PROMS is a test which involves relatively low cognitive load, i.e., only two tasks must be remembered at any given time, which possibly makes it easy and gives it a "ceiling effect" with older children and adolescents. And, in fact, preliminary data on the PROMS did show a considerable age effect. It is difficult to determine whether the variables such as glycemic control and length of disease process are responsible for the lack of differences seen in prospective memory scores in the participants aged 12-18 years, or if these results are only because the mastery level of the PROMS test occurs by twelve years of age and subjects need to be provided with a more difficult prospective memory task to see further delineation in their scores. While the prospective memory screen used in our study was specifically developed with a pediatric population in mind and has face validity, it is not a standard tool used in psychometric evaluation, and needs further validation. While this is clearly a limitation of the current study, a thorough review of the literature at the study onset revealed that there were no readily reproducible clinical measurements of pediatric prospective memory available. A further limitation is the applicability of one's prospective memory score in a brief laboratory setting to real life, day to day functioning. However, as no studies have attempted to look at prospective memory differences within a pediatric diabetic population this study served as a foundation for future research studies.

From a demographic perspective, our participants were not representative of a broader T1DM population, and this sampling bias was, very likely related to their solid overall performance on most cognitive measures including the PROMS Stated more specifically, our final study population consisted primarily of academically high-achieving children from well-educated, middle to upper class families. As prospective memory is an integral component of daily functioning and success, this self-selected group likely has better prospective memory skills compared to a more general population of families with children with T1DM. Second, the majority of the participants used intensive insulin regimens and maintained desirable HbA1Cs. It is possible that the prescribing physicians unknowingly assessed aspects of prospective memory skills of these children and their parents and deemed them capable of remembering to carry out the tasks needed for success with an intensive insulin regimen. Third, patients with lower HbA1C, and arguably better prospective memory, may have been more willing to volunteer for the study. Patients with poor glycemic control often failed to come to appointments, potentially due to deficits in prospective memory, and thus had fewer opportunities to be asked to participate. Generally these patients and their families are seen as "unmotivated" to care for T1DM by health care providers; this lack of motivation may actually represent poor prospective memory skills which make diabetic care that much more challenging for these families.

Mean HbA1C of the 20 consented children who ultimately did not participate in the study despite reminder phone calls and opportunities to reschedule was 9% compared to 7.9% of those who completed the study. As the reminder phone calls were directed to the parents, one must question the adults' prospective memory and its role in the children's glycemic control. Future examination of this relationship is warranted, particularly in younger patients in whom adults generally assume responsibility for providing the child's diabetic care.

The lack of significant relationships between frequency of hypoglycemia and prospective memory, academic achievement, and full-scale IQ may not be generalizable to a more diverse sample of children with higher rates of hypoglycemia. Only 20% of the families reported one or more episode of severe hypoglycemia. The accuracy of this occurrence rate is limited by parental recall and individual interpretation of severe hypoglycemia. Additionally, recent studies involving streptozotocin-induced juvenile diabetic rats found that cognitive deficits were cumulative over time, as evident by poorer performance on the passive avoidance box test, Morris water maze, and elevated plus maze in rats with twenty days of diabetes (comparable to 2 years of human life) compared to those ten days from diagnosis (Rajashree *et al.,* 2011, 2012). As these rats were not treated with insulin and their mean fasting blood glucose increased over time, Rajashree *et al.,* attributed these differences to longer exposure to hyperglycemia. Some of the children in our study likely were still in the honeymoon period of diabetes. To qualify for study participation, children only had to be three months out from diagnosis and while the mean duration since diagnosis was 4.9 years the standard deviation was rather wide. Typically children with diabetes in the honeymoon period have not had prolonged hyperglycemia. Our study only looked at the relationship between the PROMS test and the HbA1C value the day the testing was done; we do not have a record of overall glycemic control since diagnosis. Given the characteristics of the final study population, it is quite possible that even those with long-standing diabetes have minimized their exposure to hyperglycemia by maintaining tight control of their diabetes. This, combined with the ceiling effect of the PROMS test itself, could explain the lack of association between PROMS score and duration of disease process. Lastly, the lack of association between lower SES and cognitive functioning may also be due to the homogeneity of our sample, with virtually all of the families earning well above our national poverty threshold.

6   Conclusions

Our study introduces the idea that prospective memory and glycemic control may be interrelated in children with T1DM. The association between the 20 minute EBT score and hemoglobin A1C and not the 20 minute TBT raises the possibility that diabetic control only affects event based prospective memory. Further studies need to be conducted to determine causality. It is equally plausible that a high hemoglobin A1C negatively impacts one's prospective memory or if one's baseline prospective memory is poor that person will not be able to remember to carry out the tasks needed to maintain good diabetic control. As research in prospective memory is rapidly advancing, validated, clinically reproducible tests of prospective memory encompassing the developmental differences in the pediatric population will likely become available. Such tests should be used to determine if deficits in EBT prospective memory as seen here are reproducible, and to determine how disease duration and fluctuations in HbA1C serially influence this aspect of prospective memory. Until such tools are available the PROMS test can be used in elementary-school aged children with diabetes to minimize the ceiling effect. Repeating the same study in a more diverse population in terms of socioeconomic status, glycemic control, method of insulin delivery, duration of disease, and frequency of hypoglycemic episodes is important to increase the generalizability of the study results.

Acknowledgements

The authors would like to thank Patricia Noren, LPN for administering the PROMS and cognitive tests and Drs. Janet Fischel and Catherine Messina for their invaluable contributions in reviewing the manuscript.

Abbreviations

BG: Blood Glucose
EBT: Event Based Task
GCRC: General Clinical Research Center
HbA1C: Hemoglobin A1C
IQ: Intelligence Quotient
PROMS: Prospective Memory Screening Test
SED: Self-efficacy for Diabetes
SES: Socioeconomic Status
TBT: Time Based Task
T1DM: Type One Diabetes Mellitus

References

Association AD. 2008. Economic Costs of Diabetes in the U.S. in 2007. Diabetes Care 31:596-615.

Bjorgaas M, Gimse R, Vik T, and Sand T. 1997. Cognitive function in type 1 diabetic children with and without episodes of severe hypoglycaemia. Acta Paediatr 86(2):148-153.

Brands AM, Biessels GJ, de Haan EH, Kappelle LJ, and Kessels RP. 2005. The effects of type 1 diabetes on cognitive performance: a meta-analysis. Diabetes Care 28(3):726-735.

Corporation P. 1999. Wechsler Abbreviated Scale of Intelligence (WASI). San Antonio Texas.

Corporation P. 2002. Wechsler Inidivual Achievement Test- Second Edition (WIAT 2). San Antonio Texas.

Corporation P. 2004. Wechsler Intelligence Scale for Children- Fourth Edition (WISC 4). San Antonio, Texas.

Cukierman-Yaffee T, Gerstein, H.C., Williamson, J.D., Lazar, R.M., Lovato, L., Miller, M.E., Coker, L.H., Murray, A., Sullivan, M.D., Marcovina, S.M., Launer, L.J. 2009. Relationship Between Baseline Glycemic Control and Cognitive Function in Individuals with Type 2 Diabetes and Other Cardiovascular Risk Factors: The Action to Control Cardiovascular Risk in Diabetes-Memory in Diabetes (ACCORD-MIND) trial. Diabetes Care 32:221-226.

Delis D, Kramer, J.H., Kaplan, E. and Ober, B.A. 1994. California Verbal Learning Test- Children's Version (CVLT-C). San Antonio, Texas: Psychological Corporation.

Gaudieri PA, Chen R, Greer TF, and Holmes CS. 2008. Cognitive function in children with type 1 diabetes: a meta-analysis. Diabetes Care 31(9):1892-1897.

Gioia GA, Isquith, P.K., Guy, S.C., and Kenworthy, L. 2000. Behavior Rating Inventory of Executive Function. Lutz, Florida: Psychological Assessment Resources.

Gschwend S, Ryan C, Atchison J, Arslanian S, and Becker D. 1995. Effects of acute hyperglycemia on mental efficiency and counterregulatory hormones in adolescents with insulin-dependent diabetes mellitus. J Pediatr 126(2):178-184.

Hagen JW, Barclay C.W.,Anderson, B.J., Feeman, D.J., Segal, S.S., Bacon, G., Goldstein, G.W. 1990. Intellective Functioning and Strategy Use in Children with Insulin-dependent Diabetes Mellitus. Child Dev 61:1714-1727.

Hannonen R, Tupola S, Ahonen T, and Riikonen R. 2003. Neurocognitive functioning in children with type-1 diabetes with and without episodes of severe hypoglycaemia. Dev Med Child Neurol 45(4):262-268.

Hershey T, Bhargava N, Sadler M, White NH, and Craft S. 1999. Conventional versus intensive diabetes therapy in children with type 1 diabetes: effects on memory and motor speed. Diabetes Care 22(8):1318-1324.

Hershey T, Craft, S., Bhargava, N., and White, N.H. 1997. Memory and insulin dependent diabetes mellitus (IDDM): Effects of childhood onset and severe hypoglycemia. J Int Neuropsychol Soc 3:509-520.

Holmes CS, Cant, M.C., Fox, M.A., Lampert, N.L., Greer, T. 1999. Disease and Demorgraphic Risk Factors for Disrupted Cognitive Functioning in Children with Insulin-Dependent Diabetes Mellitus. The School Psychology Review 28:215-227.

Holmes CS, Chen R, Streisand R, Marschall DE, Souter S, Swift EE, and Peterson CC. 2006. Predictors of youth diabetes care behaviors and metabolic control: a structural equation modeling approach. J Pediatr Psychol 31(8):770-784.

Katai S, Maruyama T, Hashimoto T, and Ikeda S. 2003. Event based and time based prospective memory in Parkinson's disease. J Neurol Neurosurg Psychiatry 74(6):704-709.

Kaufman FR, Epport K, Engilman R, and Halvorson M. 1999. Neurocognitive functioning in children diagnosed with diabetes before age 10 years. J Diabetes Complications 13(1):31-38.

Kliegel M, McDaniel, M.A., and Einstein, G.O., editor. 2008. Prospective Memory: Cognitive, Neuroscience, Developmental, and Applied Perspectives. New York: Lawrence Erlbaum Associates. 452 p.

Kodl CT, and Seaquist ER. 2008. Cognitive dysfunction and diabetes mellitus. Endocr Rev 29(4):494-511.

Kovacs M, Ryan C, and Obrosky DS. 1994. Verbal intellectual and verbal memory performance of youths with childhood-onset insulin-dependent diabetes mellitus. J Pediatr Psychol 19(4):475-483.

Kvavilashvili L, Kyle, FE, Messer, DJ. 2008. Prospective memory in children: Methodological issues, empirical findings, and future directions. In: M Kliegel MM, GO Einstein, editor. Prospective Memory: Cognitive, Neuroscience, Developmental, and Applied Perspectives. Mahwah, NJ: Erlbaum. p 115-140.

Lezak M, Howieson DB, Bigler ED, Tranel D. 2012. Neuropsychological Assessment. 5th Edition. New York: Oxford.

McCarthy AM, Lindgren S, Mengeling MA, Tsalikian E, and Engvall JC. 2002. Effects of diabetes on learning in children. Pediatrics 109(1):E9.

McDaniel MaE, GO, editor. 2007. Prospective Memory: An Overview and Synthesis of an Emerging Field. Thousand Oaks, CA: Sage Publications.

Naguib JM, Kulinskaya E, Lomax CL, and Garralda ME. 2008. Neuro-cognitive Performance in Children with Type 1 Diabetes--A Meta-analysis. J Pediatr Psychol.

Northam EA, Anderson PJ, Jacobs R, Hughes M, Warne GL, and Werther GA. 2001. Neuropsychological profiles of children with type 1 diabetes 6 years after disease onset. Diabetes Care 24(9):1541-1546.

Okuda J, Fujii T, Ohtake H, Tsukiura T, Yamadori A, Frith CD, and Burgess PW. 2007. Differential involvement of regions of rostral prefrontal cortex (Brodmann area 10) in time- and event-based prospective memory. Int J Psychophysiol 64(3):233-246.

Osipoff JN, Dixon D, Wilson TA, and Preston T. 2012. Prospective memory and glycemic control in children with type 1 diabetes mellitus: a cross-sectional study. Int J Pediatr Endocrinol 2012(1):29.

Perantie DC, Lim A, Wu J, Weaver P, Warren SL, Sadler M, White NH, and Hershey T. 2008. Effects of prior hypoglycemia and hyperglycemia on cognition in children with type 1 diabetes mellitus. Pediatr Diabetes 9(2):87-95.

Preston TaE, P. 2011. Prospective Memory in Clinically Referred and Nonreferred Children. 39th Annual Meeting of the International Neuropsychological Society. Boston, MA.

Prevention CfDCa. 2008. National diabetes fact sheet: general information and national estimates on diabetes in the United States, 2007. Atlanta: U.S. Department of Health and Human Services, Centers for Disease Control and Prevention.

Rankins D, Wellard RM, Cameron F, McDonnell C, and Northam E. 2005. The impact of acute hypoglycemia on neuropsychological and neurometabolite profiles in children with type 1 diabetes. Diabetes Care 28(11):2771-2773.

Rovet J, and Alvarez M. 1997. Attentional functioning in children and adolescents with IDDM. Diabetes Care 20(5):803-810.

Rovet JF, and Ehrlich RM. 1999. The effect of hypoglycemic seizures on cognitive function in children with diabetes: a 7-year prospective study. J Pediatr 134(4):503-506.

Rovet JF, Ehrlich RM, and Hoppe M. 1988. Specific intellectual deficits in children with early onset diabetes mellitus. Child Dev 59(1):226-234.

Ryan C, Vega A, and Drash A. 1985. Cognitive deficits in adolescents who developed diabetes early in life. Pediatrics 75(5):921-927.

Skyler JS, Bergenstal R, Bonow RO, Buse J, Deedwania P, Gale EA, Howard BV, Kirkman MS, Kosiborod M, Reaven P et al., . 2009. Intensive glycemic control and the prevention of cardiovascular events: implications of the ACCORD, ADVANCE, and VA diabetes trials: a position statement of the American Diabetes Association and a scientific statement of the American College of Cardiology Foundation and the American Heart Association. Diabetes Care 32(1):187-192.

Sohlberg MM, Mateer, C.A. and Geyer S. 1985. Prospective Memory Survey. Puyallup: Assocation for Neuropsychological Research and Development.

Sohlberg MMM, C.A. . 1989. Introduction to Cognitive Rehabilitation. New York: Guilford.

Soutor SA, Chen R, Streisand R, Kaplowitz P, and Holmes CS. 2004. Memory matters: developmental differences in predictors of diabetes care behaviors. J Pediatr Psychol 29(7):493-505.

Strudwick SK, Carne C, Gardiner J, Foster JK, Davis EA, and Jones TW. 2005. Cognitive functioning in children with early onset type 1 diabetes and severe hypoglycemia. J Pediatr 147(5):680-685.

Warren RE, Zammitt NN, Deary IJ, and Frier BM. 2007. The effects of acute hypoglycaemia on memory acquisition and recall and prospective memory in type 1 diabetes. Diabetologia 50(1):178-185.

Wolters CA, Yu SL, Hagen JW, and Kail R. 1996. Short-term memory and strategy use in children with insulin-dependent diabetes mellitus. J Consult Clin Psychol 64(6):1397-1405.

Wysocki T, Harris MA, Mauras N, Fox L, Taylor A, Jackson SC, and White NH. 2003. Absence of adverse effects of severe hypoglycemia on cognitive function in school-aged children with diabetes over 18 months. Diabetes Care 26(4):1100-1105.

Hepatitis C Virus among Patients with Mental Disorders

Mohamed Ali Daw

Department of Medical Microbiology and Immunology, Faculty of Medicine
Tripoli University, Tripoli-Libya

1   Introduction

1.1   Background

Mental disorder or mental illness is a complex entities of a unique psychological anomalies reflected immensely on personnel behavior of a patients characterized by such illness. Such reflection is associated with tremendous consequences hence then special demands has to be taken in consideration by society and hospital care sectors to overcome the problems of these patients. Mental disorders vary greatly in types and prevalence all over the world and even within each country itself. Due the complexity of these disorders and its association with personnel and community behavior such patients are particularly prone to a variety of infectious diseases. Incarceration, substance and alcohol abuse, homelessness, sexual behavior, negligence and many other related factors has driven them to be more vulnerable to infectious disease associated with such circumstances particularly viral hepatitis and Human Immune Deficiency Virus (HIV). Indeed such infectious diseases are considered to endemic among this particular group of patients.

Different schemes and categorization has been used to classify mental disorders or psychiatric nosology. Either based on established system of classifying mental disorders or even rational concepts based ritual and social[cultural] believes which varies greatly among societies and communities. The widely accepted and commonly used classification as those produced by the World Health Organization (WHO,2004,2005) called Chapter V of the International Classification of Diseases (ICD-10) as shown in Table 1 and the Diagnostic and Statistical Manual of Mental Disorders (DSM-V)(American Psychiatric Association; 1994) as illustrated in Table 2.

The International Classification of Diseases (ICD) is an international standard diagnostic classification for a wide variety of health conditions. Chapter V focuses on "mental and behavioral disorders" and consists of 10 main groups:
•   F0: Organic, including symptomatic, mental disorders
•   F1: Mental and behavioral disorders due to use of psychoactive substances
•   F2: Schizophrenia, schizotypal and delusional disorders
•   F3: Mood [affective] disorders
•   F4: Neurotic, stress-related and somatoform disorders
•   F5: Behavioral syndromes associated with physiological disturbances and physical factors
•   F6: Disorders of personality and behavior in adult persons
•   F7: Mental retardation
•   F8: Disorders of psychological development
•   F9: Behavioral and emotional disorders with onset usually occurring in childhood and adolescence
•   In addition, a group of "unspecified mental disorders"

*** Within each group there are more specific subcategories

Table 1: WHO Classification of Mental Disorders- ICD-10.

The DSM-V, produced by the American Psychiatric Association, characterizes mental disorder as "a clinically significant behavioral or psychological syndrome or pattern that occurs in an individual

The DSM-V-TR (Text Revision, 2000) consists of five axes (domains) on which disorder can be assessed. The five axes are:

Axis I: Clinical Disorders (all mental disorders except Personality Disorders and Mental Retardation)

Axis II: Personality Disorders and Mental Retardation

Axis III: General Medical Conditions (must be connected to a Mental Disorder)

Axis IV: Psychosocial and Environmental Problems (for example limited social support network)

Axis V: Global Assessment of Functioning (Psychological, social and job-related functions are evaluated on a continuum between mental health and extreme mental disorder)

Table 2: Classification of Mental Disorders according to Diagnostic and Statistical Manual of Mental Disorders (DSM-V).

There are many different categories of mental disorder, and many different facets of human behavior and personality that can become disordered. Some disorders are transient, while others may be more chronic in nature. Anxiety or fear, phobias panic disorder, agoraphobia, obsessive-compulsive disorder and post-traumatic stress disorder, depression schizophrenia, and delusional disorder, eating disorders, sleep disorders various behavioral addictions, such as gambling addiction, may be classed as (including alcohol), when it persists despite significant problems related to its use, may be defined as a mental disorder. The DSM incorporates such conditions under the umbrella category of substance use disorders, which includes substance dependence and substance abuse.

1.2   Etiology

Different hypothesis and speculations have been postulated regarding the etiology of mental disorders. However no evident proofs have been established. Infectious agents may play a role in some of these diseases to some unknown degree. Mental disorders may have an infectious disease component within their pathological foundation. A link between psychopathology and infectious disease has been speculated. Lyme disease, syphilis, babesiosis, ehrlichiosis, mycoplasma pneumonia, toxoplasmosis, borna virus, AIDS, CMV, herpes, streptococcal infections and other unknown infectious agents were found to play a rule in the etiology of Mental disorders (Rosenberg *et al.,* 2003). A better understanding of the [such] role of infection may speed treatment and prevention efforts and reduce the degree of disability and stigma associated with mental illness. Vaccines and antimicrobial agents might enhance current therapeutic options for mental illnesses. Even if infectious diseases were a primary factor in only 1% of neuropsychiatric illnesses, some 10 million persons might benefit from antimicrobial therapies. Stigma and discrimination can add to the suffering and disability associated with mental disorders (or with being diagnosed or judged as having a mental disorder), leading to various social movements attempting to increase understanding and challenge social exclusion.

1.3   Mental Disorders Worldwide

An estimated 14% of total global burden of disease and about a third of total adult disability are attributable to neuropsychiatric conditions. Worldwide more than one in three people in most countries report sufficient criteria for at least one at some point in their life. The World Health Organization estimates that

1.5 billion people worldwide suffer from a neuropsychiatric disorder. Of the 10 leading causes of disability in 1990, four were psychiatric disorders: unipolar depression, manic depression, schizophrenia, and obsessive-compulsive disorders. The Rates of such disorders varied by region,- A 2004 cross-Europe study found that approximately one in four people reported meeting criteria at some point in their life for at least one of the DSM-IV disorders assessed. - A 2005 review of surveys in 16 European countries found that 27% of adult Europeans are affected by at least one mental disorder in a 12 month period - Approximately one in ten met criteria within a 12-month period (Murray and Lopez 1996).

People with severe mental illness represent approximately 2.6% of the US population. Furthermore, 46% of the Americans qualify for a mental illness at some point - A US survey that incidentally screened for personality disorder found a rate of 14.79%. The National Institute of Mental Health recently estimated that as many as 20% of young Americans ages 7 to 14—approximately 10 million children—have mental health problems severe enough to compromise their ability to function . The Substance Abuse and Mental Health Services Administration found that annual visits to mental health specialists (i.e., psychiatrists and psychologists) increased by 50 percent between 1992 and 2000. The National Ambulatory Medical Care Survey found that the number of people receiving treatment for depression tripled between 1987 and 1997. The Robert Wood Johnson Foundation Community Tracking Survey found that the number of people with a serious mental illness who were treated by a specialist increased by 20 percent between 1997 and 2001.

The picture is more complex in the developing countries, the burden of neuro psychiatric conditions in low-income and middle-income countries accounts for an estimated three-quarter of the global burden for these conditions. The disease burden attributable to these conditions exceeds that for infectious, cardiovascular, or neoplastic diseases—neuropsychiatric disorders are already the most important causes of illness in men and women. In China alone mental disorder in adults was greater than 17% in 2001–05. This figure is more rigorous in India and African countries.

Although the rates of psychological disorders are often the same for men and women, women and younger people of either gender showed more cases of disorder. Women tend to have a higher rate of depression. Each year 73 million women are afflicted with major depression, and suicide is ranked 7th as the cause of death for women between the ages of 20-59. Depressive disorders account for close to 41.9% of the disability from neuropsychiatric disorders among women compared to 29.3% among men. There is a lack of published information on the prevalence of microbial disease among patients with mental disorders particularly hepatitis C virus. Hence then Planning to overcome such problems requires accurate data on the prevalence and rate of treatment of HCV among such patients.

1.4   Dissemination of Microbial diseases in Mental Disorders

Along with their psychiatric impairment, persons with severe mental illness are at increased risk for several comorbid conditions such as substance use disorder. They are also likely to be overrepresented in high-risk categories for infection not only with HIV but also with other pathogens with similar routes of transmission, such as hepatitis B virus (HBV) and hepatitis C virus (HCV).

Relative to the general population, women with severe mental illness appear to be at particularly elevated risk (estimated infection rates of 5% vs. 0.17%). Despite the data regarding elevated prevalence rates of HIV/AIDS in people with severe mental illness, and despite reported elevations of infectious hepatitis in psychiatric patients in other countries, there is a dearth of published information on the prevalence of HBV and HCV among people with severe mental illness worldwide. Several explanations have been advanced to account for the increased prevalence of such diseases in persons with severe mental illness. Both the direct (e.g., affective liability) and indirect (e.g., homelessness) effects of severe mental illness have been hypothesized to increase high-risk behavior and result in elevated rates of HIV infection.

In general, people with severe mental illness appear to have increased rates of sexually transmitted diseases (STDs), and they are likely to engage in high-risk behaviors such as using injection drugs, having multiple sexual partners and high-risk partners, infrequently using condoms, engaging in same-sex sexual activity, trading sex for money or drugs, and engaging in sex while using psychoactive substances. These risk factors, along with the poverty characteristic of people with severe mental illness, raise the concern that this population is also at elevated risk for HBV and HCV infection (Daw *et al*, 2000 & 2002). Although these two infections are much more prevalent than HIV in the US population (estimated rates of 4.9% and 1.8%, respectively) and share key risk factors, no enough data were published on the prevalence of HBV and HCV among people with severe mental illness worldwide.

Individuals with severe mental illness are at a high risk for blood-borne infectious diseases, such as HIV and hepatitis B. Hepatitis C virus shares risk factors for transmission with these viruses; 1.8% of the general population has been exposed to the hepatitis C virus and is therefore at risk for the long-term health consequences of chronic infection. Ominously, recent studies found the seroprevalence of hepatitis C virus to be 19.6% among mentally ill patients, approximately 11 times that of the general adult population. The prevalence of HBV was almost five times and HCV showed the highest elevation among, adult population with mental disorders.

In general, it appears that the risk factors operants for HIV, HBV, and HCV in people with severe mental illness are very similar to the risk factors present in the general population. Elevated rates within several risk categories may reflect the poverty, risky environments, and overall poor health and medical care services are common in people with severe mental illness.

2   Hepatitis C Virus infection

2.1   Biology of Hepatitis C Virus

Hepatitis C virus (HCV) is a member of the Hepacivirus genus, within the *Flaviviridae* family, responsible for non-A non-B hepatitis, affecting about 3% of the human population worldwide. Hepatitis C virus (HCV) is a small single-stranded RNA of positive polarity with a lipid envelope (E) containing glycoproteins (E1 and E2) and a core with a genome consisting of 9500 nucleotides. AS illustrated in Figure 1, HCV components are both structural (core, E1, and E2) and nonstructural (NS; P7, NS2, NS3, NS4A, NS4B, NS5A, and NS5B). The nonstructural genes encode various enzymes including a polymerase responsible for replication of HCV.

HCV infection is a highly dynamic process with a viral half-life of only a few hours and production and clearance of an estimated 1012 virions per day in a given individual. This high replicative activity, together with the lack of a proof-reading function of the viral RdRp, is the basis of the high genetic variability of HCV. These properties are similar to those of HIV infection and provide a strong rationale for the development and implementation of antiviral combination therapies. HCV isolates can be classified into genotypes and subtypes. There are 6 major genotypes that differ in their nucleotide sequence by 30–35%. Such genotypes were determine the epidemiology of HCV virus worldwide and guide the responses of clinical therapy against HCV.

structure of HCV

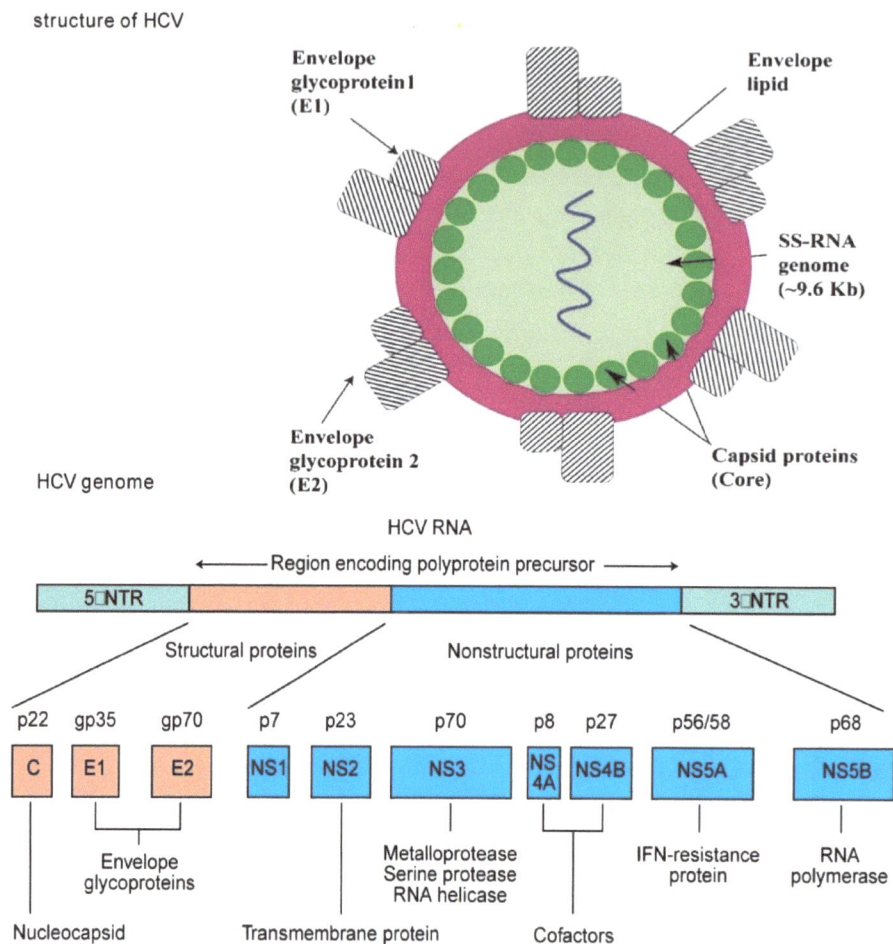

Figure 1: Viral Structure and the Genomic Organization of HCV.

2.2   Laboratory Diagnosis of Hepatitis C Virus

Diagnosis of Hepatitis C involves confirmation of the diagnosis of Hepatitis C virus (HCV) infection and assessment of the severity of liver disease. In addition, evaluation of patients with Hepatitis C should include determination of the patients' suitability for treatment. Diagnostic tests for hepatitis C as shown in Table 3 can be divided into the following two general categories:

1.   Serological assays that detect antibody to hepatitis C virus (anti-HCV).

2.   Molecular assays that detect, quantify, and/or characterize HCV RNA genomes within an infected patient.

Serological assays have been subdivided into screening tests for anti-HCV, such as the enzyme immunoassay (EIA), and supplemental tests such as the recombinant immunoblot assay (RIBA). Three generations of anti-HCV tests have been developed, and each generation has resulted in an improvement in the sensitivity of detecting anti-HCV Third-generation anti-HCV tests (EIA-3 and RIBA-3, respectively) contain antigens from the HCV core, non- structural 3, nonstructural 4, and nonstructural 5 genes.

Type of the Test:

1 - Anti-HCV (antibody)
   - EIA (enzyme immunoassay)
   - Recombinant immunoblot assay (e.g. RIBA™)
   Uses
   Verify if necessary positive EIA with HCV RNA detection Indicates past or present infection, but does not differentiate between acute, chronic or past infection.

2 - HCV RNA (virus)
   Qualitative tests
       PCR - Amplicor HCV™
       Transcription-mediated amplification" (TMA)
   - Versant HCV
   To: Detect presence or absence of virus. Detect virus 1-3 weeks after exposure. Detection of HCV RNA during course of infection may be intermittent. A single negative PCR is not conclusive.
   Quantitative tests
       PCR - Amplicor HCV Monitor™
       Branched DNA signal amplification
   - Quantiplex™ HCV RNA (bDNA)
   - Versant HCV RNA Quantitative Assay
   Other tests
   - Super Quant, LCx, real-time PCR…
   To: Determines *titre of HCV. Used to monitor patients on antiviral therapy.

3 - HCV core antigen EIA, Trak-C;
   To: Detect presence or absence of virus. Detect virus 1-3 weeks after exposure. Under evaluation for the monitoring of patients on antiviral therapy.

4 - Genotype;
   To: Groups isolates of HCV into 6 genotypes based on genetic differences. With new therapies, length of treatment varies based on genotype.

Table 3: Diagnostic tests for hepatitis C virus

Detection of HCV RNA in patient specimens by polymerase chain reaction (PCR) provides evidence of active HCV infection and is potentially useful for confirming the diagnosis and monitoring the antiviral response to therapy.

Currently, the second-generation enzyme immunoassay (EIA-2) for antibodies to HCV (anti-HCV) is the most practical screening test for HCV infection. The diagnosis of HCV infection can be supported or confirmed by the recombinant immunoblot assay (RIBA) or tests for HCV RNA. Nowadays, the second-generation enzyme immunoassay (EIA-2) for antibodies to HCV (anti-HCV) is the most favorite practical screening test for HCV infection. The diagnosis of HCV infection can be supported or confirmed by the recombinant immunoblot assay (RIBA) or tests for HCV RNA. RIBA detects antibodies to individual HCV antigens and confers increased specificity compared to EIA-2. Qualitative reverse transcription- polymerase chain reaction (RT-PCR) assays for HCV RNA are simpler than quantitative tests and sufficient for confirmation of the diagnosis of HCV infection.

While the vast majority of anti-HCV- positive patients who present with chronic liver disease have ongoing HCV infection as confirmed by the presence of HCV RNA in serum, only 35 percent and 25 percent of anti-HCV-positive blood donors are RIBA- and HCV RNA-positive, respectively. The proportion of anti-HCV-positive blood donors who are confirmed to be HCV RNA-positive varies from 70 percent for those who are RIBA-positive to 2-25 percent for those who are RIBA- indeterminate and none for those who are RIBA-negative. Thus, supplementary and confirmatory tests for HCV infection should always be performed in asymptomatic low-risk subjects who are found to be anti-HCV-positive, particularly if they have normal aminotransferase (ALT) levels; but these tests may not be necessary in all anti-HCV-positive patients who present with chronic liver disease.

Severity of liver disease is best assessed by liver biopsy. There is in general a poor correlation between serum ALT level and activity of liver disease. More importantly, several recent studies found that significant liver disease can be found in anti-HCV-positive patients despite normal ALT levels. These studies reported that 70 percent of RIBA- positive blood donors who had persistently normal ALT levels have chronic hepatitis or cirrhosis on biopsy. Although most donors (77 percent) who had abnormal liver histology were HCV RNA-positive, significant liver disease was also found in 30 percent of RIBA- positive donors who were HCV RNA- negative and had normal ALT levels on three separate occasions. This may be related to the fluctuating course of chronic HCV infection with intermittently normal ALT levels and undetectable levels of viremia. It may also reflect variations in sensitivities of "home-made" RT-PCR assays for HCV RNA. Liver biopsy should be always recommended except in elderly patients, patients with severe concomitant medical problems, and those with neither coagulopathy, since neither serum HCV RNA nor ALT level can reliably predict activity or degree of fibrosis. HCV genotyping could be used to monitor the clinical response of HCV therapy, it could only be recommended as a research tool rather than a routine diagnostic test. Such diagnostic tests for HCV infection were found to have a high sensitivity, specificity and feasibility among individuals with mental disorders.

2.3   Epidemiology of Hepatitis C Virus

Hepatitis C virus is the most ongoing important viral hepatitis that appears to be endemic in most parts of the world. There are, however, substantial geographic and temporal variations in the incidence and prevalence of HCV infection, largely due to differences in regional risk factors for the transmission of HCV (Daw & Dau 2012). The overall world prevalence of HCV was estimated to be 3% as over 170 million persons were infected. **Figure 2** shows the geo-epidemiolgy of hepatitis C worldwide. Such prevalence varies greatly from one country to another and even among the province within the same country.

Most of the studies however were based on testing of selected populations such as blood donors. However, population-based surveys are rarely available for most parts of the world. Low rate area (0.1-0.9%) such as Northern Europe to 0.1–0.5% in Western Europe, North America, parts of Central and South America,, intermediate area (1-5%), have been reported from Brazil, Eastern Europe, the Mediterranean area, the Indian subcontinent, and parts of Africa and Asia, High rate area > 5% such Arabian peninsula, Africa and China. The highest prevalence of HCV has been found in Egypt (17–26%) Table 4 shows the Global Prevalence of HCV and its genotypes worldwide.

The major risk factors for HCV infection are blood transfusions from unscreened donors and intravenous drug use. However, exposure to HCV-infected blood from other health-care-related procedures and regional cultural practices are increasingly recognized as having an important function in HCV transmission in some parts of the world. Since the introduction and improvement in the 1990s of the screening of blood donors, HCV transmission by blood transfusions is now exceedingly rare (around or less than one per million) in developed countries.

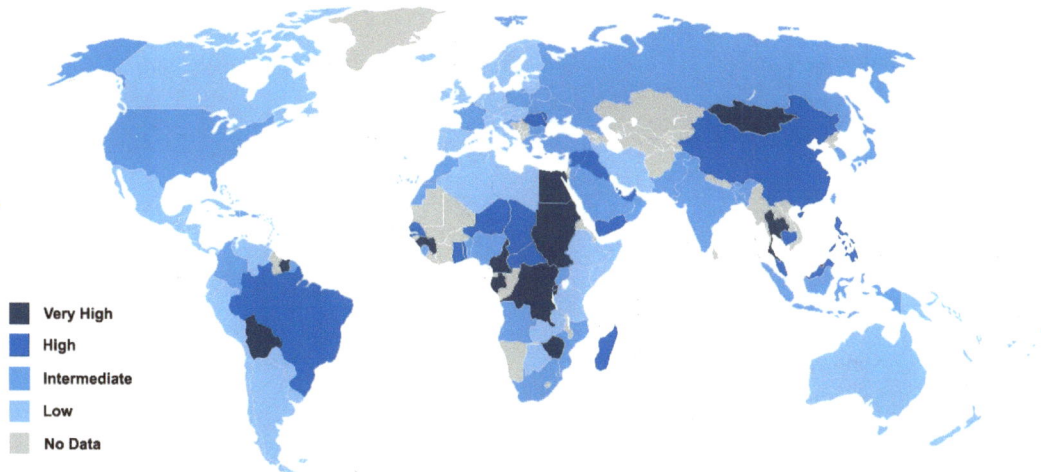

Figure 2: Geo-epidemiology of hepatitis C virus worldwide.

Unfortunately, the screening of blood donors for HCV is not yet routinely performed by some blood banks in developing countries. Most new cases in developed countries are related to intravenous drug use. Health-care-related procedures leading to nosocomial HCV transmission are not restricted to hemodialysis facilities. Several reports from Western countries have clearly documented nosocomial transmission of HCV through inadvertent sharing of multidose vials or unsterilized instruments, among others. Similar nosocomial transmission of HCV outside dialysis units is certainly not less likely to occur in developing countries but has not been reported until now. Additional risk factors for HCV transmission include occupational exposure, especially by accidental needle stick, as well as perinatal transmission (about 6%), whereas the transmission of HCV by sexual activity appears relatively inefficient.

The clinical history of HCV is a unique, usually its mild and rarely patients need a clinical consultation and thus it's usually discovered at the chronic stage. Chronicity rates range from 50 to 90%, with somewhat lower rates in children and young healthy women (50–60%) and higher rates in older individuals and African descents. The major long-term complications of chronic HCV infection are liver fibrosis and cirrhosis, portal hypertension and liver failure, and a high risk for hepatocellular carcinoma. Interferon-a (IFN-a) and long-acting pegylated IFNs were the most commonly approved acceptable treatment of HCV infections (Daw *et al.,* 2013), though new and more efficient therapy has been recently introduced including HCV protease inhibitors such as Boceprevir and Telaprevir. Table 5 summarizes the most commonly approved therapeutic agents used to treat hepatitis C infected patients.

2.4 Mental Health and Neurocognitive (Neurocognition) Associated with Hepatitis C Virus Infections

Chronic hepatitis C infection is frequently associated with mental Health concerns. Such mental health problems include depression, anxiety post substance use disorders, bibolar disorder, post-traumatic stress disorder (PTSD). Another common issue for patients with HCV is problems with thinking and memory which called *neurocognition*. Such phenomenon may be associated with the direct effect of HCV on the brain or direct effect of substance on the brain. Patients with HCV often complain of depression, fatigue and impairments in quality of life. Individuals with HCV appear to perform below expected level on tests of attention, concentration and planning.

Region	Prevalence of HCV(%)	Common Genotypes
North America	0.1 – 0.5	1a, 1b, 2a, 2b, 3a
South America	1 – 5	1a, 1b, 2, 3a
Europe		
North Europe	0.1 – 0.5	1a, 1b, 2b, 2a, 3a
South Europe	0.5 – 7	1b, 2c
Australia	0.1 – 0.5	1a, 1b, 2a, 2b, 3a.
Africa		
South Africa	1 – 5	1, 2, 3, 5a
North & Central Africa	1.2 – 7	1a, 4a
Egypt	17 – 26**	4a
Asia		
Pacific & Fareast	0.2 – 3%	1b, 2a, 2b, 6a
Indian Peninsula	1 – 5%	1b, 2a
Arabian Peninsula	1.3 – 7%	4a, 1b

** The highest in the world

Table 4: Global Prevalence of Hepatitis C Virus and Worldwide distribution of the genotypes.

1	**Type I interferons-Subcutaneous injection**
	A - Pegylated interferon α-2a (Pegasys®)
	B - Pegylated interferon α-2b (PEGIntron®)
	C - Interferon α-2a (Roferon®)
	D - nterferon α-2b (Intron A®)
	E - Consensus Interferon (Infergen®)
2	**Ribavirin- Oral tablets or capsules**
	A - Ribavirin (Copegus®)
	B - Ribavirin (Rebetol®)
3	**HCV protease inhibitors- Oral tablets or capsules**
	A - Boceprevir (Victrelis®)
	B - Telaprevir (Incivek®, Incivo®)

Table 5: Clinically Approved drugs for treating of chronic hepatitis C infection

Indirect Effects of HCV those were associated with HCV consequences as liver damage or which could result in hepaticencephalopathy that affects their thinking and memory. This as a result of neurotoxins as ammonia and Manganese which gets in the brain and thus effect its proper function. HCV therapy is usually associated with depression termed as (interferon-induced depression which more likely related to activation of immune system). This more likely represented by irritability, fatigue, slowed movement and changes in sleep and eating habits.

3   Prevention of hepatitis C virus among mental disorders

3.1   Epidemiology and Risk Factors

Individuals with severe mental illness are at a high risk for blood-borne infectious diseases, such as HIV and hepatitis B. Hepatitis C virus shares risk factors for transmission with these viruses; 1.8% of the general population has been exposed to the hepatitis C virus and is therefore at risk for the long-term health consequences of chronic infection. Different studies found that the sero-prevalence of hepatitis C virus among mentally ill patients, approximately 11 times that of the general adult population. Table 6 summarizes the demographic and clinical characteristic of HCV among patients with mental disorder.

Characteristics	Prevalence of HCV(%)
Clinical Characteristics of Mental Disorder	
Schizophrenia	5.0 – 11
All non-affective psychoses	5.0 – 10
Major depression	14 – 20
Any depressive illness	25 – 31
Bipolar affective disorder	21 – 25
Any mood disorder	50 – 53
Any anxiety or adjustment disorder	5.0 – 9.0
Any psychoactive substance abuse or dependence	64 – 68
Any personality disorder	0 – 4.0
Any organic mental disorder	0 – 2.0
Other diagnoses	
Ethnic grouping	
Blacks	11 – 17
Whites	7 – 11
Marital Status	
Single	55 – 60
Married	15 – 19
Others	25 – 29
Gender	
Male	75 – 79
Female	19 – 24

Table 6: Demographic, Clinical characteristics and prevalence of hepatitis C virus among patients with Mental Disorders.

In terms of risk factors, epidemiological studies showed that mental disorders were involved in high risk behaviors or the unfortunate circumstance they may bring in further to lack of care to such group of people. This brought them to be more vulnerable of acquiring HCV. Table 7 summarizes most of the potential risk associated with the increasing risk of HCV among patients with mental disorders.

A - Personal moderating factors	
♦ Help seeking	♦ Barrier to risk reduction
♦ Treatment compliance	♦ Benefits of risk reduction
♦ HIV health beliefs	♦ Cues to action
♦ Perceived severity	♦ Perceived susceptibility
B - Psychiatric disorders	
♦ Substance abuse	♦ Level of functioning
♦ Symptoms	♦ Comorbid illness
♦ Severe mental illness or substance abuse diagnosis	
C - Social or contextual moderating factors	
♦ Residential stability	♦ Urban or rural
♦ Socioeconomic status	♦ Insurance status
♦ Race	♦ Social support
♦ HIV & HBV prevalence	♦ Violence
♦ Drug use	♦ Victimization

Table 7: Potential Risk factors associated with increased risk of HCV among individuals with mental disorders.

3.2   Homelessness

Individuals with mental disorders are most often unable to acquire and maintain regular, safe, secure, and adequate housing, or lack "fixed, regular, and adequate night-time residence and even refereed as street people who may be accommodated in shelters or warming centers. It is estimated that 20-25% of home-less people, compared with 6% of the non-homeless, have severe mental illness (Fischer *et al* 1986). Others estimate that up to one-third of the homeless suffer from mental illness. Studies have found that there is a correlation between homelessness and incarceration. Those with mental illness or substance abuse problems were found to be incarcerated at a higher frequency than the general population. Homeless persons are at high risk of HCV as a result of injecting drug use, unprotected sex, prostitution and victimization. Studies conducted with homeless people found that 73 to 80 % report a life time history of drug use with 13to 20 % involved in injecting drug use. Over 70 % of homeless adult report unprotected sex with multiple partners.

3.3   Alcohol and Drug Abuse

There is a very high prevalence of HCV antibodies among I.V drug addicts as they due share contaminat-ed needles and syringe, the rates were found to be higher than 50% and close 100 % in some population. Surprisingly HCV infection has been found in patients with alcohol abuse. Anti-HCV antibodies were detected in 16 % of unselected patients; it varies from 7to49 % among alcoholics, particularly those with advanced cirrhosis and hepatocellular carcinoma as it raises the possibility that HCV and alcohol abuse are additive in causing liver injury. Alcohol abusers have also been found to be at increased risk in some studies in which no other risk factors existed. Other studies found alcohol users to be at greater risk particularly of injection drug use.

3.4   Sexual and Habitual Behaviors

HCV may well be sexually transmitted and should therefore also be taken into account at regular STD screenings. The extent to which HCV is sexually transmissible remains an important concern among Mental Disorders. They involved in high risk behavior by having multiple sexual partners and high-risk partners, infrequently using condoms, engaging in same-sex sexual activity, trading sex for money or drugs, and engaging in sex while using psychoactive substances. Further to negligence and not seeking medical advice. However further studies on sexual transmission as well as other potential risk factors together with habitual behavior such as sharing of toothbrushes, razors should be investigated.

3.5   Symptoms and Signs of Hepatitis C Infection among Patients with Mental Disorder

Chronic hepatitis C infection is usually hidden among individuals with mental disorders not only due to the asymptomatic nature of the disease but also due to the special circumstance of such patients. The absence of symptoms and abnormal clinical signs, and lack of complain therefore, does not exclude significant liver disease. However, early diagnosis and offering treatment may improve prognosis. Overlapping of such symptoms are common in MD patients, these symptoms may include:

- Early progressive liver disease
- Progressive liver disease
- Advanced disease complications
- Extra-hepatic manifestations

People with Mental disorders who have chronic HCV infection score poorly on many quality-of-life parameters, including a range of physical and psychological measures of wellbeing. In reality, mental disorders patients with chronic hepatitis C shown little or no correlation between biochemical parameters such as ALT level and presence of symptoms. Furthermore, the stage of liver disease (prior to liver failure) and the viral load in chronic hepatitis C have a poor association with the extent of symptoms. People often progress to cirrhosis without development of significant symptoms and different factors may be associated with the progressive of the disease as shown in Table 8.

Peripheral stigmata of chronic liver disease, such as spider naevi, liver nails and palmar erythema, may develop if there is progression to cirrhosis. Advanced liver disease complications of HCV infection consist of liver failure (decompensated cirrhosis), often in association with signs of portal hypertension such as refractory ascites and variceal bleeding as illustrated in Figure 3 and 4.

3.6   Consequence of Hepatitis C Virus Infection

Data suggest that people with severe mental illness, who exhibit elevated rates of both HBV and HCV and who also have very high lifetime prevalence rates of alcohol use disorder, are at unusually high risk for developing severe liver disease. Both HBV and HCV are major causes of liver disease, including cirrhosis and hepatocellular carcinoma. However, the latter generally develops 1 to 3 decades after initial

> • Age at acquisition of infection (> 40 years)
> • Heavy alcohol intake (> 40 grams/day)
> • Male gender
> • Longer duration of infection
> • Moderate to severe hepatic fibrosis on baseline liver biopsy
> • Coinfection with HIV and/or chronic hepatitis B
> • Obesity

Note: There is no evidence for an association.

Table 8: Factors associated with progression to advanced liver disease in chronic hepatitis C.

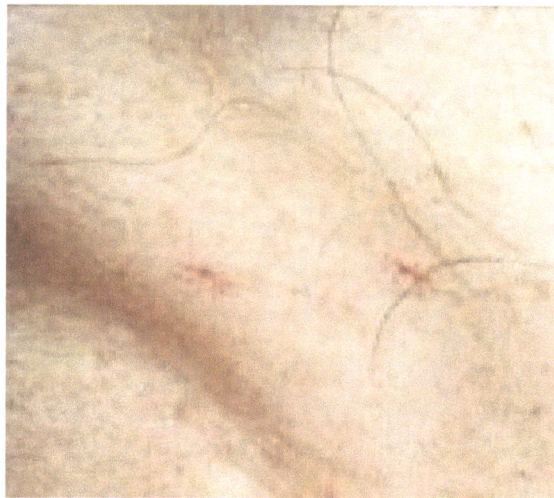

Figure 3: Spider naevi in chronic hepatitis C infection.

infection. The increasing number of cases of hepatocellular carcinoma is but one indicator of the importance of identifying high-risk groups and individuals infected with either or both of these forms of hepatitis.

4 Management of Hepatitis C Infection among Patients with Mental Disorders

4.1 Approaches and Barriers

Therapeutic intervention, treatment policies and management approaches are aimed to improve the quality of the infected patients and supersede the progress of the disease among them. Hence then treatment outcomes for hepatitis C include preventing the spread of the disease; treating symptoms; preventing the development of cirrhosis, hepatocellular carcinoma, and end-stage liver disease; and decreasing morbidity and preventing mortality. Additionally, the primary goals of therapy are to normalize hepatic ami-

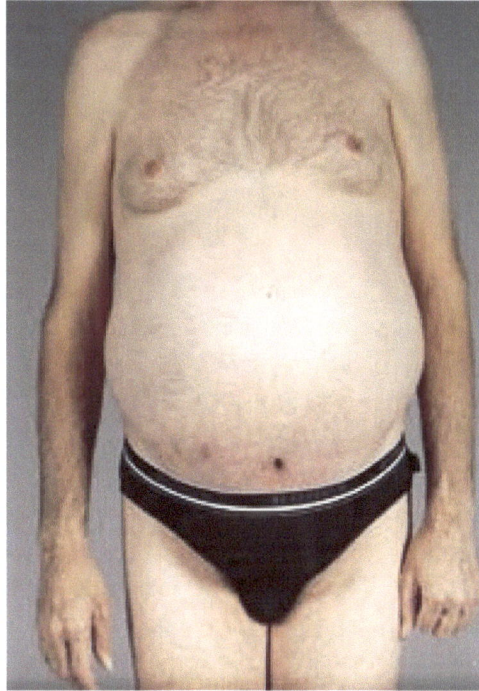

Figure 4: Decompensate cirrhosis secondary to hepatitis C infection

notransferases and improve histology, and ultimately to suppress and have undetectable viral replication by sustained virologic response (SVR) 24 weeks following treatment discontinuation. Such goals are not easy to chive particularly among mentally disorientated persons (Demyttenaere *et al.,* 2004). Therefore a comprehensive plan and a major strategy has be formulated and designed for such specific group of people.

Antiviral therapy is at present is expensive, associated with significant side effects, ineffective in a substantial number of cases, and in this particular population likely to be difficult to administer because of the need for ongoing compliance and the lack of coordination between public health and mental care health systems. Moreover, since most psychotropic drugs are hepatically metabolized, chronic hepatitis C may complicate pharmacotherapy in this population. Previously mental illness, considered to be a contraindication to treatment with IFN. Data about treatment of persons with mental disorders are scant and the effectiveness of antiviral treatment in this population is unknown. Good Interaction and cooperation between health care provider and these patients becomes a priority in order to achieve a management successful outcome.

Patients with Mental disorders do face many challenges in gaining access to health care, including logistical hardships (e.g., lack of transportation) and distrust of the health-care system. Prejudice and inexperience in treating such patients may contribute to health care provider physicians' reluctance or limited ability to provide adequate care. Although a variety of factors may minimize the efficacy of treatment and managements among these patients, every effort should be taken to overcome such barriers (Daw, Dau & Agnan 2012). Table 9, summarizes most of these barriers.

4.2   Patients Associated Factors

Pharmacological responses, histological markers, eradication of HCV and diminishing the progress of disease have been used as major determinants for successful HCV therapy. However, amelioration of symptoms or improvement in the quality of life of infected patients is rarely mentioned as a part of such therapy.

Despite all the progress that has been made in preventing HCV worldwide, antiviral therapy however, remains the main sole in preventing serious HVC associated liver diseases. Hence then compiling with such treatment becomes the mile stone in curing HCV and preventing any further complications associated with. Such target becomes more complicated among patients with Mental Disorders. As the concept of accepting treatment is lacking among this group, further to lack of understanding to the consequences and complication of HC infections. Hence then, HCV prevention, care and treatment program must recognize community specific epidemiology, which varies greatly by setting and level of economic development among Mental disorders comparable to other risk groups prone to HCV infections. Despite the data regarding elevated prevalence rates of HCV in people with severe mental illness, and reported elevations of other infectious hepatitis in psychiatric patients, relative to the general population, women with severe mental illness appear to be at particularly elevated risk (estimated infection rates of 5% vs. 0.17%). Medical factors such as genetic status of the patients, progress of disease, its clinical stage, side effects and adherence of the used therapy and co-infection with other viruses has great influence of the success of HCV therapy. Further studies were needed regarding the effect of such variables on the SVR either independently or in combinations with other factors.

- **Barriers associated with individual patients**
    - Communications & Lack of feeling and responsibility
    - Medical condition &co-morbidities
    - Alcohols
    - Patient preference
    - Appointments & follow up
- **Barriers associated with Health care or providers factors**
    - Health services
    - Reluctance and hesitation
    - Treatment perceptions and contraindications
    - Lack of team work &Organization
- **System factors**
    - Social factors
    - Insurance coverage
    - Quality of life
    - Psychological well being
    - Communications with Medical specialists
- **Miscellaneous [Combined] barriers**
    - Environmental factors, Toxic
    - Quality of life
    - Social factors

Table 9: Barriers influencing the efficacy of treatment of hepatitis C virus.

Quality of life and sexual health has been found to be diminished among patients with mental disorder infected with hepatitis C. Such functioning and satisfaction is associated with the degree of hepatic fibrosis or cirrhosis. Lower sexual summary scores were highly associated as well with female gender, older age, history of cholesterol medication use, and concomitant use of antidepressant or anxiolytic medications.

Such deterioration in the quality of health among patients with chronic hepatitis C can be improved, at least in part, by successful antiviral therapy. Patients who achieve an SVR may feel less stigmatized and concerned about potential transmission of HCV to their sexual partners, which has been a factor associated with lower quality of life. Furthermore ribavirin is highly teratogenic, hence then patients expecting pregnancy which is usually uncontrolled among these patients and receiving therapy must diligently observe two forms of birth control during treatment and for six months after stopping.

Health care providers should make decisions about treatment together, after a thorough discussion of the need for adherence to the treatment regimen and the risks of adverse effects and re-infection. The patient's current and previous adherence to medical regimens and his or her mental health and risk of depression should be considered, as should access to safe injection equipment and knowledge of safe injection practices, such discussions may not lead to treatment for injection-drug users. This however, will not cover most of the patients as they are more likely to have poor adherence to treatment regimens, uncontrolled depression, or unsafe injection practices may remain obstacles to therapy. Hence then, further studies are needed to overcome such barriers.

4.3   Social and Environmental Factors

Poor social circumstances, environmental barriers, Incarceration - poor housing may further compromise a person's desire and ability to seek care. Factors such as these have been shown to substain the use of antiretroviral treatments for mentally disoriented patients infected with HCV. Therefore, one important of a comprehensive care program is patients' orientation, as many of them decline treatment as they were not aware of the consequence of HCV disease and/or treatment. Furthermore, HCV incidence is greater where structural factors like poverty, stigma, or lack of services impede individuals from protecting themselves. Hence then heuristic social models that accounts for the dynamic and interactive nature of structural factors that may impact HCV prevention behaviors should be designed and implemented to account for social factors associated with HCV particularly with other concomitant infections as HIV. Few studies have examined associated risk factors, such as IDU exposure, incarceration patterns, and other high risk behaviors among patients with mental disorders. Assessment of the sources of risk behaviors will facilitate decision-making about how to screen for HCV, prevent further spread of the disease, and provide appropriate care to such patients. The prevalence of HCV among this group is eleven times higher than general population. Hence the development of policies for systematic HCV screening among these patients may be implemented. This could improve resource planning, education, and health care within corrections systems and for parolees reentering the community. Furthermore, specific universal programs with general approach may actually be a more appropriate and realistic setting for treatment of this high-risk population than the general community, where health care is fragmented and access to it is limited.

4.4   Economic Burdens Associated with Hepatitis C Infection

The effect of hepatitis C treatment response on medical costs has not been well studied. HCV infection however, costs the health care system in developed countries a heavy burden and that expected to be doubled in the near futures. The average lifetime cost (i.e., medical costs and economic losses) for an affected patient has been estimated to at one million dollars under normal conditions. This however is more complex and expensive if it's applicable on individuals with mental disorders. Such medications may include costs for prescription, nonprescription, and complementary medications which may relate to antiviral therapy, adverse effect and other co-morbid conditions. Financial constrains which an obvious phenomena among this particular group of patients, however, may lead to lack of persistence and adherence with medication use, poor health outcomes, and higher overall health care costs. Health care profession hence then should be vigilant for such factors and use specific strategy to help the patients to overcome such barriers. Further studies are needed to explore the cost effectiveness of the medication with special attention the costly ones among psychiatric patients infected with HCV.

4.5   Influence of Alcohol on Hepatitis C Infection

Alcohol intake has a major effect in liver associated diseases particularly viral hepatitis. Such consumption may not only damage the liver itself but also influence the behavior of such patients. Individuals with HCV continue to seriously jeopardize their health by using and abusing alcohol. These individuals experience more rapid disease progression and more -related complications as a result of alcohol use. HCV-infected people who use alcohol excessively may also engage in risky sexual behaviors while under its influence, exposing both themselves and their partners to sexually transmitted infections. Different studies have shown that the use of various substances can have an effect on antiviral medication adherence. Although not all studies examining the relationship between alcohol use and medication adherence, such speculation still exist and further studies are needed to clarify such correlation.

Alcohol has great concern in HCV patients co-infected with HIV with the consequence that end-stage liver disease accelerated as a result of alcohol use among those co-infected and accelerates the illness and death among these individuals. Furthermore, HCV treatment is less effective in people with HIV co-infection, and its effectiveness is limited even more by ongoing alcohol use.

5   Treatment of Hepatitis C Infection among patients with Mental Disorders

5.1   Concept of Treatment

Treatment of such group becomes a priority and new concept of management has merged. The arguments for excluding these patients from treatment often do not stem from the results of suitable prospective and controlled clinical studies that included patients who were drug users or had psychiatric disorders. There is a pressing need to develop improved therapeutic and management approaches to ensure that patients with HCV and comorbid psychiatric illness complete a full, uninterrupted course of HCV IFN treatment.

The management of patients with HCV infection who have psychiatric illness also poses unique challenges because psychotropic medications (e.g., antidepressants, antipsychotics, and mood stabilizers) are metabolized by the liver and can be hepatotoxic. The combination of HCV-induced liver disease, alcohol use, and psychotropic drugs may hasten the progression to cirrhosis. Patients with HCV and psychiatric illness who progress to cirrhosis and end-stage liver disease may also be less likely to receive a liver transplant because of the perceived difficulties they might have adhering to the rigorous post-transplant regimen (Schaefer, *et al.,* 2003). With the exception of a few recent studies on the use of IFN in patients with substance use disorders, Table 10 shows the commonly used approaches to improve the quality of treatment among patients with mental disorders.

Different studies have confirmed that patients with psychiatric disorders, methadone-treated patients, and patients with a history of drug addiction had response rates and adherence during treatment of chronic hepatitis C with standard IFN, and ribavirin similar to those of patients in a nonpsychiatric control group.

-Universal approaches

- Pretreatment intervention scheme may be applied

- Multidisciplinary management caring team [Nurse, Infectious disease physician, social care worker, psychiatrist]

- High professional level of management regarding diagnosis, treatment regimens and follow up

- Educational scheme for patients

- Cooperative and family-like relationship with patients regarding mutual respect, acknowledgement, avoid frustration, palming and expectation

-Specific approaches

- Patients con-infected with HIV

- Patients with IDUs

- Women seeking pregnancy undergoing treatment

- Alcoholic Patients

- Patients with underlying depilated diseases

- Introduction Case based management

Table 10: Approaches to overcome factors influencing hepatitis C treatment.

5.2   Minimizing Risk Factors

Several explanations have been advanced to account for the increased prevalence of HCV in persons with severe mental illness. Both the direct (e.g., affective lability) and indirect (e.g., homelessness) effects of severe mental illness have been hypothesized to increase high-risk behavior and result in elevated rates of HIV infection. Evidence-based patient selection is paramount when attempting to minimize the morbidity and mortality associated with IFN treatment of HCV patients with comorbid psychiatric illnesses. Though much remains to be learned about primary prevention and effective provision of treatment in this group, a universal consensus among health care providers indicated that people who have viral hepatitis with mental health disorders should take several actions to improve clinical outcome, these may include:

- Not to drink alcoholic beverages, and if necessary, get into treatment, because alcohol makes liver disease worse.

- IDUs should stop injecting drugs and get into and stay in substance abuse treatment. If they can't stop, they should follow safe injection practices (always use a sterile syringe; do not share drug solution, syringes, or drug preparation equipment).

- People with Mental disorders particularly individuals with chronic liver disease should be immunized against hepatitis A and hepatitis B.

- Individuals with chronic HCV infection should be under medical supervision.

- Implement a role for more routine screening. Particularly for Hepatitis B and C and HIV.

- Heightened awareness of potential hepatotoxicity when prescribing drugs.

- The high prevalence of the HCV virus in this population places. Mental health care workers at higher risk for HCV infection, and thus they should implement universal precautions protocols.

5.3   Assessment and Evaluation

A baseline clinician evaluation should be conducted for all patients who are anti-HCV positive. At minimum, this evaluation should include the following:

Targeted history taking and physical examination: Evaluate for signs and symptoms of liver disease, quantify prior alcohol consumption, and determine risk behaviors for acquiring HCV infection. Attempt to estimate and document the earliest possible date of infection, including when risk factors for exposures started and stopped, e.g., the time period in which the inmate engaged in injection drug use. Evaluate for other possible causes of liver disease, especially alcoholism, nonalcoholic steatohepatitis (NASH), iron overload, and autoimmune hepatitis. Inquire about prior treatment for HCV infection, specific medications used, dosages and duration of treatment, and outcomes, if known.

Laboratory diagnostic tests: Recommended baseline laboratory tests as shown in Table 3 based on the clinical situation of each patient. These should include Routine Laboratory Studies such as: complete white blood cell count with differential, platelet count, prothrombin time (international normalized ratio), comprehensive metabolic panel (that includes serum creatinine, alanine aminotransferase [ALT], aspartate aminotransferase [AST], total bilirubin, serum albumin), hepatitis B surface antigen (HBsAg), thyroid stimulating hormone (TSH), and a fasting lipid panel. In addition, cryoglobulin levels should be obtained in patients with any signs or symptoms that suggest cryoglobulinemia (palpable purpura, arthralgias, renal disease, or peripheral neuropathy). Candidates for anti-HCV therapy should undergo HCV genotype testing. Otherwise, until it is clinically needed an HCV RNA, or an HCV genotype, or a liver biopsy are not routinely performed.

Individual Cases Assessment: Each HCV positive case should be evaluated individually, patients with chronic HCV who have not received treatment for HCV and are not planning to start treatment for HCV should have ongoing monitoring for complications related to their liver disease. Health care providers should counsel these patients to abstain from alcohol use, and advice to be given to certain food supplement intake and drugs that may complicate such cases. They have to be evaluated regularly for consideration of HCV treatment further to development and implementation of a plan to assist patients in HCV treatment readiness. All patients with HCV should be interviewed about their past and current alcohol and other substance use which may affect the decision to initiate HCV treatment, as well as their response to therapy.

Psychiatric evaluation: Patients with mental disorders infected with HCV do require referral to a psychiatrist or mental health professional for evaluation and therapy before initiation of antiviral treatment. HCV infected patients should be evaluated for psychiatric disorders, such as depression. Uncontrolled depression or active suicidal ideation is an absolute contraindication to HCV IFN-based therapies. Patients with psychiatric disorders that are stable or in remission may receive antiviral therapy. Standardized depression scales (e.g., Beck Depression Inventory or Patient Health Questionnaire) serve as useful tools for baseline and on-treatment psychiatric assessment.

5.4 Initiating of Hepatitis C Virus Therapy

Health care providers particularly clinicians remain hesitant to initiate treatment in HCV patients with psychiatric illness because of concerns about precipitating or worsening psychiatric symptoms. The practice of excluding patients with psychiatric illness from HCV treatment clinical trials is itself stigmatizing and can result in substantial morbidity and mortality for such a vulnerable population (Edlin *et al.,* 2001).

Despite the absence of a consensus on the use of INF and when it should be used or withheld clinicians and health care providers must undertake an individualized and balanced risk-benefit analysis for each patient before offering IFN treatment, incorporating not only factors specific to HCV disease and the potential for psychiatric complications but also the patient's preferences and the psychosocial support available.

The risk-benefit analysis for an HCV patient with evidence of liver cirrhosis and psychiatric illness may justify IFN treatment. Furthermore, patients with psychiatric illness who receive IFN treatment without achieving SVR may achieve normalization of liver function tests and improvement in liver pathology. However, long-term follow-up studies are needed to determine whether this benefit for IFN non-responders would translate into a reduction in the incidence of liver cirrhosis or hepatocellular carcinoma. If such a benefit is confirmed, it would strengthen the argument for treating patients with HCV and psychiatric illness with IFN. Models of care should be introduced to improve the quality of life of mental disorders infected with HCV, this include introducing holistic approaches by incorporating all discipline of health care providers. Such intervention programs may be of use in inpatient, outpatient, and community-based settings. Figure 5 shows a flow diagram that illustrates the co-management and integration of care for patients with HCV, substance use disorders, and psychiatric illnesses.

There are currently neither practice guidelines nor programs for screening, testing, or treating people with severe mental illness who have contracted hepatitis C virus. This increases the likelihood that many patients with severe mental illness, particularly those at an elderly age with chronic, HCV, are in the process of developing cirrhotic liver disease or have asymptomatic hepatocellular carcinoma. The following guide lines may be helpful in the treatment HCV patient with Mental Disorders:

1. Refer to- Mental Health Crisis Assessment Team [General Practitioners / Psychologist / Accident and Emergency]

2. Refer to mental health service for assessment or Accident and Emergency within six hours if urgent/within 24 hours if non-urgent to a private psychiatrist/psychologist.

3. Monitoring: Psychiatric monitoring is recommended for people who have a history of mental illness with hepatitis C Virus or Treatment.

4. Risk factors analysis: such as medication to be considered.

5. Psychiatric Screening: Primary health care practitioners can screen for depression when symptoms suggest. Many simple screening instruments are available for this purpose.

6. Determine treatment on case-by-case bases.

7. If interferon indicated monitor for Psychiatric symptoms.

8. Ongoing psychiatric follow-up indicated.

9. Proceed on the bases of patient preference.

10. Delay or stop interferon treatment based on psychiatric analysis.

11. Invasive or specific clinical tests such as Liver biopsy should be considered.

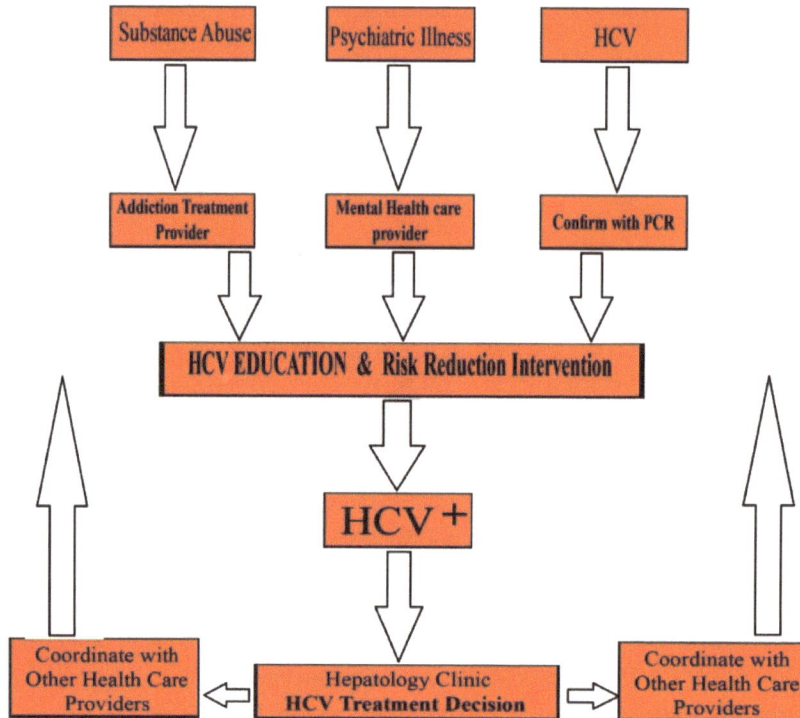

Figure 5: Flow diagram that illustrates the co-management and integration of care for patients with HCV, substance use disorders, and psychiatric illnesses.

5.5   Monitoring of Treatment

Health care provider should assess the risk of underlying diseases such coronary heart disease, to control preexisting medical problems, such as uncontrolled diabetes and hypertension, and to pre-screen all candidates for symptoms of depression prior to iniating therapy, further to a preliminary assessment of depression.

HCV infected Patients should be monitored during therapy to assess the response to treatment and for the occurrence of side effects. A reasonable schedule would be established on time wise schedules to follow up during treatment and thereafter until the end of therapy. HCV monitoring should include measurement of the complete blood count, serum creatinine and ALT levels, and HCV RNA by a sensitive assay at weeks 4, 12, 24, 4 to 12 week intervals thereafter, the end of treatment, and 24 weeks after stopping treatment. Thyroid function should be monitored every 12 weeks while on treatment.

Patients under treatment who achieve an SVR usually have improvement in liver histology and clinical outcomes. Others who achieve an SVR but who have cirrhosis are at risk for hepatic decompensation and HCC and death in the short term (5 years) and therefore should continue to be monitored periodically, including screening for HCC (See AASLD guidelines on Management of Hepatocellular Carcinoma).There is no role for a post treatment liver biopsy among those who achieve an SVR. Patient should be evaluated regularly regarding the presence of side effects. Further to compliance and adherence to treatment.

General Recommendations

- A liver biopsy should be considered in patients with chronic hepatitis C infection if the patient and health care provider wish information regarding fibrosis stage for prognostic purposes or to make a decision regarding treatment (Class IIa, Level B).

- Currently available noninvasive tests may be useful in defining the presence or absence of advanced fibrosis in persons with chronic hepatitis C infection, but should not replace the liver biopsy in routine clinical practice (Class IIb, Level C).

- Treatment decisions should be individualized based on the severity of liver disease, the potential for serious side effects, the likelihood of treatment response, the presence of comorbid conditions, and the patient's readiness for treatment (Class IIa, Level C).

- For patients in whom liver histology is available, treatment is indicated in those with bridging fibrosis or compensated cirrhosis provided they do not have contraindications to therapy (Class I, Level B).

- The optimal therapy for chronic HCV infection is the combination of peginterferon alfa and ribavirin (Class I, Level A).

- HCV RNA should be tested by a highly sensitive quantitative assay at the initiation of or shortly before treatment and at week 12 of therapy.

6   Strategy and Future Planning

6.1   Future Prospects

A relatively brief, skills-focused on prevention programs of HCV among psychiatric patients and yet analysis of such programs and further efforts are needed. This should include legal, ethical and policy issues. Further to immediate intervention planning and Long run strategies. Practice guidelines for mental health providers to address HCV is needed as there is a lack of information and concern about HCV particularly when Co-infected with HIV and HBV on the part of both providers and patients with severe mental illness.

6.2   Development of New Therapeutic Regimens

With continued efforts to gain more knowledge of the HCV life cycle and its viral structure, the first generation of drugs known as specifically targeted antiviral therapy for hepatitis C (STAT-C) or direct-acting antivirals (DAAs) have emerged to improve SVR cure rates and reduce the treatment duration of therapy. FDA-approved DAA drugs for HCV genotype 1 disease are the protease inhibitors boceprevir and telaprevir. Such therapy was found to be efficient in treating patients infected with HCV particularly when combined with interferon. This should have place in treating these patients and further clinical trials were needed to analyze the benefits of such therapy among patients with mental disorders.

6.3   Emerging New Models of Care

Hepatitis C virus infection among patients with mental disorder is a complex phenomenon associated with multi-disciplinary factors both with the infected patients and their surroundings. Further they are particularly prone to HIV and HBV which complicated the clinical status of the patients and make the management comprehensive more demanding. New model of treatment further to evidence-based approach should emerge which may include MD and Co-infection clinics and new concepts of treatment approaches mimicking that in chronic illness.

6.4   Vaccination

Vaccines are among the most efficacious means to control infectious diseases. However, the development of vaccines against highly heterogeneous viruses such as HCV and human immunodeficiency virus (HIV) is considerably hampered by variant-specific neutralizing immune responses. Classical approaches to vaccine development are yet to produce broadly protective vaccines against HCV and HIV. Novel vaccine strategies recently developed to cope with viral antigenic diversity focus either on using epitopes with limited heterogeneity, generating a concoction of heterogeneous epitopes or mimotopes, or predicting consensus sequences, center of tree variants or phylogenetic ancestors. Such promising prospect will definitely influence epidemiology of HCV among this particular group of patients.

References

Diagnostic and Statistical Manual of Mental Disorders, Fourth Edition. Washington, DC: American Psychiatric Association; 1994.

Daw MA, Dau AA. Hepatitis C virus in Arab world: a state of concern. Scientific World Journal. 2012; 2012:719494.

Daw MA, Siala IM, Warfalli MM, Muftah MI Seroepidemiology of hepatitis B virus markers among hospital health care workers. Analysis of certain potential risk factors. Saudi Med J. 2000; 21:1157-60.

Daw MA, Elkaber MA, Drah AM, Werfalli MM, Mihat AA, Siala IM. Prevalence of hepatitis C virus antibodies among different populations of relative and attributable risk. Saudi Med J. 2002 Nov, 23(11):1356-60.

Daw MA, Elasafier H. Dau AA, Agnan MM. The role of hepatitis C virus genotyping in evaluating the efficacy of INF-based therapy used in treating hepatitis C infected patients in Libya. Virology Discovery 2013;in press] http://www.hoajonline.com/journals/pdf/2052-6202-1-3.pdf.

Daw MA, Dau AA, Agnan MM. Influence of healthcare-associated factors on the efficacy of hepatitis C therapy. Scientific World Journal. 2012; 2012:580216.

Demyttenaere K, Bruffaerts R, Posada-Villa J, et al., (June 2004). "Prevalence, severity, and unmet need for treatment of mental disorders in the World Health Organization World Mental Health Surveys". JAMA 291 (21).

Edlin BR, Seal KH, Lorvick J, Kral AH, Ciccarone DH, Moore LD, et al., Is it justifiable to withhold treatment for hepatitis C from illicit-drug users? N Engl J Med 2001;345:211-215.

Fischer, Pamela J., Breakey, William R. (Winter 1985-86). "Homelessness and Mental Health: An Overview". International Journal of Mental Health 14 (4): 10.

Murray CJL, Lopez AD. The global burden of disease: a comprehensive assessment of mortality and disability from diseases, injuries, and risk factors in 1990 and projected to 2020. Cambridge: Harvard School of Public Health, 1996.

Rosenberg SD, Swanson JW, Wolford GL, et al: The Five-Site Health and Risk Study of Blood-Borne Infections Among Persons With Severe Mental Illness. Psychiatric Services 54:827–835, 2003.

Schaefer M, Schmidt F, Folwaczny C, Lorenz R, Martin G, Schindlbeck N, et al., Adherence and mental side effects during hepatitis C treatment with interferon alfa and ribavirin in psychiatric risk groups. HEPATOLOGY 2003;37:443-451.

World Health Organization (2005). WHO Resource Book on Mental Health: Human rights and legislation (PDF). ISBN 924156282 Check |isbn= value (help).

WHO. The global burden of disease: 2004 update. Geneva: World Health Organization, 2008.

Early Intervention to Improve Clinical and Functional Outcome in Patients with First Episode-Psychosis

Marcelo Valencia
Division of Epidemiological and Psychosocial Research
National Institute of Psychiatry Ramon de la Fuente, Mexico City, Mexico

Francisco Juarez
Division of Epidemiological and Psychosocial Research
National Institute of Psychiatry Ramon de la Fuente, Mexico City, Mexico

Marcela Delgado
Division of Epidemiological and Psychosocial Research
National Institute of Psychiatry Ramon de la Fuente, Mexico City, Mexico

Alejandro Díaz
Division of Clinical Services
National Institute of Psychiatry Ramon de la Fuente, Mexico City, Mexico

1 Introduction

During the last two decades significant advances in the long-term clinical management of schizophrenia have demonstrated the importance of early treatment for first-episode psychosis. When early treatment is not provided the long duration of untreated psychosis has been associated with poor clinical and functional outcome (Melle *et al.*, 2004; Norman & Malla 2001; Perkins *et al.*, 2006); psychosocial decline (Jones *et al.*, 1993; Lieberman *et al.*, 2001), some degree of behavioral deterioration (McGlashan, 1988), lower overall functioning, lower quality of life, more severe positive and negative symptoms and as a consequence a reduced possibility of achieving remission (Marshall *et al.*, 2005). These young individuals are usually actively psychotic for one o two years before they receive treatment (Beiser *et al.*, 1993), 30% experience an onset of psychotic symptoms by age 18 (McGrath *et al.*, 2008) and 70% can be expected to relapse after the first episode (Mueller, 2004), mostly related to non-adherence to medication (Robinson *et al.*, 1999; Verdoux *et al.*, 2000).

Over the last 20 years a new postulate has emerged, based upon studies of first episode psychosis that indicates that early intervention may result in better treatment outcome (Guo *et al.*, 2010; Malla & Norman, 2002; Mattai *et al.*, 2010). As a result, a new field of study has emerged known as "Early Psychosis" (Birchwood & Spencer, 2001), or "Early intervention for psychosis" (McGorry *et al.*, 2007). In addition, numerous Early Psychosis Programs have been designed and implemented for first-episode psychotic patients and their relatives (Alvarez-Jimenez *et al.*, 2008; Bird *et al.*, 2010). The parameters of a model of treatment should advocate a broader approach considering that evidence-based treatment has recommended that individuals suffering from schizophrenia should be provided with a combination of various essential interventions: 1) optimal dose of antipsychotic medication, 2) psychosocial treatment, psychoeducation and family therapy for patients and for their caregivers, and 3) case management to resolve, prevent and handle crisis such as: exacerbation of symptoms, relapse and rehospitalizations (Dixon *et al.*, 2010; Falloon *et al.*, 2004).

Clinical research indicates that antipsychotic medications have shown to be effective in reducing positive psychotic symptoms (Emsley *et al.*, 2007; Robinson *et al.*, 2005) and now they are the mainstay of treatment for patients with schizophrenia (Freedman, 2003; Lieberman *et al.*, 2005). However, these medications have limitations in their ability to improve overall outcome; therefore, adjunctive psychosocial interventions for first-episode psychosis have been recommended, since they have demonstrated when combined with medication that they may produce greater improvement in functional outcome compared with medication treatment alone (Addington *et al.*, 2011; Power *et al.*, 2007; Ruhrmann *et al.*, 2010; Tang *et al.*, 2010; Uzenoff *et al.*, 2012).

Early treatment for first-episode psychosis can be divided in two categories: single and multi-element interventions (Edwards & McGorry, 2002). Single interventions include one component such as: pharmacotherapy, or individual cognitive behavior therapy, while multi-element interventions include multiple services components such as case management, community outreach, in-and out patients, and various therapeutic approaches that would constitute a comprehensive intervention.

In addition to low-dose antipsychotic medication, first-episode psychotic patients may benefit from a great array of psychosocial approaches: social skills training, cognitive behavioral therapy, housing, assertive community treatment, supportive therapy, psychoeducation, vocational assistance, case management, family therapy, supported employment, cognitive remediation, peer support and weight management (Henry *et al.*, 2010; Bertelsen *et al.*, 2008; Malla & Payne, 2005; Penn *et al.*, 2005; Petersen *et al.*, 2005). These services can be delivered considering each patient´s needs, during hospitalization or when patients are living in the community using individual, couples, group or family format. Each intervention sets goals, evaluating improvements in specific components: cognitive functioning and quality of life (Malla & Norman, 2002), social functioning (Addington & Young, 2003) compliance with medication (Hudson *et al.*, 2008), prevention of relapse (Bebbington *et al.*, 2006), and reducing trauma secondary to psychosis and hospitalization (McGorry *et al.*, 1996).

Taking into account all these previous considerations, it is worth mentioning that outcome has been a main issue in schizophrenia. Research outcome has been a key concern since it involves assessing several specific domains including clinical symptoms, response to treatment, remission, quality of life, social functioning, cognitive function, employment, recovery, and family burden. Maintained symptomatic remission and appropriate functioning should be considered as desirable therapeutic outcome (Figueira & Brissos, 2011). Three domains of outcome measurement have been included in this chapter: symptomatic remission, psychosocial functioning, and functional outcome as a result of the implementation of pharmacological and psychosocial treatments for first-episode psychosis patients. Remission was measured using the operational definition of symptomatic remission proposed by the Remission in Schizophrenia Working Group (Andreasen *et al.*, 2005) that covers two components: 1) a threshold of symptom severity with a score of mild or less using eight key schizophrenia symptoms of the Positive and Negative Syndrome Scale (PANSS) (Kay *et al.*, 1990), that represent the "core features" of the illness, and 2) a duration criteria of 6 months that must be maintained to achieve remission. On the other hand, psychosocial functioning has been considered as a necessary outcome criterion to measure success of pharmacological and psychosocial treatments of schizophrenia patients (Harvey & Bellack, 2009; Juckel & Morosini, 2008). Although, numerous scales have been developed to assess psychosocial functioning, the most frequently used is the Global Assessment of Functioning (GAF) (American Psychiatric Association, 1994; Burns & Patrick, 2007; Goldman *et al.*, 1992). Good, adequate, appropriate or normal psychosocial functioning has been measured with the GAF using means scores of > 50 (Whitehorn *et al.*, 2002), > 61 (Harding *et al.*, 1987), > 65 (Torgalsboen, 1999), > 80 (Bobes *et al.*, 2009) and at least 81 (San *et al.*, 2007). Psychosocial functioning was measured with the GAF. To determine the effects of a multi-element intervention: Integrated treatment versus a single element intervention: Standard treatment, symptomatic remission and psychosocial functioning were assessed as indicators of functional outcome. A recent review that included 13 studies of first-episode psychosis showed that remission rates vary between 17% and 88% (Emsley *et al.*, 2011) according to the "Remission in Schizophrenia Working Group" criteria. Rates of functional outcome for first-episode psychotic patients have been reported at 48% (Whitehorn *et al.*, 2002); 50% (Harrison *et al.*, 2001); 19.2% (Wunderinck, *et al.*, 2009), and 31% (Henry *et al.*, 2010).

We chose as an operational definition of functional outcome the combination of two elements: 1) symptomatic remission according to the "Remission in Schizophrenia Working Group" criteria with the use of the PANSS, plus 2) psychosocial functioning within a "normal range" according to the Torgalsboen criteria with a GAF score above 65 (Torgalsbøen, 1999; Torgalsbøen & Rund, 2010). The fulfillment of the definition of functional outcome was considered as favorable, otherwise unfavorable. The six-month time period of treatment was considered to be the duration criterion to achieve functional outcome. Assessments were at baseline and at 6 months follow-up. Additional clinical variables were measured, such as; relapse, re-hospitalization, medication compliance and therapeutic adherence. In this chapter, we report the results of a six-month randomized controlled trial of an early psychosis integrated program consisting of pharmacotherapy and psycho-social intervention for patients, and psycho-education for relatives, compared with a standard care of pharmacological treatment alone.

The aim was to compare a single versus multi-element interventions according to the two categories described by Edwards & McGorry, (2002) to determine clinical and functional outcome improvements. We hypothesize the following; a) that a greater proportion of patients receiving integrated treatment would meet remission criteria and would show higher psychosocial functioning improvement when compared to those receiving standard treatment; b) patients who fulfilled both criteria: symptomatic remission and a better level of psychosocial functioning, and as a result would be achieving functional outcome, will be significantly higher in the integrated treatment group.

2   Methods

2.1   Design of the Study and Participants

Antipsychotic-naive patients who met eligibility criteria participated in the study protocol. These were out-patients receiving pharmacological treatment for their first time at the Schizophrenia Clinic of the Hospital of the National Institute of Psychiatry in Mexico City. One hundred and twenty patients who fulfilled inclusion criteria were included in the study, all patients voluntarily accepted to participate. Patients were randomly assigned, in an alternate order, to two treatment conditions: 60 patients to integrated treatment and 60 to standard treatment (medication alone). Of the 120 patients who initiated treatment, six from integrated treatment (10%), (one started a full time job; two returned to school, three moved out of Mexico City for family reasons), and twelve patients from standard treatment (20%) (four moved out of Mexico City for family reasons; two returned to school, two started a full time job, and four decided to receive treatment in another psychiatric hospital) failed to complete the study protocol with a total of 18 patients (15%) for the total sample. The final sample was 102 patients: $n = 54$ in integrated treatment and $n = 48$ in standard treatment. Patients were recruited into the study when they met the following inclusion criteria: never been hospitalized for psychiatric reasons, taking anti-psychotic medication for the first time, allowing a period of no more than 15 days to demonstrate clinical stability in terms of psychotic symptoms (corroborated by a score lower than 60 in the PANSS), their diagnoses verified according to DSM-IV (American Psychiatric Association, 1994) criteria and corroborated with the CIDI (Robins *et al.*, 1988), had completed at least six years of elementary education, range age between 16 to 50 years old, with no substance (drug or alcohol) abuse verified with their relatives before and during treatment, living in Mexico City's metropolitan area, and participation of at least one relative in psychoeducation and family sessions. The participant relative was the one with closest contact to the patient, the relative and the patients, both, should be living in the same household.

2.2   Procedures

The study protocol was approved by the Research Committee and the Ethics Committee of the National Institute of Psychiatry. A session was held where patients and relatives were informed about all therapeutic procedures. Afterwards, they voluntarily expressed in a written informed consent document their desire to participate in the research project.

Measures of outcomes were administered to patients: symptomatology, symptom remission, and psycho-social functioning at baseline and at the end of treatment. Independent interviewers that were blind to the two treatment conditions completed the assessments. The last procedure consisted that, patients and their relatives were randomly assigned either to integrated treatment or to continue with standard treatment (antipsychotic medication alone).

2.3 Integrated treatment

The integrated treatment can be defined as a comprehensive model including socials skills training, psychoeducation for relatives, family therapy and pharmacotherapy.

2.3.1 Social skills training

Social skills training focused on four areas: a) medication management, b) symptom management, c) social relations, and d) family relations. Learning certain skills was set as a goal that included: learning about the illness, compliance with medication, identifying warning signs of relapse, developing a relapse preventive plan, learning skills to manage social relations, and learning problem-solving skills for better family relations. A therapist´s manual describes the areas including the skills corresponding to each area, and the training strategies for each session (Valencia et al., 2001). Two therapists were in charge of teaching patients skill acquisition using the "learning activities". Six learning activities were utilized: 1) introduction and explanation of skills to be learned in each session; 2) skill demonstration by therapists that included a question-and-answer segment for clarification of skills to be learned; 3) patient practice of skills using role playing and other techniques; 4) feedback allowing patients to identify resources needed to use skills in the real world; 5) practice skills in the community; and, 6) each session began with verification of skills registered in a learning check-list. Of the seven originally proposed learning activities (Kopelowicz et al., 2003; Liberman & Corrigan, 1993; Wallace et al., 1992), six were utilized excluding video technology as it is being used in the United States since this type of technology has not yet been developed in Mexico. As a substitute of video technology live demonstration of the learning skills by the therapists were carried out during sessions.

A therapist evaluation form was used to verify that all treatment areas were conducted properly. Therapists´ competency during treatment was assessed by a specially trained research assistant. Before treatment, competency levels had to be demonstrated with at least a 90 percent level of efficacy. Monitoring for maintenance of fidelity occurred throughout the study. Group sessions, eight patients per group, were conducted weekly by two therapists with a time limit of 90 minutes during six-month of treatment.

Goals of the interventions included: 1) training patients to acquire social skills; 2) improving psychosocial functioning, 3) preventing relapse and rehospitalization, 4) promoting treatment compliance, and 5) achieving functional outcome measured by symptomatic remission and psychosocial functioning.

2.3.2 Psycho-education

Eight multi-family group sessions were held where relatives received information about schizophrenia, symptoms, medication management, side effects, compliance with medication, keeping appointments, and recognition and management of warning signs of relapse. As it was requested in the inclusion criteria, at least one relative per family had to participate, but if more relatives expressed their desire to participate, they were welcomed to psychoeducation and family sessions. Family therapy included four sessions for each patient and his family focused on problem solving and improving communication skills. Two family therapists were in charge of psycho-education and family sessions.

Integrated treatment included the following professionals: two psychiatrists for medication management, two clinical psychologists in charge of psychosocial treatment, and two family therapists for psycho-education and family sessions.

2.3.3   Standard treatment

Standard treatment consisted of the usual service provided to patients: pharmacological treatment that was provided at the Schizophrenia Clinic of the National Institute of Psychiatry. Patients of both groups under study attended 20-minute monthly consultations given by two clinical psychiatrists, who were blind to the two treatment conditions. In addition of controlling prescribed antipsychotic medication, the treating psychiatrists were in charge of registering attendance to consultations and verifying medication compliance with patients´ and their corresponding relatives during consultations.

2.4   Measures of outcome

Symptomatology was assessed with a validated Spanish adaptation of the Positive and Negative Syndrome Scale (PANSS) (Kay *et al.*, 1990) composed of three subscales: positive (7 items), negative (7 items) and general psychopathology (GPS) (16 items). Each item is scored from 1 (absence of psychopathology) to 7 (extremely severe).

Symptomatic remission was assessed according to the Remission in Schizophrenia Working Group (RSWG) criteria (Andreasen *et al.*, 2005) using eight core symptoms in psychotisism, disorganization and negative symptoms of the Positive and Negative Syndrome Scale (PANSS). Maintenance of all scores has to be 3 (mild) for at least six months.

Psychosocial functioning was assessed with the Global Assessment of Functioning Scale (GAF) (American Psychiatric Association., 1994). This scale measures the combination of symptom severity and the level of impairment in psychological, social and occupational functioning on a mental health-illness continuum which indicates the level of functioning ranging from 1-100. Scores above 65 are considered within the "normal psychosocial functioning" range (Torgalsbøen, 1999; Torgalsbøen & Rund, 2010).

Independent raters evaluated the two groups under study at baseline and at the end of treatment. They were properly trained for the application of all research instruments. Raters had no participation in the treatment team and had no knowledge of the research project. Hence, they were blind to the two treatment conditions.

Another set of clinical variables were assessed during treatment such as relapse, and rehospitalization rates, compliance with medication and therapeutic adherence. When patients experienced significant exacerbation of psychotic symptoms considered as warning signs of relapse they received immediate consultation from their treating psychiatrist, who then made necessary adjustments in their antipsychotic medication to avoid relapse. A psychotic relapse was considered when patients had at least a 20% worsening on the PANSS total score from baseline evaluation. Similar criteria have been utilized by other researcher when assessing relapse (Csernansky & Schuchart, 2002; Lipkovitch *et al.*, 2007). Patients were hospitalized when psychotic symptom exacerbation could not be controlled nor stabilized with antipsychotic medication. Compliance with antipsychotic medication was assessed by the treating psychiatrist during monthly consultations for pharmacological management. Compliance was assessed as a result of a consensus between the patient and a relative participating in psycho-education. Compliance was registered when patients had at least taken 90 percent of prescribed antipsychotic medication; otherwise, non-adherence was assessed.

2.5   Statistical Analysis

Data handling and analysis were carried out using the Statistical Package for Social Sciences for Windows version 20 (IBM SPSS Statistics, 2010). We performed descriptive and Chi square analysis to compare percentages, Student t tests to verify that there were no significant differences between the two groups under study in their initial levels of symptomatology, and psychosocial functioning. At baseline, Student t tests were used to verify that no statistically significant differences existed between the two groups regarding the PANSS and GAF scores. Analysis of variance for repeated measures (ANOVA) was used to detect pre-post differences within and between the two study groups. We calculated the standardized estimate of effect sizes using Cohen´s d formula defined as: $d = (x_1 - x_2)/ s$ where x_1 and x_2 are the means at baseline and at end of treatment of the two groups under study, and s is the pooled within-group standard deviation (SD) (Cohen, 1977). Three levels of effect size were considered: small = 0.25, medium = 0.50 and large = 1.00 irrespective of the sign (+ or −) of the number (Kazdin, 1999).

3   Results

Demographic and clinical characteristics of the sample are shown in Table 1. Patients in both treatment conditions were similar with no demographic differences for any of these variables. No statistically significant differences were found at study entry between the two groups under study in symptomalogy, (PANSS) or psychosocial functioning (GAF).

	Integrated treatment ($n = 54$)	Standard Treatment ($n = 48$)
Gender, n (%)		
Male	42 (77.8)	37 (77.1)
Female	12 (22.2)	11 (22.9)
Marital status, n (%)		
Single	54 (100)	46 (95.8)
Married	--	1 (2.1)
Speratated/divorced	--	1 (2.1)
Occupation, n (%)		
Employed	10 (18.5)	10 (20.8)
Unemployed	44 (81.5)	38 (79.1)
Age, years, $\bar{x}$ (s)	26.9 (4.8)	26.7 (5.0)
Education, years, $\bar{x}$ (s)	11.1 (2.0)	10.9 (2.2)
Age at onset, years, $\bar{x}$ (s)	19.5 (3.5)	20.8 (4.1)

Table 1: Demographic and clinical characteristics of the study sample.

Significantly statistical improvements in symptomatology were found over 6 months of treatment according to mean changes scores, as rated by the PANSS, in positive and negative symptoms, general psychopathology and in total PANSS score for both groups under study. Group-by-time analysis demonstrated significantly greater improvement in patients of integrated treatment when compared with patients receiving medication alone. Comparison of the effect sizes were large for integrated treatment patients on the total PANSS score, positive scale, negative scale, and in the general psychopathology scale. Effect sizes were medium for all score scales of the standard treatment group. Significant improvement in psychosocial functioning was also found for patients of integrated treatment but not for patients of standard treatment since they remained at the same level of functioning (41 − 50) as rated by the GAF, from baseline to post treatment assessment. Standard treatment patients improved two levels of functioning from 41 – 50 at baseline to 61 – 70 at the end of treatment. Effect size was large for integrated treatment and small for standard treatment (Table 2).

	Integrated treatment $n = 54$	Standard treatment $n = 48$	Statistics [b]		
			Main effect for time	Main effect for group	Interaction of group and time
PANSS[a] overall score, $\bar{x}$ (s)					
Baseline	90.1 (39.8)	81.4 (34.1)	$p < .001$	--	$p < .01$
Post	41.6 (10.0)	54.0 (15.9)			
Effect size	-1.2	-0.8			
PANSS positive[a], $\bar{x}$ (s)					
Baseline	20.4 (11.0)	17.7 (10.0)	$p < .001$	--	$p < .01$
Post	8.8 (2.1)	11.0 (4.2)			
Effect size	-1.1	-0.7			
PANSS negative[a], $\bar{x}$ (s)					
Baseline	23.7 (10.9)	21.8 (9.6)	$p < .001$	--	$p < .01$
Post	10.8 (4.2)	14.5 (6.1)			
Effect size	-1.2	-0.8			
PANSS GPS[a, c], $\bar{x}$ (s)					
Baseline	46.0 (19.7)	41.9 (16.2)	$p < .001$	--	$p < .01$
Post	22.0 (4.8)	28.6 (8.3)			
Effect size	-1.2	-0.8			
Psychosocial functionig[d] (GAF) , $\bar{x}$ (s)					
Baseline	43.6 (6.4)	43.6 (6.7)	$p < .001$	$p < .001$	$p < .001$
Post	67.0 (8.9)	44.8 (9.4)			
Effect size	3.7	0.2			

[a] Higher scores indicate more severe symptoms.
[b] Analysis of variance for repeated measures.
[c] GPS, General Psychopathology Scale.
[d] Higher scores indicate better global functioning.

Table 2: Symptomatology (PANSS) and psychosocial functioning (GAF) outcomes.

Other variables such as relapse and re-hospitalization rates, medication compliance and therapeutic adherence were measured during treatment. Integrated treatment patients had lower relapse: 9.3%, ($p < .01$) and re-hospitalization rates: 5.6%, at the end of treatment compared to 32.5% and 10% respectively for the standard treatment group that received medication alone. Antipsychotic medication compliance was higher in the integrated treatment group: 88.9% compared to 82.5% of the standard treatment group. Therapeutic adherence to the social skills training sessions was 86.4%, which means a higher adherence level according to the therapeutic adherence levels: excellent: 90 – 100; high: 80 – 89; good: 70 – 79; regular: 60 – 69; poor: 50 – 59; and bad: 40 – 49.

The assessment of symptomatic remission, psychosocial functioning and functional outcome demonstrated at baseline that remission was achieved by 29.6% of the integrated treatment group compared with 20.8 % of standard treatment. At the end of the interventions, integrated treatment patients showed a 96.3% of symptomatic remission compared to 56.3% of standard treatment. Psychosocial functioning within a "normal range" (GAF score above 65) was not achieved by either group under study at baseline. At the end of treatment psychosocial functioning was achieved by 50% of patients of integrated treatment compared to 2.5% of standard treatment. The two groups under study did not achieve functional outcome at baseline, while, 50% of the standard treatment group met both criteria: symptomatic remission and psychosocial functioning within a "normal range" at the end of treatment and were considered to have achieved functional outcome (favorable outcome) compared to 2.1% of the standard treatment group (unfavorable outcome) (Table 3).

	Integrated treatment n = 54	Standard treatment n = 48	McNemar
Symtomatic remission at baseline	16 (29.6%)	10 (20.8%)	p < .01
Symtomatic remission after treatment	52 (96.3%)	27 (56.3%)	
Psychosocial functioning at baseline	--	--	p < .01
Psychosocial functioning after treatment	27 (50%)	1 (2.5%)	
Functional outcome at baseline	--	--	p < .01
Functional outcome after treatment)	27 (50%)	1 (2.1%)	

Table 3: Symptomatic remission, psychosocial functioning and functional outcomes

4   Discussion

The present findings provide evidence that early integrated treatment in first episode psychosis is positively linked with statistically significant improvements in symptomatology, psychosocial functioning, lower relapse rate, high compliance with medication and high therapeutic adherence. Effect sizes in symptomatology and psychosocial functioning were large for integrated treatment. These results indicate that outcome can be improved through early intervention after the onset of psychosis. The maintenance of a stable clinical state is no longer considered as the ultimate therapeutic goal of treatment. New proposals indicate that the focus of treatment should include the achievement of symptomatic remission, and good psychosocial functioning that would lead to functional outcome as it was measured in the present study. Results indicate that a high proportion of patients that participated in integrated treatment achieved remission at the end of treatment: above than 95% compared to less than 60% of standard treatment. Psychosocial functioning within a normal range was accomplished by half of patients of integrated treatment compared to less that 3% of standard treatment. Functional outcome was achieved by half of patients of integrated treatment (favorable outcome) compared to less than 2.5% of standard treatment (unfavorable outcome). The aim of the study was to compare a single versus multi-element interventions indicated that the latter determined a favorable clinical and functional outcome. Remission achieved in the present study was higher than remission rates reported in the international literature: 17% – 88% (Emsley *et al.*, 2011) according to the Schizophrenia Working Group criteria. Functional outcome that was observed in half of the patients of integrated treatment was similar (Harding *et al.*, 1987; Harrison *et al.*, 2001), and higher as other studies (Harrison *et al.*, 2001; Whitehorn *et al.*, 2002). Achieving and maintaining remission has been related to a better clinical status and functional outcome as reported in various studies (Docherty *et al.*, 2007; Emsley *et al.*, 2007; Hellding *et al.*, 2007). Symptomatic remission can be considered as a good indicator of better clinical and psychososocial functioning (Brissos *et al.*, 2011), and it has been associated with good functioning (Bodén *et al.*, 2009)

Although, there is not an international accepted consensus definition for symptomatic remission, the operational definition proposed by the Schizophrenia Working Group, has been useful to measure symptomatic remission as it has been verified in a great number of studies (Gorwood & Peuskens, 2012). Using eight items of the PANSS, the remission criteria are very easily to apply by a trained clinician, and could be considered as a good example of the need of shorter and simpler instruments. Even though, the operational definition is not related to any improvements in functioning, symptomatic remission has been associated with higher levels of social functioning (Bodén *et al.*, 2009). Usually, remission and functioning have been assessed separately. For the present study, we included these two variables to assess functional outcome, as it has been considered that functional outcome should include various domains. There is not a consensus either on how to measure functional outcome, since the rates and definitions vary considerably across studies from "poor", "fair" or "good" outcome (Henry *et al.*, 2010; Salokangas *et al.*, 2013). As it has been found in the present study, favorable outcome has been reported in developing countries (Hooper *et al.*, 2007; Novick *et al.*, Teferra *et al.*, 2012)

Early treatment for schizophrenia should go beyond the measurement of symptom change. Psychosocial functioning can be considered as a very serious concern that should be included in the assessment of clinical and psychosocial effectiveness of interventions, these two variables should encompass functional outcome. The primary goal of schizophrenia treatment, in addition of symptom relief, should be the restoration of functioning, that is, the ability to function adequately in the community. First episode psychosis individuals present impairments in psychosocial functioning before the first psychotic episode; hence, these impairments must be addressed in initial treatment (Grant *et al.*, 2001).

The great majority of patients that participated on this research project, 95% of them (Valencia *et al.*, 2003) were living at home with their families. The experience of family caregivers to manage a person with a first-episode psychosis was a complicated burden since they had no knowledge of how to handle the illness. Relatives very clearly manifested the need for more information about the disease that would help them to cope with the burden and lower the stress related to living with a person with psychosis. These issues were included as components of the integrated treatment approach. The purpose was connecting patients and relatives needs with treatment strategies. At first, relatives were eager to believe that their needs and opinions would be taken into account as components of treatment, since they manifested that final decisions about treatment are only made by doctors. However, when these issues were incorporated and verified by them during treatment, they were satisfied since they felt that their needs were being accomplished by learning new skills that helped them to cope with the burden and illness management. These positive experiences increased involvement and commitment to treatment by relatives. A particular strength of this study should be explained by the fact that patients of integrated treatment experienced a significant lower relapse rate (10%). It seems that patients and relatives learned to identify the warning signs to prevent relapse which might be associated with high compliance with antipsychotic medication (88.9%). Considering that medication compliance was high and relapse rate was low, this might indicate that patients and relatives were aware of the benefits of medication as a protective factor to avoid relapse. Therefore, it appears that they learned the necessary skills about symptom management, and the importance of taking antipsychotic medication. It seems that high medication compliance was helpful for preventing relapse, and learning how to prevent relapse has been considered a priority in schizophrenia (Gleeson *et al.*, 2009; Mueser & Bellack, 1992). These favourable results can be explained by the fact that all efforts by patients, their corresponding relatives and the treatment team were oriented towards functional improvements. The work with patients and relatives, using an integrated treatment approach, can be considered as an effective way to promote functional outcome for first episode psychosis patients (Bertelsen *et al.*, 2008; Petersen *et al.*, 2005).

Participation of relatives in a psychoeducational multi family group intervention and later on in family therapy sessions for each patient and his family were beneficial (Rossberg & Johannssen, 2010), and essential as it has been established for family interventions (Pitschel-Walz *et al.*, 2001). Participation of family caregivers was considered a strategic treatment issue since we pursued establishing a therapeutic alliance between patients, their relatives and the treatment team. Strong therapeutic alliance is related to better outcome in early treatment of schizophrenia (Johansen *et al.*, 2013). Psychoeducation promoting a positive therapeutic alliance might be helpful in reducing the burden experienced by relatives, improving family relations and preventing the exacerbation of psychotic symptoms (Smerud & Rosenbarb, 2008)

At the National Institute of Psychiatry, in Mexico City, there has been a long term tradition of using a single-element treatment model such as pharmacotherapy as standard treatment. However, in the last twenty years, research protocols have been conducted including in addition to medication, psychosocial, psychoeducational, family therapy and rehabilitation approaches. Two components were considered for designing these treatment programs: 1) evidence based practices re-commendations (Falloon *et al.*, 2004; Shean, 2009) and 2) the situation, needs and demands from our patients and their relatives. Several experimental and clinical trials have been conducted with a duration of six or twelve months of treatment in chronic patients (Valencia *et al.*, 2007; 2010; Valencia, Diaz *et al.*, 2012; Valencia, Liberman *et al.*, 2012) but also with first-episode psychotic patients during one year (Valencia, Juarez *et al.*, 2012), and another study, during six months as reported in this chapter.

It is worth mentioning that in a previous study, first episode patients that received integrated treatment during one year demonstrated statistically significant improvements in symptomatology, psychosocial functioning, lower relapse and re-hospitalization rates, higher compliance with medication and high therapeutic adherence (Valencia, Juarez *et al.*, 2012). In the present study significant improvements were not found in variables such as re-hospitalizations and compliance with medication. Although, six months of treatment proved its effectiveness, we wonder if a one year treatment would be more suitable for first-episode psychosis patients, which leads to the question that needs to be addressed referring to how long patients should remain in early treatment interventions for schizophrenia. Therefore, a limitation of the present study could be the short duration of the intervention as well as the difficulty to determine what components of the integrated treatment were relevant for clinical and functional improvements.

First-Episode psychosis patients need prompt diagnosis and early intervention for improving long-term outcome that will lead them to live productive lives in the real world. Early intervention, at this critical period, could lead to a more favorable outcome to prevent clinical and psychosocial deterioration.

References

Addington, J. & Young, J. (2003). *Social outcome in early psychosis. Psychological Medicine, 33, 1119-1124.*

Addington, J., Epstein, I., Liu, L., French, P., Boydell, K.M., & Zipursky, R. B. (2011). *A randomized controlled trial of cognitive therapy for individuals at clinical risk of psychosis. Schizophrenia Research, 125, 54-61.*

Alvarez-Jimenez, M., Hetrick, S. E., Gonzalez-Blanch, C., Gleeson, J. F., & McGorry, P. D. (2008). Non-pharmacological management of antipsychotic-induced weight gain: Systematic review and meta-analysis of randomized controlled trials. British Journal of Psychiatry, 193, 101-107.

American Psychiatric Association. (1994). Diagnostic and Statistical Manual of Mental Disorders (Fourth Edition). Washington, D. C.: American Psychiatric Association.

Andreasen, N., Carpenter, W., Kane, J., Lasser, R. A., Marder, S. R., & Weinberger, D. R. (2005). Remission in schizophrenia: proposed criteria and rational for consensus. The American Journal of Psychiatry, 162, 441-449

Bebbington, P. E., Craig, T., Garety, P., Fowler, D., Dunn, G., Colbert, S.,... Kuipers, E. (2006). Remisssion and relapse in psychosis: operational definition based on case-note data. Psychological Medicine, 36, 1551-1556.

Beiser, M., Erickson, D., Fleming, J.A., & Jacono, W. G. (1993). Establishing the onset of psychotic illness. The American Journal of Psychiatry, 150, 1349-1354.

Bertelsen, M., Jeppesen, P., Petersen, L., Thorup, A., Øhlenschlaeger, J., Le Quach, P.,... Nordentoff, M. (2008). Five-year follow-up of a randomized multicenter trial of intensive early intervention vs standard treatment for patients with a first episode of psychotic illness: the OPUS trial. Archives of General Psychiatry, 65, 762-771.

Birchwood, M. & Spencer, E. (2001). Early intervention in psychotic relapse. Clinical Psychological Review, 21, 1211-1226.

Bird, V., Premkumar, P., Kendal, T., Whittington, C., Mitchell, J., & Kuipers E. (2010). Early intervention services, cognitive-behavioural therapy and family interventions in early psychosis: Systematic review. British Journal of Psychiatry, 197, 350-356.

Bobes, J., Ciudad, A., Alvarez, E., San, L., Polavieja, P., & Gilaberte I. (2009). Recovery from Schizophrenia: Results from a 1-year follow-up observational study of patients in symptomatic remission. Schizophrenia Research, 115, 58-66.

Bodén, R., Sunström, J., Lindström, E., & Lindström, L. (2009). Association between symptomatic remission and functional outcome in first-episode schizophrenia. Schizophrenia Research, 107, 232-237.

Brissos, S., Dias, V. V., Balanzá-Martinez, V., Carita, A.I., & Figueira, M. L. (2011). Symptomatic remission in schizophrenia patients: Relationship with social functioning, quality of life, and neurocognitive performance. Schizophrenia Research, 129, 133-136.

Burns, T. & Patrick, D. (2007). Social functioning as an outcome measure in schizophrenia studies. Acta Psychiatrica Scandinavica, 116(6), 403-418.

Cohen, J. (1977). Statistical Power Analysis for the Behavioral Sciences. New York, NY, USA., Academia Press.

Csernansky, J. G. & Schuchart, E. K. (2002). Relapse and rehospitalization rates in patients with schizophrenia: Effects of second generation antipsychotics. CNS Drugs, 16, 473-484.

Dixon, L.B., Dickerson, F., Bellack, A. S., Benett, M., Dickinson, D., Goldber, R. W.,... Kreyenbuhl, J. (2010). The 2009 schizophrenia PORT psychosocial treatment recommendations and summary statements. Schizophrenia Bulletin, 36, 48-70.

Docherty, J. P., Bossie, C. A., Lachaux, B., Bouhours, P., Zhu, Y., Lasser, R., & Gharabawi, G. M. (2007). Patient-based and clinician-based support for the remission criteria in schizophrenia. International Clinical Psychopharmacology, 22 (1), 51-55. doi: 10.1097/01.yic.0000224791.06159.88

Edwards, J. & McGorry, P.D. (2002). Implementing early interventions in psychosis: A guide to establishing early psychosis services. Martin Dunitz. London.

Emsley, R., Bonginkosi, C., Asmal, L., & Lehloenya, K. (2011). The concepts of remission and recovery in schizophrenia. Current Opinion in Psychiatry, 24, 114-121.

Emsley, R., Rabinowitz, J., & Medori, R. (2007). Remission in early psychosis: rates, predictors, and clinical and functional outcomes correlates. Schizophrenia Research, 89, 129-139.

Falloon, I., Montero, I., Sungur, M., Mastroeni, A., Malm, U., Economou, M.,... Gedye, R. (2004). Implementation of evidence-based treatment for schizophrenic disorders: two-year outcome of an international field trial of optimal treatment. World Psychiatry, 3(2), 104-109.

Figueira, M. L. & Brissos, S. (2011). Measuring psychosocial outcomes in schizophrenia patients. Current Opinion Psychiatry, 24, 91-99.

Freedman, R. (2003). Schizophrenia: New England Journal of Medicine, 349(18), 1738-1749.

Gleeson, J. F., Cotton, S. M., Alvarez-Jimenez, M., Wade, D. Gee, D., Crisp, K.,... McGorry, P.D. (2009). A randomized controlled trial of relapse prevention therapy for first-episode psychosis patients. Journal of Clinical Psychiatry, 70(4), 477-486.

Goldman, H. H., Skodol, A. E., & Lave, T. R. (1992). Revising axis V for DSM-IV: A review of measures of social functioning. The American Journal of Psychiatry, 149, 1148-1156.

Gorwod, P. & Peuskens, J. (2012). Setting new standards in schizophrenia outcomes: symptomatic remission 3 years before versus after the Andreasen criteria. European Psychiatry, 27(3), 170-175.

Grant, C., Addington, J., Addington, D., & Konnert, C. (2001). Social functioning in first-and multiepisode schizophrenia. Canadian Journal of Psychiatry, 46, 746-749.

Guo, X., Zhai, J., Liu, Z., Fang, M., Wang, B., Wang, C.,... Zhao, J. (2010). Effect of antipsychotic medication alone vs combined with psychosocial intervention on outcomes of early-stage schizophrenia. Archives of General Psychiatry, 76(9), 895-904.

Harding, C. M., Brooks, G. W., Ashikaga, T., Strauss, J. S., & Breier, A. (1987). The Vermont longitudinal study of persons with severe mental illness: II. Long-term outcome of subjects who retrospectively met DSM-III criteria for schizophrenia. The American Journal of Psychiatry, 144, 727-735.

Harrison, G., Hopper, K., Craig, T., Laska, E., Siegel, C., Wanderling, J.,... Wiersma, D. (2001). Recovery from psychotic illness: a 15- and 25- year international follow-up study. British Journal of Psychiatry, 178(6), 506-517.

Harvey, P. D. & Bellack, A. S. (2009). Toward a terminology for functional recovery in schizophrenia. Schizophrenia Bulletin, 35(2), 300-306.

Helding, LN., Kane, J.M., Karilampi, U., Norlander, T., &Archer, T. (2007). Remission in prognosis of functional outcome: A new dimension in the treatment of patients with psychotic disorders. Schizophrenia Research, 93, 160-168.

Henry, L. P., Amminger, G. P., & Harris, M.G. (2010). The EPPIC follow-up study of first episode psychosis: longer term clinical and functional outcome 7 years after index admission. Journal of Clinical Psychiatry, 71, 716-728.

Hooper, K., Harrison, G., Janca, A., & Sartorius, N. (2007). Recovery from schizophrenia: An international perspective-results from the WHO-Coordinated International Study of Schizophrenia. New York, Oxford: Oxford University Press.

Hudson, T. J., Owen, R. R., Thrush, C. R., Armitage, T. L., & Thapa, P. (2008). Guideline implementation and patient-tailoring strategies to improve medication adherence for schizophrenia. Journal of Clinical Psychiatry, 69(1), 74-80.

IBM SPSS Statistics (version 20) [Computer software]. (2010). New York, E. U.: IBM Corporation, SPSS Inc.

Johansen, R., Iversen, V. C., Melle, I., & Hestad, K. A. (2013). Therapeutic alliance in early schizophrenia spectrum disorders: a cross-sectional study. Annals of General Psychiatry, 12, 1-14.

Jones, P. B., Bebbington, P., Foerster, A., Lewis, S. W., Murray, R. M., Russle, A.,... Wilkins, S. (1993). Premorbid social underachievement in schizophrenia: results of the Camberwell Collaborative Psychosis Study. British Journal of Psychiatry, 162, 65-71

Juckel, G. & Morosini, P. (2008). The new approach: psychosocial functioning as a necessary outcome criterion for therapeutic success in schizophrenia. Current Opinion in Psychiatry, 21, 630-639.

Kay, S. R., Fiszbein, A., Vital-Herne, M., & Fuentes, L.S. (1990). The positive and negative syndrome scale-Spanish adaptation. The Journal of Nervous and Mental Disease, 178, 510-517.

Kazdin, A. (1999). The meanings and measurement of clinical significance. Journal of Consulting and Clinical Psychology, 67(3), 332-339.

Kopelowicz, A., Zarate, R., Gonzalez Smit, V. Mintz, J. & Liberman, R.P. (2003). Disease management in Latinos with schizophrenia: A family assisted, skills training approach. Schizophrenia Bulletin, 29(2), 211-227.

Liberman, R. P. & Corrigan, P. W. (1993). Designing new psychosocial treatments for schizophrenia. Psychiatry, 56, 238-249.

Lieberman, J. A., Perkins, D., Belger, A., Chakos, M., Jarskog, F., Boteva, K., & Gilmore, J. (2001). The early stages of schizophrenia: speculations on pathogenesis pathophysiology, and therapeutic approaches. Biological Psychiatry, 50(11), 884-897.

Lieberman, J. A., Stroup, T. S., McEvoy, J. P., Swartz, M. S. Rosenheck, R. A., Perkins, D. O.,... Hsiao, J.K. (2005). Effectiveness of antipsychotic drugs in patients with chronic schizophrenia. New England Journal of Medicine, 353, 1209-1223.

Lipkovitch, I., Debert, W., Csernansky, J. G., Buckley, P., Peuskens, J., Kollack-Walker, S.,... Houston, J.P. (2007). Predictors of risk relapse in patients with schizophrenia or schizoaffective disorder during olanzapine. Journal of Psychiatric Research, 41, 305-310.

Malla, A. K. & Norman, R. M. G. (2002). Early intervention in schizophrenia and related disorders: advantages and pitfalls. Current Opinion in Psychiatry, 15(1), 17-23.

Malla, A. K. & Payne, J. (2005). First.episode psychosis: Psychopathology, quality of life, and functional outcome. Schizophrenia Bulletin, 31(3), 650-7611.

Marshall, M., Lewis, S., Lockwood, A., Drake, R., Jones, P., & Crouder, T. (2005). Association between duration of untreated psychosis and outcome in cohorts of first-episode patients. Archives General of Psychiatry, 62, 975-983.

Mattai, A. K., Hill, J., & Lenroot R.K. (2010). Treatment of early-onset schizophrenia. Current Opinion in Psychiatry, 23, 304-310.

McGlashan, T. H. (1988). A selective review of recent North American long-term follow-up studies of schizophrenia. Schizophrenia Bulletin, 14(4), 515-542.

McGorry, P. D., Edwards, J., Mihalopoulos, C., Harrigan, S.M., & Jackson, H.J. (1996). EPPIC: an evolving system of early detection and optimal management. Schizophrenia Bulletin, 22(2), 305-326.

McGorry, P. D., Killackey, E., & Yung, A.R. (2007). Early intervention in psychotic disorders: detection and treatment of the first-episode and critical early stages. Medical Journal of Australia, 187, S8-S10.

McGrath, J., Salva, S., Chant, D., & Welham, J. (2008). Schizophrenia: a concise overview of incidence, prevalence, and mortality. Epidemiology Review, 30, 67-78.

Melle, J., Larsen, T. K., Haahr, U., Friss, S., Johannssen, J. O., Opjordsmoen, S.,... McGlashen, T. (2004). Reducing the duration of untreated first-episode psychosis: effects on clinical presentation. Archives of General Psychiatry, 61, 143-150.

Mueller, N. (2004). Mechanisms of relapse prevention in schizophrenia. Pharmacopsychiatry, 37(2), S141-S147.

Mueser, K. T. & Bellack, A. (1992). An assessment of the educational needs of chronic psychiatric patients and their relatives. British Journal of Psychiatry, 160, 674-680.

Norman, R. M. & Malla, A. K. (2001). Duration of untreated psychosis: a critical examination of the concept and its importance. Psychological Medicine, 31, 381-400.

Novick, D., Haro, J.M., Hong, J., Brugnoli, R., Lepine J.P., Bertsch, J.,... Alvarez, E. (2012). Regional differences in treatment response and three year course of schizophrenia across the world. Journal of Psychiatric Research, 46, 856-864.

Penn, D. L., Waldheter, E. J., Perkins, D. O., Mueser, K. T., & Lieberman, J. A. (2005). Psychosocial treatment for first-episode psychosis: A research update. The American Journal of Psychiatry, 162, 2220-2232.

Perkins, D. O., Gu, H. Boteva, K., & Lieberman J.A. (2006). Relationship between duration of untreated psychosis and outcome in first-episode schizophrenia: a critical review and meta-analysis. The American Journal of Psychiatry, 162, 1785-1804.

Petersen L, Jeppesen P, Thorup A, Abel MJ, Ohlenschlaeger J, Christensen TO, et al. (2005). A randomised multicentre trial of integrated versus standard treatment for patients with a first episode of psychotic illness. British Medical Journal, doi: 10. 38565.415000. E01.

Pitschel-Walz, G., Leucht, S., Bäuml, J., Kissling, W., & Engel, R.R. (2001). The effect of family interventions on relapse and rehospitalization in schizophrenia- A meta-analysis. Schizophrenia Bulletin, 27(1), 73-92.

Power, P., Mcguire, P., Lacoponi, E., Garety, P., Morris, E., Valmaggia, L.,... & Craig, T. (2007). Early onset (LEO) and outreach & support in south London (OASIS) service. Early Intervention Psychiatry, 1, 97-113.

Robins, L. N., Wing, J. K., & Witchen, H.U. (1988). The composite international diagnostic interview; an epidemiological instrument suitable for use in conjunction with different diagnostic systems and in different cultures. Archives of General Psychiatry, 45, 1069-1077.

Robinson, D., Woemer, M. G., Alvir, J. M., Bilder, R., Goldman, R., Geisler, S.,... Lieberman, J.A. (1999). Predictors of relapse following response from a first episode of Schizophrenia or schizoaffective disorder. Archives of General Psychiatry, 56(3), 241-247.

Robinson, D. G., Woerner, M. G., Delman, H. M., & Kane, J. M. (2005). Pharmacological treatment for first-episode schizophrenia. Schizophrenia Bulletin, 31, 705-722.

Rossberg, J. I., Johannssen, J. O., Klungsoir, O., Opjordsmoen, S., Eversen, J., Fjell, A, McGlashan, T. (2010). Are multi family groups appropriate for patients with first episode psychosis? A 5-year naturalistic follow-up study. Acta Psychiatrica Scandinavica, 122, 484-394.

Ruhrmann, S., Schultze-Lutter, F., Salokangas, R., Heinimaa, M., Linszen, D., Dingemans, P.,... Klosterkötter, J. (2010). Prediction of psychosis in adolescents and young adults at high risk. Results from the prospective European prediction of psychosis study. Archives of General Psychiatry, 67(3), 241-251.

Salokangas, R. K. R., Nieman, D. H., Heinimaa, M., Svirskis, T., Luutonen, S., From, T.,... EPOS group. (2013). Psychosocial outcome in patients at clinical high risk of psychosis: a prospective follow-up. Social Psychiatry and Psychiatric Epidemiology, 48(2), 303-311.

Shean, D. G. (2009). Evidence-Based Psychosocial Practices and Recovery from Schizophrenia. Psychiatry, 72(4), 307-320

Smerud, P. E. & Rosenfarb, I. S. (2008). The therapeutic alliance family psychoeducation in the treatment of schizophrenia: an exploratory prospective change process study. Journal of Consulting and Clinical Psychology, 76(3), 505-510.

Tang, Y., Wong, G., Hui, C., Lam, M. M., Chiu, C. P., Chan, S. K.,... Chen, E.Y. (2010). Early interventions for psychosis in Hong Kong the EASY program. Early Intervention Psychiatry, 4(3), 214-219.

Teferra, S., Shibre, T., Fekadu, A., Medhin, G., Wakwoya, A., Alem, A., & Jacobsson, L. (2012). Five-year clinical course and outcome of schizophrenia in Ethiopia. Schizophrenia Research, 136, 137-142.

Torgalsbøen, A. K. & Rund, B. R. (2010). Maintenance of recovery from schizophrenia at 20 year follow-up: What happened? Psychiatry, 73(1), 70-83.

Torgalsbøen, A. K. (1999). Full recovery from schizophrenia: The prognostic role of premorbid adjustment, symptoms at first admission, precipitating events and gender. Psychiatry Research, 88(2), 143-152.

Uzenoff, S. R., Penn, D. L., Graham, K. A., Saade, S., Smith, B. B., & Perkins, D. O. (2012). Evaluation of a multi element treatment center for early psychosis in the United States. Social Psychiatry and Psychiatric Epidemiology, 47, 106-115.

Valencia, M., Díaz, A., & Juárez, F. (2012). Integration of pharmacological and psychosocial treatment for schizophrenia: the case of a developing country proposal. In: Pharmacotherapy. Badria, F. (Editor). Rijeka, Croatia. InTech Publishers,

Valencia, M., Juárez, F., & Ortega, H. (2012). Integrated treatment to achieve functional recovery for first-episode psychosis. Schizophrenia Research and Treatment, Article ID 962371, 9 pages, doi: 10.1155/2012/962371.

Valencia, M., Liberman, R. P., Rascón, M. L., & Juárez, F. (2012). Habilidades psicosociales para la esquizofrenia. En Alternativas terapéuticas para la esquizofrenia. Valencia, M, (Edit). Mexico City. Herder.

Valencia, M., Rascón, M. L., & Quiroga, H. (2003). Research contributions on psychosocial Treatment and family therapy for patients with schizophrenia. Salud Mental, 26(5), 1-18.

Valencia, M., Rascón, M. L., Juárez, F., & Murow, E. (2007). A psychosocial skills training approach in Mexican outpatients with schizophrenia. Psychological Medicine, 37, 1393-1402.

Valencia, M., Rascón, M. L., Juárez, F., Escamilla, R., Saracco, R., & Liberman, R.P. (2010). Application in Mexico of psychosocial rehabilitation with schizophrenia patients. Psychiatry, 73(3), 248-263.

Valencia, M., Rascon, M. L., & Ortega, H. (2001). Psychosocial treatment in patients with schizophrenia. In Schizophrenia: Current Views and Perspectives. Ortega, H & Valencia, M (Eds.). México City: Editorial Lasser.

Verdoux, H., Lengronne. J., Liraud, F., Gonzales, B., Assens, F., Abalan, F., & van Os, J. (2000). Medication adherence in psychosis: predictors and impact outcome. A 2 year follow-up of first admitted subjects. Acta Psychiatrica Scandinavica, 102(3), 203-210.

Wallace, C. J., Liberman, R. P., MacKain, S. J., Blackwell, G., & Eckman, T. A. (1992) Effectiveness and replicability of modules for teaching social and instrumental skills to the severely mentally ill. The American Journal of Psychiatry, 149(5), 654-658.

Whitehorn, D., Brown, J., Richard, J., Rui, Q., & Kopala, L. (2002). Multiple dimensions of recovery in early psychoses. International Review of Psychiatry, 14(4), 273-283.

Wunderinck, L., Sytema, S., Fokko, J. N., & Wiersma, D. (2009). Clinical recovery in first-episode psychosis. Schizophrenia Bulletin, 35(2), 362-369.

Current Status of Treatment Options and New Availability of Cognitive Behavioral Therapy for Social Anxiety Disorder

Naoki Yoshinaga
Organization for Promotion of Tenure Track
University of Miyazaki, Japan

1   Introduction

1.1   Pathology of Social Anxiety Disorder

Social anxiety disorder (SAD; also known as social phobia) is classified in the current Diagnostic and Statistical Manual of Mental Disorders (DSM-IV-TR) (4th ed., text rev., American Psychiatric Association, 2000) and is characterized by a persistent fear of social situations in which individuals fear and avoid the scrutiny of others. In such situations, patients are apprehensive of saying or doing something that will result in embarrassment or humiliation. These concerns can be so pronounced that they shun most interpersonal encounters or endure such situations only with intense discomfort. Once largely neglected, SAD came to the attention of the general medical community a decade ago (Stein, 1996), and is now garnering increased attention and recognition as a widespread and impairing, but treatable condition (Schneier, 2006). SAD is one of the most prevalent psychiatric disorders, with a life time prevalence of 12.1% in developed and developing countries; it is even more frequent among women. The mean age of onset is usually in the mid-teens, although it can occur at an early age of five years (Kessler *et al.*, 2005; Stein *et al.*, 2010b; Grant *et al.*, 2005; Fredrikson *et al.*, 1996). If left untreated, SAD increases the risk of major depressive disorder, substance abuse, and other mental health problems. Therefore, SAD is a functional disability that can impair quality of life and incur a significant economic burden (Stein *et al.*, 2005b; Wang *et al.*, 2005; Sareen *et al.*, 2006). Risk factors for SAD include the female gender, family history of SAD, and early childhood shyness or behaviorally inhibited temperament (Kessler *et al.*, 2005; Grant *et al.*, 2005; Hirshfeld-Becker *et al.*, 2008).

Individuals with SAD are typically shy when meeting new people, quiet in groups, and withdrawn in unfamiliar social settings. When they interact with others, they may or may not show overt evidence of discomfort (e.g., blushing and avoiding eye contact), but they invariably experience intense emotional or physical symptoms or both (e.g., fear, heart racing, sweating, trembling, and difficulty concentrating). They may crave the company of others but still shun social situations for fear of being perceived as stupid, unlikable, or boring. Accordingly, they avoid speaking in public, expressing opinions, or even fraternizing with peers; this can lead to such individuals being mistakenly labeled as snobs. The disorder has two subtypes: generalized and non-generalized SAD. In generalized SAD, distressing fears are experienced in most social situations (e.g., in conversations, presentations, meetings, parties, and other interactions). In non-generalized or circumscribed SAD, fears are limited to one or a few specific social situations.

Cultural factors may be related to the pathology of SAD. For instance, *taijin kyofusho* (in Japanese, *taijin* means "interpersonal," *kyofu* means "fear," and *sho* means "syndrome"), listed in the appendix of the DSM-IV (1994), is a culture-bound syndrome unique to East Asian countries. Although fear of interpersonal relations has been considered a culture-bound syndrome (Prince & Tcheng-Laroche, 1987; Russell, 1989; Kleinknecht *et al.*, 1997), it can also be classified under existing categories in the DSM-IV-TR (APA, 2000; Suzuki *et al.*, 2003; Choy *et al.*, 2008; Hofmann *et al.*, 2010). Moreover, the notion that fear of interpersonal relations is purely a culture-bound syndrome is not always true. Despite some differences between the conceptualizations of SAD and *taijin kyofusho*, patients suffering from SAD in different parts of the world have many features in common, and similar assessments and interventions have been utilized across the world (Stein, 2009).

1.2   Overview of Psychological and Pharmacological Treatments for Social Anxiety Disorder

Pharmacotherapy and psychotherapy have been recommended as first-line treatments for SAD (Bandelow *et al.*, 2008; Stein *et al.*, 2010a; Blanco *et al.*, 2013). Several randomized controlled trials have demonstrated the efficacy and tolerability of selective serotonin reuptake inhibitors (SSRIs) (Blanco *et al.*, 2013). Similarly, cognitive behavioral therapy (CBT) has shown significant efficacy in randomized controlled trials (Hofmann & Smits, 2008). Despite the lack of conclusive evidence that the combination of SSRIs and CBT is more effective than single-modality intervention (Blomhoff *et al.*, 2001; Davidson *et al.*, 2004), CBT has several potential advantages over pharmacotherapy for the treatment of anxiety disorders, such as longer-term effects, higher acceptability, fewer adverse events, lower relapse rates (Gelernter *et al.*, 1991; Heimberg *et al.*, 1998; Hofmann *et al.*, 1998), and obviation of the potential disadvantages of pharmacotherapy such as drug side effects and relapse upon discontinuation (Lepola *et al.*, 2004; Liebowitz *et al.*, 2005a & b). The rest of this chapter is organized as follows. First, recommended treatment options for SAD and their drawbacks will be described. Second, a preliminary study of CBT for patients with SSRI-resistant SAD is reported.

2   Recommended Treatment Options

As of this writing, there is no standard treatment protocol for SAD. Thus, the following summary is based on the primary literature, systematic reviews, meta-analyses, ongoing clinical experience, and the current state of clinical practice (Bandelow *et al.*, 2008; Baldwin *et al.*, 2005; Swinson *et al.*, 2006; Stein *et al.*, 2010a). An overview of treatment options is provided at the end of this section (see Figure 1).

2.1   First-Line Cognitive Behavioral Therapy

Randomized controlled trials have consistently demonstrated the efficacy of CBT as first-line treatment for SAD (Fedoroff & Taylor, 2001). There are three basic types of CBT: individual, group based, and internet based. Recent studies have demonstrated the superiority of individual CBT over group based CBT (Mörtberg *et al.*, 2007; Stangier *et al.*, 2003), while internet CBT has shown effectiveness comparable to group CBT (Hedman *et al.*, 2011). In addition, SAD patients often prefer psychological treatment to pharmacotherapy; this preference is also often reported in depression studies (Dwight-Johnson *et al.*, 2000). Despite patient preference and the aforementioned advantages, CBT is used much less frequently in clinical practice than pharmacotherapy due to the limited availability of specialized practitioners and, possibly, limited promotion of pharmacotherapy by pharmaceutical companies (Insel, 2009). As a result, pharmacotherapy has become the most common first choice treatment for SAD, even in countries with initiatives to improve access to psychological therapies (e.g., the UK and Australia) (Department of Health, 2011a & b; Pirkis *et al.*, 2004).

Various cognitive models have been proposed to explain the pathological thought processes that lead to and sustain SAD. One widely regarded cognitive model of SAD (e.g., Clark & Wells, 1995) proposes a set of interacting maladaptive thoughts and behaviors that prevent individuals with SAD from disproving their (mistaken) beliefs. First, when individuals with SAD enter a social situation, they shift their attention to the monitoring and observation of themselves. Second, they engage in behaviors to reduce the risk of rejection and provide a sense of safety. Third, they show an anxiety-induced deficit in performance and overestimate how negatively other people evaluate their performance. Fourth, before and after a social event, they think about the social situation in detail and primarily focus on past failures, negative self-images in the situation, and negative predictions of one's performance and rejection. Specific CBT techniques differ slightly depending on the treatment model or protocol. However, common elements may include psychoeducation, cognitive restructuring, and exposure practices or behavioral experiments that test and repudiate these maladaptive thoughts. Please see the "**3.2.3 Interventions**" section for an example of a procedure based on the Clark and Wells model.

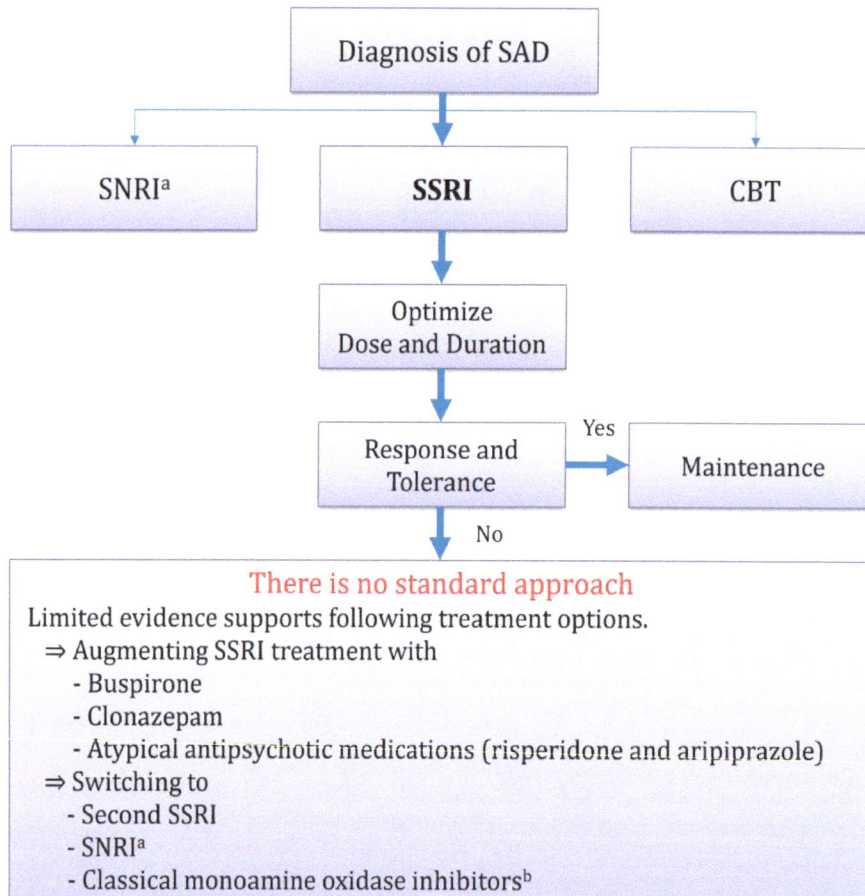

Figure 1: Overview of treatment options and algorithm for generalized social anxiety disorder. [a]Venlafaxine. [b]Phenelzine. Abbreviations: SAD, social anxiety disorder; SSRI, selective serotonin reuptake inhibitor; SNRI, serotonin-noradrenaline reuptake inhibitor; CBT, cognitive behavioral therapy.

2.2   First-Line Pharmacotherapy

The choice of pharmacotherapy often depends on whether SAD is considered generalized or non-generalized. In non-generalized SAD, symptoms are limited to specific circumstances. Therefore, medication is often prescribed on an "as needed" basis. Several small clinical trials have found that beta-blockers (e.g., pindolol) and benzodiazepines (e.g., alprazolam and clonazepam) reduce performance anxiety (Liebowitz *et al.*, 1985; James *et al.*, 1983; Hartley *et al.*, 1983; Schneier, 2006). Moreover, these drugs achieve anxiolytic effects within 30 to 60 minutes. However, the potential for benzodiazepines abuse, particularly in persons with a history of alcohol or other substance abuse, should also limit the use of benzodiazepine for SAD. In the following summary, we focus primarily on treatment options for generalized SAD because there is currently very limited clinical trial-based evidence for the treatment of non-generalized SAD (Liebowitz *et al.*, 1992; Davidson *et al.*, 1993). Selective serotonin reuptake inhibitors are currently the predominant first-line pharmacotreatment for SAD, and several randomized controlled trials have demonstrated that SSRIs are effective (Stein *et al.*, 2004; Blanco *et al.*, 2003a; Ipser *et al.*, 2006). Further, there is strong evidence that SSRIs are effective for treating many comorbid conditions (e.g., major depression) frequently associated with SAD.

Serotonin-noradrenaline reuptake inhibitors are also recommended for first-line pharmacotherapy, but comparatively few studies have been conducted on this class of drugs compared with those on SSRIs, and only venlafaxine has been showed to be effective (Liebowitz *et al.*, 2005a & b; Stein *et al.*, 2005a). Thus, fewer countries have approved serotonin-noradrenaline reuptake inhibitors for SAD (e.g., they have not been approved in Japan).

In general, SSRIs have relatively flat dose–response curves (van der Linden *et al.*, 2000). Nevertheless, evidence suggests that a superior response in SAD patients may be obtained with higher doses (Lader *et al.*, 2004). Clinical experience also suggests that some patients may require higher-than-normal starting doses to achieve an optimal response, and may even require maximum doses (Table 1). Administration of SSRIs should continue for at least 12 weeks before efficacy is assessed (Stein *et al.*, 2002). In addition, SSRI treatment usually includes some type of non-specific psychotherapy (e.g., supportive counseling) from the general practitioner.

A meta-analysis (Hansen *et al.*, 2008) concluded that various antidepressants (including escitalopram, paroxetine, fluvoxamine, sertraline, and venlafaxine) are more effective than placebo for treating SAD. Although effect sizes differed slightly, no significant difference in efficacy (e.g., reduction of anxiety, disability, and global impression) between these medications was demonstrated in this meta-analysis.

The most commonly reported adverse events of these drugs in SAD patients were nausea, insomnia, loss of energy, and fatigue, although the side-effects profile of specific drugs was not analyzed. In an earlier meta-analysis of depression treatments, the overall incidence of adverse events and discontinuation rates was similar among antidepressants, but the side-effects profile did differ among drugs (Hansen *et al.*, 2005). Antidepressant response should thus be monitored closely in the initial weeks, because side effects are most likely to emerge during this period (Schneier, 2011).

Type	Drug	Dose range (mg/d)
SSRI	Citalopram	20–60
	Escitalopram	10–20
	Fluoxetine	20–60
	Fluvoxamine	50–300
	Paroxetine	20–60
	Sertraline	50–200
SNRI	Venlafaxine	75–225

Table 1: Selective serotonin and serotonin-noradrenaline reuptake inhibitors currently approved or used for the treatment of generalized social anxiety disorder as of 2013.

2.3   Second-Line Treatment Options for SSRI Resistant Cases

A significant proportion of SAD cases fail to respond to initial SSRIs (Stein & Stein, 2008). The presence of residual symptoms is associated with higher relapse rates, lower quality of life, and greater functional impairment (Fava & Tomba, 2009); however, there is no standard approach to their management. Conventional second-line treatment is based on the clinician's own judgment. It is of increasing importance to establish therapeutic alternatives for patients with SAD who demonstrate resistance to SSRIs. A systematic review has suggested a few treatment options with limited evidence supporting efficacy, including augmentation with another pharmacological agent or switching to another antidepressant, if patients show little or no response to the initial SSRIs after 12 weeks (Stein *et al.*, 2002).

Limited evidence supports the effectiveness of augmenting SSRIs with buspirone (Van Ameringen *et al.*, 1996), clonazepam (Seedat & Stein, 2004), or atypical antipsychotic medications such as risperidone and aripiprazole (Simon *et al.*, 2006; Worthington *et al.*, 2005). A few studies have also shown positive results when SAD patients were switched to a second SSRI or to a serotonin-noradrenaline reuptake inhibitor (Pallanti & Quercioli, 2006; Kelsey, 1995; Altamura *et al.*, 1999). Similarly, classical monoamine oxidase inhibitors are effective for SAD and are also thought to have a useful role in the management of SSRI-refractory SAD patients (Aarre, 2003).

3   Efficacy of CBT as Second-Line Treatment

3.1   Background

While there is some evidence for the effectiveness of combined pharmacotherapy and CBT, evidence for an additive effect is mixed; furthermore, there is no evidence for the effectiveness of combined therapy in SSRI-resistant cases (Blomhoff *et al.*, 2001; Davidson *et al.*, 2004; Blanco *et al.*, 2010). Previously published systematic reviews (including case reports with ≥11 cases) indicated that there are no available studies regarding the use of CBT as a next step for SSRI non-remitters among SAD patients (Rodrigues *et al.*, 2011). In our previous study (Yoshinaga *et al.*, 2013a), most patients with SAD exhibited substantial resistance to SSRIs; however, 73% of the participants in the study were judged to be CBT treatment responders, with 40% meeting the criteria for remission. The within-group effect size between pre- and post-CBT Liebowitz Social Anxiety Scale (LSAS) total scores was also large (Cohen's $d = 1.71$). Thus, this study suggested that CBT has potential as a next-step strategy, even for SSRI-resistant SAD. This section reports preliminary outcomes of CBT in patients with SSRI-resistant SAD from our routine clinical practice.

3.2   Methods

3.2.1   Study Design

This study was conducted as an uncontrolled open trial to report preliminary outcomes and test the feasibility of CBT intervention for SSRI-resistant SAD in a clinical setting. After enrollment, participants received CBT for 14–16 weeks. Concomitant medications were permitted if the dose had been stable for at least 4 weeks prior to study entry and remained stable throughout the study. Assessments were conducted at pre-CBT (baseline), mid-CBT (halfway point), and post-CBT (post-intervention) time points.

This study was conducted at the psychiatric outpatient section of Chiba University Hospital, and the study protocol was approved by the Ethics Committee of the Chiba University Graduate School of Medicine (reference number: 1216).

3.2.2 Participants

Inclusion criteria for patients were a primary diagnosis of at least moderately severe SAD according to the DSM-IV and a score of 50 or over on the LSAS (Liebowitz, 1987; Raj, 2001), age 18–65 years, and intolerance (because of drowsiness, nausea, sleep disturbances, sexual dysfunction, appetite change, or other effects) or resistance to SSRIs. The definition of SSRI resistance was at least one SSRI found to be inadequate for treatment despite administration at the maximum dose for at least 12 weeks. Comorbid diagnoses were permitted if clearly secondary (i.e., if the SAD symptoms were both the most severe and the most impairing), so that the study population would reflect routine clinical practice. The exclusion criteria were psychosis, pervasive developmental disorders/mental retardation, autism spectrum disorders, current high risk of suicide, substance abuse or dependence in the past 6 months, antisocial personality disorder, unstable medical condition, pregnancy, or lactation.

All participants were evaluated by a psychiatrist using the Structured Clinical Interview for Axis I Disorders (SCID-I; First, 1997a). Participants were also screened for autism spectrum disorder with the Autism Spectrum Quotient (Baron-Cohen, 2001) and the avoidant personality disorder section of the SCID-II (First, 1997b), because these measures show some overlap with social anxiety features and cannot be screened using the SCID-I. Treatment history was confirmed by the prescribing clinician and by chart review.

3.2.3 Interventions

CBT intervention was conducted over 14–16 weekly during 50–90 minute sessions with individual patients. Our CBT program was based on Clark and Wells model (Clark & Wells, 1995) because it has shown excellent treatment outcomes (Mörtberg et al., 2007; Stangier et al., 2003; Clark et al., 2003, 2006; Stangier et al., 2011). To reduce patient self-consciousness and to summarize discussions, notes were taken on a whiteboard during all sessions, and homework was assigned after every session. The main components in treatment were as follows:

(a) Developing an individualized version of the cognitive-behavioral model of SAD (see Figure 2)

(b) Conducting role play-based behavioral experiments with and without safety behaviors

(c) Restructuring distorted self-imagery using videotape feedback

(d) Practicing external focus and shifting attention

(e) Behavioral experiments to test negative beliefs

(f) Modifying problematic pre- and post-event processing

(g) Discussing the differences between self-beliefs and other people's beliefs (opinion survey)

(h) Dealing with the remaining assumptions (schema work)

(i) Rescripting early memories linked to negative images in social situations

(g) Preventing relapse

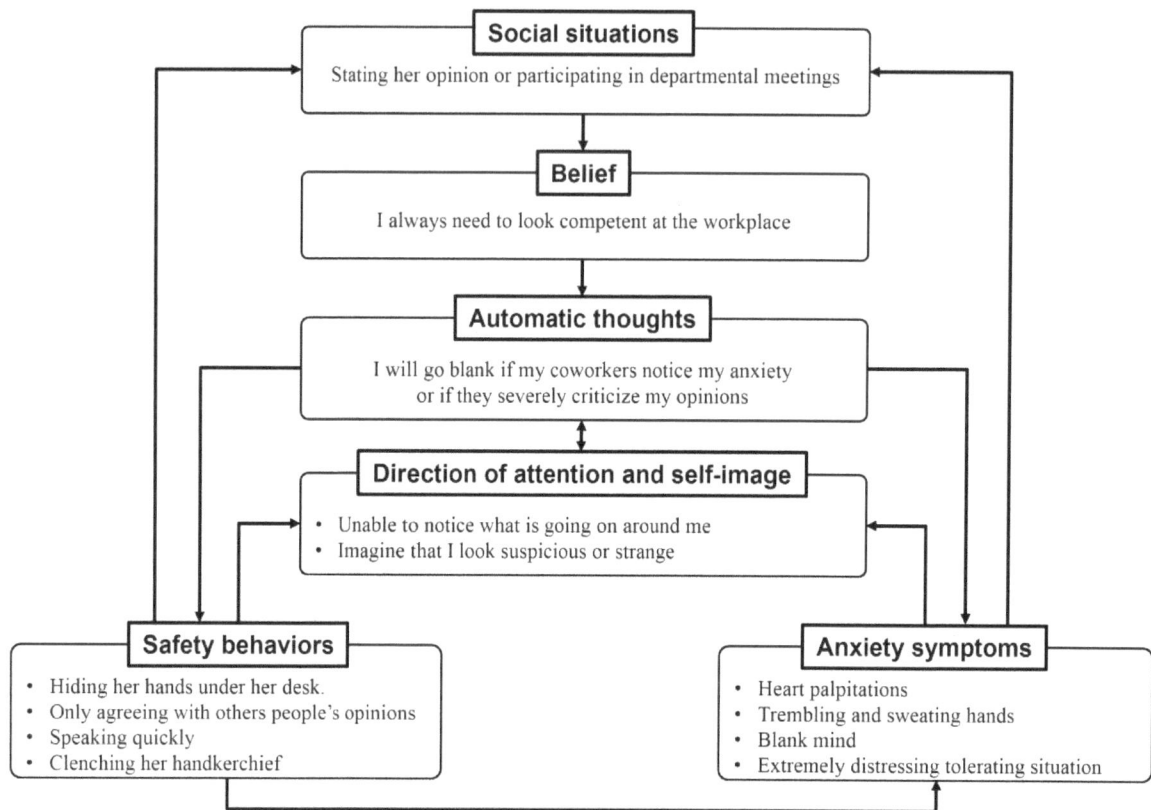

Figure 2: Case formulation demonstrating how maladaptive behaviors and cognitions maintain and exacerbate social anxiety.

Clark and colleagues devised a specialized cognitive treatment for SAD to reverse the behavioral and cognitive processes sustaining SAD. As the model places particular emphasis on self-focused attention, negative self-processing, and safety behaviors, the treatment emphasizes ways of reversing these features to reconfigure social phobic processing strategies in a way that maximizes opportunities for disconfirming negative beliefs by direct observation of the social situation, rather than observation of oneself. Further expositions of the treatment can be found in Clark and Wells (1995), Wells and Clark (1997), Clark (1997), and Wells (1997, 1998).

3.2.4   Therapist and Quality Control

CBT intervention was delivered by 9 therapists (4 clinical psychologists, 2 nurses, 2 psychiatrists, and 1 psychiatric social worker) experienced in the use of CBT for anxiety disorders and who had completed the CBT training program at Chiba University (Chiba Improving Access for Psychological Therapies project). To check adherence to the protocol and assist with planning future sessions for each treatment, all therapists attended weekly group supervision sessions with other therapists and supervision sessions with a senior supervisor. The senior supervisor also checked the quality of their CBT using the Cognitive Therapy Scale-Revised (Blackburn *et al.*, 2001). The CTS-R is the most commonly used measure of CBT competence. The competence of the CBT therapist was assessed on the CTS-R by reviewing randomly selected videotaped sessions.

3.2.5   Outcomes

The primary outcome measure was self-reported symptoms of social anxiety as reported on the LSAS (Liebowitz, 1987), the most frequently used scale for the assessment of SAD. It is a 24-item scale that provides separate scores for fear (0–3 indicates *none, mild, moderate*, and *severe*, respectively) and avoidance (0–3 indicates *never, occasionally, often*, and *usually*, respectively) of social interactions and performance situations, thus providing scores on four subscales: Fear of Performance, Avoidance of Performance, Fear of Social Interaction, and Avoidance of Social Interaction. Good reliability and validity have been reported for the Japanese versions (Asakura *et al.*, 2002).

3.2.6   Statistical Analysis

The analysis was by intention-to-treat, and the last obtained data points for non-completers (because of adverse events, lack of compliance, and so on.) were carried forward until the endpoint assessment. All statistical tests were two-tailed, and an α of .05 was considered significant in multiple comparisons. All data were analyzed using IBM SPSS Statistics for Windows Version 20.0 (IBM Inc., Armonk, New York, USA).

Pre-CBT, mid-CBT, and post-CBT scores were compared within groups by single-factor (time) repeated-measures analysis of variance (ANOVA) using Greenhouse–Geisser correction. Pair-wise differences were measured using paired *t*-tests with Bonferroni correction to control for Type I errors. The adjusted α value was α = .05/4 = .013.

The mean changes in our primary outcome measure (LSAS) were calculated among patients showing both symptomatic response and remission. We established the following threshold for response and remission (Bandelow et al., 2006): treatment-responder status was defined as a 31% or greater reduction in LSAS scores over the course of treatment; remission was defined as a score of ≤36 on the LSAS. Patient remission was confirmed by SCID-I interviews conducted by a psychiatrist experienced with SAD who was not a CBT therapist. The magnitude of the treatment effect is expressed by the effect size $((M_{pre-CBT} - M_{post-CBT})/SD_{pre-CBT})$ for LSAS. According to Cohen (1988), effect sizes are categorized as follows: small (.20–.49), medium (.50–.79), and large (≥.80).

3.3   Results

3.3.1   Therapist Competence

All therapists conducting CBT treatment also participated in the training program (Chiba Improving Access for Psychological Therapies project) for 2 years and were able to adhere to the treatment protocol under weekly supervision. The mean CTS-R rating (adjusted for caseload) was 42.7 (on the basis of 15 randomly selected sessions; average SD = 4.6), which is greater than the threshold of competence expected in UK CBT training programs (Blackburn *et al.*, 2001).

3.3.2   Baseline Data

Eighteen participants were eligible for the study based on the inclusion and exclusion criteria (Section **3.2.2 Participants**). All participants met the core DSM-IV diagnostic criteria for SAD and were defined as SSRI resistant. The baseline demographic and clinical variables of this patient group are shown in Table 2.

Variable		Value
Gender female, *n* (%)		11 (61)
Age, years, Mean (SD)		30.3 (9.2)
Subtype generalized, *n* (%)		16 (89)
Comorbid axis I diagnosis, *n* (%)	No comorbid condition (SAD only)	11 (61)
	Mood disorder (major depression)	5 (28)
	Other anxiety disorder (panic)	2 (11)
Duration of SAD, years, Mean (SD)		16.7 (8.6)
Length of education, years, Mean (SD)		14.4 (1.9)
Current Medication, *n* (%)	Benzodiazepine (BZ)	3 (17)
	Antidepressant (AD)	7 (39)
	Both BZ and AD	6 (33)
	No medication	2 (11)

Table 2: Baseline demographic and clinical characteristics ($N = 18$)

3.3.3   Treatment Outcomes

Figure 3 presents the mean pre-CBT, mid-CBT, and post-CBT raw LSAS scores. No patient dropped out during the study. Single-factor repeated-measures ANOVA revealed a significant main effect of time on outcome measure after the completion of treatment ($p < .001$). Pair-wise comparisons indicated that CBT led to a significant reduction in LSAS score at the middle stage of treatment (pre–mid-CBT; $p < .05$) and a further significant reduction after treatment completion (mid–post -CBT; $p < .05$). On the basis of our primary outcome measure (LSAS), 14 patients (78%) were judged as responders, of which 9 (50% of the total) met the criteria for SAD remission at the post-CBT evaluation. Moreover, our pre- to post-CBT effect size was large (1.75)

3.4   Discussion

This study demonstrated that individual CBT could lead to a significant reduction in SAD severity even for SSRI-resistant patients. Moreover, our individual CBT demonstrated high acceptability as evidenced by the lack of dropouts. Our study was designed to recruit patients similar to those seen in routine clinical practice; therefore, 39% had comorbid disorders, as is typical in clinical practice (Stein & Stein 2008).

Our pre- to post-treatment effect size of 1.75 was comparable to the 1.29–1.94 range of previous studies of individual CBT for SAD using the model of Clark and Wells and LSAS as the principal outcome measure (Clark *et al.*, 2003; Clark *et al.*, 2006; Mörtberg *et al.*, 2007; Stangier *et al.*, 2011). The average score on LSAS at baseline among our recruited patients was higher than that observed in these studies (more severe SAD), and the average post-treatment LSAS score was also above the recommended cut-off of 36 (Bandelow *et al.*, 2006). The people of Japan are more likely to express their shyness or social anxiety than those of the West. For instance, although it is reported that a cut-off of 36 on the LSAS total score represented the best balance of specificity and sensitivity for SAD, Sugawara *et al.* (2012) reported that the mean total LSAS score was 42.4 in healthy Japanese community-dwelling subjects (Sugawara *et al.*, 2012). Thus, the severity of SAD following CBT as measured by LSAS (46.6) was close to that of the healthy Japanese.

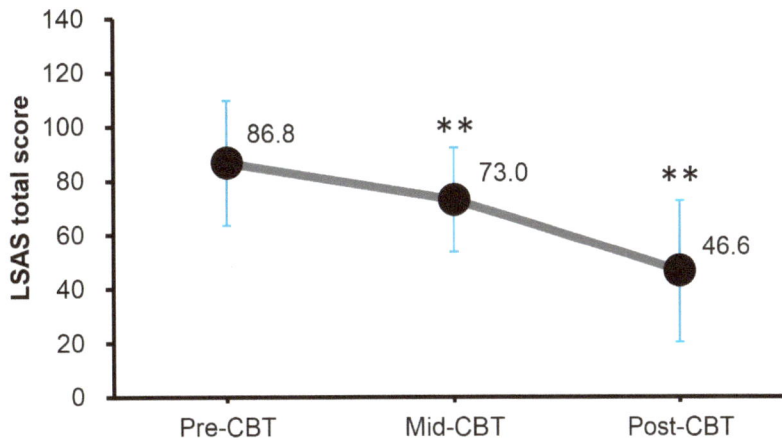

Figure 3: Changes in mean Liebowitz Social Anxiety Scale (LSAS) score before, during, and after completion of cognitive behavioral therapy ($N = 18$). Pair-wise comparisons to baseline score, ${}^{**}p < .05$. Bars: standard deviations.

We cannot directly compare the results of this study to past studies on the efficacy of CBT for SSRI-resistant SAD because outcome measures, the definition of SSRI resistance, and study design (e.g., prospective or retrospective) differ markedly. In addition, the number of patients recruited in many previous trials was less than the minimum sample size of 12 needed to estimate treatment effect (Julious, 2005). Nonetheless, our preliminary study suggests that CBT is a promising treatment for SSRI-resistant SAD.

The role of culture in treatment outcome, cross-cultural differences in SAD expression, and adaptation of CBT for Japanese patients may have also influenced the outcome of this study. Offensive-subtype SAD (most notably *taijin kyofusho*) is a clinical subtype more frequently seen in collectivist cultures such as those in Asia and the Pacific Islands. In collectivist cultures, harmony within the group is a higher priority than fulfilling individual goals, and norms and role expectations have a considerable impact on behavior. Although SAD and *taijin kyofusho* have many features in common (Stein, 2009), offensive-subtype SAD is concerned primarily with offending or embarrassing another person or otherwise disturbing the group atmosphere, and not with embarrassing oneself. Patients with offensive-subtype SAD often struggle to find the right things to say, when to say it, and whose opinion they should not disagree with; they fear diverging from group norms or disrupting the group atmosphere. Therefore, when planning a behavioral experiment, therapists may want to ask what the worst-case scenario would be if the patient diverged from the group norms or disrupted the group atmosphere. Further clinical research and case presentations are required to design behavioral experiments and adapt CBT for offensive-subtype SAD so as to better serve patients from collectivist societies. In East Asian cultures, eye contact during social interaction (e.g., while speaking) is considered less important compared with Western cultures (Argyle *et al.*, 1986). East Asians make less eye contact compared with Western people during business negotiations and maintain less eye contact when formulating answers to questions (Hawrysh & Zaichkowsky, 1991; McCarthy *et al.*, 2006 & 2008). These cultural differences may be partly explained by the fact that avoidance of eye contact is a sign of respect or deference within East Asian culture. In contrast, maintaining eye contact is a sign of respect and interest in what is said in Western cultures (Sue

& Sue, 1977). Therefore, it is not necessary for East Asian patients with SAD to be able to make eye contact as a social skill during social situations. However, avoiding eye contact increases self-focused attention and makes it difficult to maintain external focus. Thus, therapists treating East Asian SAD patients need not focus on making eye contact as a communication skill, but making eye contact is nonetheless a useful behavioral manipulation to prevent self-focused attention. If an East Asian SAD patient has a strong fear of making eye contact, the therapist may encourage the patient to look at the communicator's mouth region to maintain external focus.

Although the present study provides evidence for the efficacy of CBT for moderately severe and SSRI-resistant SAD patients, our design imposes several limitations. (1) This study included only a small sample, and the patient population was heterogeneous with regard to comorbidity, treatment history, and current medication (Table 2). (2) This was a single-center study, so our participants are not necessarily representative of those encountered in routine clinical practice. (3) While a significant fraction of patients achieved remission according to the LSAS, the follow-up period was limited, so we have no estimate of long-term relapse. This is an important consideration in evaluating the effectiveness of CBT because CBT generally has longer-term effects and lower relapse rates. (4) Psychotropic medication intake could not be discontinued before the start of this study. (5) This was no controlled condition. Therefore, we cannot conclude definitively that CBT was effective. Whether the observed improvement in SAD severity is related to the natural course of SAD remains unknown.

Future studies, including randomized controlled trials with homogenous patient populations, are required to replicate these findings, further improve the cultural adaptation of CBT, and address relapse rates during long-term follow-up. Despite these limitations, this study suggests that individual CBT is beneficial for patients with SAD who have failed to respond adequately to SSRI treatment.

4   Summary

Pharmacotherapy and CBT are both effective as first-line treatments for SAD. Nevertheless, pharmacotherapy is more often the first choice in clinical practice. In many countries, the first line pharmacotherapy is the administration of a SSRI. Although a significant proportion of patients with SAD fail to respond to the first SSRI prescribed, there is no standard approach to the management of SSRI-resistant SAD. Much more work needs to be done to establish guidelines for the treatment of SSRI-refractory SAD. Although we focused on the preliminary outcome of a single-arm study, our individual CBT program appears feasible and may achieve favorable treatment outcomes even for SSRI-resistant SAD. Further controlled trials are required to address the limitations of this study. Currently, our research team is running a randomized controlled trial of CBT in combination with conventional treatment for SSRI-resistant SAD (Yoshinaga *et al.*, 2013b). This study reflects the use of quality practice; its results will contribute to the development of second-line treatments and future treatment algorithms.

Competing interests

The authors declare that they have no competing interests.

References

Aarre, T.F. (2003). Phenelzine efficacy in refractory social anxiety disorder: a case series. Nordic Journal of Psychiatry, 57, 313–315.

Altamura, A. C., Pioli, R., Vitto, M., & Mannu, P. (1999). Venlafaxine in social phobia: a study in selective serotonin reuptake inhibitor non-responders. International Clinical Psychopharmacology, 14(4), 239–245.

Asakura, S., Inoue, S., Sasaki, F., Sasaki, Y., Kitagawa, N., Inoue, T., Denda, K., Koyama, T., Ito, M., & Matsubara, R. (2002). Reliability and validity of the Japanese version of the Liebowitz Social Anxiety Scale. Seishin Igaku Clinical Psychiatry, 44(10), 1077–1084.

American Psychiatric Association. (2000). Diagnostic and Statistical Manual of Mental Disorders (4th ed., text rev.). Washington, DC: Author.

Argyle, M., Henderson, M., Bond, M., Iizuka, Y., Contarello, A. (1986). Cross-cultural variations in relationship rules. International Journal of Psychology, 21, 287–315. doi:10.1080/00207598608247591.

Baldwin, D.S., Anderson, I.M., Nutt, D.J., Bandelow, B., Bond, A., Davidson, J.R.T., den Boer, J.A., Fineberg, N.A., Knapp, M., Scott, J., & Wittchen, H.-U. (2005). Evidence-based guidelines for the pharmacological treatment of anxiety disorders: recommendations from the British Association for Psychopharmacology. Journal of Psychopharmacology, 19(6), 567–596. doi:10.1177/0269881105059253.

Bandelow, B., Baldwin, D. S., Dolberg, O. T., Andersen, H. F., & Stein, D. J. (2006). What is the threshold for symptomatic response and remission for major depressive disorder, panic disorder, social anxiety disorder, and generalized anxiety disorder? The Journal of Clinical Psychiatry, 67(9), 1428–1434.

Bandelow, B., Zohar, J., Hollander, E., Kasper, S., Möller, H.-J., Zohar, J., Hollander, E., Kasper, S., Möller, H.-J., Bandelow, B., Allgulander, C., Ayuso-Gutierrez, J., Baldwin, D.S., Buenvicius, R., Cassano, G., Fineberg, N., Gabriels, L., Hindmarch, I., Kaiya, H., Klein, D.F., Lader, M., Lecrubier, Y., Lépine, J.-P., Liebowitz, M.R., Lopez-Ibor, J.J., Marazziti, D., Miguel, E.C., Oh, K.S., Preter, M., Rupprecht, R., Sato, M., Starcevic, V., Stein, D.J., van Ameringen, M., & Vega, J. (2008). World Federation of Societies of Biological Psychiatry (WFSBP) guidelines for the pharmacological treatment of anxiety, obsessive-compulsive and post-traumatic stress disorders - first revision. The World Journal of Biological Psychiatry: the Official Journal of the World Federation of Societies of Biological Psychiatry, 9(4), 248–312. doi:10.1080/15622970802465807.

Blackburn, I.-M., James, I. A., Milne, D. L., Baker, C., Standart, S., Garland, A., & Reichelt, F. K. (2001). THE REVISED COGNITIVE THERAPY SCALE (CTS-R): PSYCHOMETRIC PROPERTIES. Behavioural and Cognitive Psychotherapy, 29(04). doi:10.1017/S1352465801004040.

Blanco, C., Bragdon, L. B., Schneier, F. R., & Liebowitz, M. R. (2013). The evidence-based pharmacotherapy of social anxiety disorder. The International Journal of Neuropsychopharmacology/Official Scientific Journal of the Collegium Internationale Neuropsychopharmacologicum (CINP), 16(1), 235–249. doi:10.1017/S1461145712000119.

Blanco, C., Heimberg, R.G., Schneier, F.R., Fresco, D.M., Chen, H., Turk, C.L., Vermes, D., Erwin, B.A., Schmidt, A.B., Juster, H.R., Campeas, R., & Liebowitz, M.R. (2010). A placebo-controlled trial of phenelzine, cognitive behavioral group therapy, and their combination for social anxiety disorder. Archives of General Psychiatry, 67(3), 286–295. doi:10.1001/archgenpsychiatry.2010.11.

Blanco, C., Schneier, F. R., Schmidt, A., Blanco-Jerez, C.-R., Marshall, R. D., Sánchez-Lacay, A., & Liebowitz, M. R. (2003). Pharmacological treatment of social anxiety disorder: a meta-analysis. Depression and Anxiety, 18(1), 29–40. doi:10.1002/da.10096.

Blomhoff, S., Haug, T. T., Hellström, K., Holme, I., Humble, M., Madsbu, H. P., & Wold, J. E. (2001). Randomised controlled general practice trial of sertraline, exposure therapy and combined treatment in generalised social phobia. The British Journal of Psychiatry: the Journal of Mental Science, 179, 23–30.

Choy, Y., Schneier, F. R., Heimberg, R. G., Oh, K.-S., & Liebowitz, M. R. (2008). Features of the offensive subtype of Tai-jin-Kyofu-Sho in US and Korean patients with DSM-IV social anxiety disorder. Depression and Anxiety, 25(3), 230–240. doi:10.1002/da.20295.

Clark, D. M. & Wells, A. (1995). A cognitive model of social phobia. In R. Heimberg, M. Liebowitz, D.A. Hope, & F. R. Schneier (Eds.), Social phobia: Diagnosis, Assessment and Treatment. (pp. 69–93). New York: Guilford Press.

Clark, D. M. (1997). Panic disorder and social phobia. In D. M. Clark & C. G. Fairburn (Eds.), Science and Practice of Cognitive Behaviour Therapy (pp. 119–153). Oxford: Oxford University Press.

Clark, D.M., Ehlers, A., Hackmann, A., McManus, F., Fennell, M., Grey, N., Waddington, L., & Wild, J. (2006). Cognitive therapy versus exposure and applied relaxation in social phobia: A randomized controlled trial. Journal of Consulting and Clinical Psychology, 74(3), 568–578. doi:10.1037/0022-006X.74.3.568.

Clark, D.M., Ehlers, A., McManus, F., Hackmann, A., Fennell, M., Campbell, H., Flower, T., Davenport, C., & Louis, B. (2003). Cognitive therapy versus fluoxetine in generalized social phobia: a randomized placebo-controlled trial. Journal of Consulting and Clinical Psychology, 71(6), 1058–1067. doi:10.1037/0022-006X.71.6.1058.

Cohen, J. (1988). Statistical Power Analysis for the Behavioral Sciences (2nd ed.). London: Routledge.

Davidson, J. R., Potts, N., Richichi, E., Krishnan, R., Ford, S. M., Smith, R., & Wilson, W. H. (1993). Treatment of social phobia with clonazepam and placebo. Journal of Clinical Psychopharmacology, 13(6), 423–428.

Davidson, J.R.T., Foa, E.B., Huppert, J.D., Keefe, F.J., Franklin, M.E., Compton, J.S., Zhao, N., Connor, K.M., Lynch, T.R., & Gadde, K.M. (2004). Fluoxetine, comprehensive cognitive behavioral therapy, and placebo in generalized social phobia. Archives of General Psychiatry, 61(10), 1005–1013. doi:10.1001/archpsyc.61.10.1005.

Department of Health (2011a). No Health Without Mental Health: a Cross-Government Mental Health Outcomes Strategy For People of all Ages. London: HM Government.

Department of Health (2011b). Talking Therapies: a Four Year Plan of Action. London: HM Government.

Dwight-Johnson, M., Sherbourne, C. D., Liao, D., & Wells, K. B. (2000). Treatment preferences among depressed primary care patients. Journal of General Internal Medicine, 15(8), 527–534.

Fava, G. A., & Tomba, E. (2009). Increasing psychological well-being and resilience by psychotherapeutic methods. Journal of Personality, 77(6), 1903–1934. doi:10.1111/j.1467-6494.2009.00604.x

Fedoroff, I. C., & Taylor, S. (2001). Psychological and pharmacological treatments of social phobia: a meta-analysis. Journal of Clinical Psychopharmacology, 21(3), 311–324.

First, M.B. & Gibbon, M. (1997a). User's Guide for the Structured Clinical Interview for DSM-IV Axis I Disorders SCID-I: Clinician Version. Arlington: American Psychiatric Publishing, Inc.

First, M.B. & Gibbon, M. (1997b). User's Guide for the Structured Clinical Interview for DSM-IV Axis II Personality Disorders: SCID-II. Arlington: American Psychiatric Publishing, Inc.

Fredrikson, M., Annas, P., 1, Fischer, H., Wik, G. (1996). Gender and age differences in the prevalence of specific fears and phobias. Behaviour Research and Therapy, 34(1), 33–39.

Gelernter, C. S., Uhde, T. W., Cimbolic, P., Arnkoff, D. B., Vittone, B. J., Tancer, M. E., & Bartko, J. J. (1991). Cognitive-behavioral and pharmacological treatments of social phobia. A controlled study. Archives of General Psychiatry, 48(10), 938–945.

Grant, B.F., Hasin, D.S., Blanco, C., Stinson, F.S., Chou, S.P., Goldstein, R.B., Dawson, D.A., Smith, S., Saha, T.D., Huang, B. (2005). The epidemiology of social anxiety disorder in the United States: results from the National Epidemiologic Survey on Alcohol and Related Conditions. Journal of Clinical Psychiatry, 66(11), 1351-1361.

Hansen, R.A., Gartlehner, G., Lohr, K.N., Gaynes, B.N., Carey, T.S. (2005). Efficacy and safety of second-generation antidepressants in the treatment of major depressive disorder. Annals of Internal Medicine, 143(6), 415-426.

Hansen, R.A., Gaynes, B.N., Gartlehner, G., Moore, C.G., Tiwari, R., Lohr, K.N. (2008). *Efficacy and tolerability of second-generation antidepressants in social anxiety disorder. International clinical psychopharmacology, 23(3), 170-179. doi: 10.1097/YIC.0b013e3282f4224a.*

Hartley, L.R., Ungapen S., Davie, I., & Spencer, D.J. (1983) *The Effect of beta adrenergic blocking drugs on speakers' performance and memory. The British Journal of Psychiatry, 142, 512-517.*

Hawrysh, B.M., & Zaichkowsky, J.L. (1991). *Cultural Approaches to Negotiations: Understanding the Japanese. European Journal of Marketing, 25, 40–54. doi:10.1108/EUM0000000000626.*

Hedman, E., Andersson, G., Ljótsson, B., Andersson, E., Rück, C., Mörtberg, E., & Lindefors, N. (2011). *Internet-based cognitive behavior therapy vs. cognitive behavioral group therapy for social anxiety disorder: a randomized controlled non-inferiority trial. PloS One, 6(3), e18001. doi:10.1371/journal.pone.0018001.*

Hedman, E., Ljótsson, B., & Lindefors, N. (2012). *Cognitive behavior therapy via the Internet: a systematic review of applications, clinical efficacy and cost-effectiveness. Expert Review of Pharmacoeconomics & Outcomes Research, 12(6), 745–764. doi:10.1586/erp.12.67.*

Heimberg, R.G., Liebowitz, M.R., Hope, D.A., Schneier, F.R., Holt, C.S., Welkowitz, L.A., Juster, H.R., Campeas, R., Bruch, M.A., Cloitre, M., Fallon, B., & Klein, D.F. (1998). *Cognitive behavioral group therapy vs phenelzine therapy for social phobia: 12-week outcome. Archives of General Psychiatry, 55(12), 1133–1141.*

Hirshfeld-Becker DR, Micco J, Henin A, Bloomfield A, Biederman J, Rosenbaum J. (2008). *Behavioral inhibition. Depress Anxiety, 25(4):357-67. doi: 10.1002/da.20490.*

Hofmann, S.G., Barlow, D.H., Papp, L.A., Detweiler, M.F., Ray, S.E., Shear, M.K., Woods, S.W., & Gorman, J.M. (1998). *Pretreatment attrition in a comparative treatment outcome study on panic disorder. The American Journal of Psychiatry, 155(1), 43–47.*

Hofmann, Stefan G, Anu Asnaani, M. A., & Hinton, D. E. (2010). *Cultural aspects in social anxiety and social anxiety disorder. Depression and Anxiety, 27(12), 1117–1127. doi:10.1002/da.20759.*

Hofmann, Stefan G, & Smits, J. A. J. (2008). *Cognitive-behavioral therapy for adult anxiety disorders: a meta-analysis of randomized placebo-controlled trials. The Journal of Clinical Psychiatry, 69(4), 621–632.*

Insel, T. R. (2009). *Translating scientific opportunity into public health impact: a strategic plan for research on mental illness. Archives of General Psychiatry, 66(2), 128–133. doi:10.1001/archgenpsychiatry.2008.540.*

Ipser, J. C., Carey, P., Dhansay, Y., Fakier, N., Seedat, S., & Stein, D. J. (2006). *Pharmacotherapy augmentation strategies in treatment-resistant anxiety disorders. Cochrane Database of Systematic Reviews (Online), (4), CD005473. doi:10.1002/14651858.CD005473.pub2.*

James, I.M., Burgoyne, W., & Savage, I.T. (1983) *Effect of Pindolol on Stress-Related Disturbances of Musical Performance: Preliminary Communication. Journal of the Royal Society of Medicine, 76(3), 194-196.*

Julious, S.A. (2005). *Sample size of 12 per group rule of thumb for a pilot study. Pharmaceutical Statistics, 4(4), 287-291. doi: 10.1002/pst.185.*

Kelsey, J. E. (1995). *Venlafaxine in social phobia. Psychopharmacology Bulletin, 31(4), 767–771.*

Kleinknecht, R. A., Dinnel, D. L., Kleinknecht, E. E., Hiruma, N., & Harada, N. (1997). *Cultural factors in social anxiety: a comparison of social phobia symptoms and Taijin kyofusho. Journal of Anxiety Disorders, 11(2), 157–177.*

Kessler, R.C., Chiu, W.T., Demler, O., Walters, E.E. (2005). *Prevalence, severity, and comorbidity of 12-month DSM-IV disorders in the National Comorbidity Survey Replication. Archives of General Psychiatry, 62, 617–627.*

Lader, M., Stender, K., Bürger, V., & Nil, R. (2004). *Efficacy and tolerability of escitalopram in 12- and 24-week treatment of social anxiety disorder: randomised, double-blind, placebo-controlled, fixed-dose study. Depression and Anxiety, 19(4), 241–248. doi:10.1002/da.20014.*

Lepola, U., Bergtholdt, B., St Lambert, J., Davy, K. L., & Ruggiero, L. (2004). *Controlled-release paroxetine in the treatment of patients with social anxiety disorder. The Journal of Clinical Psychiatry, 65(2), 222–229.*

Liebowitz, M R. (1987). Social phobia. Modern Problems of Pharmacopsychiatry, 22, 141–173.

Liebowitz, M.R., Gorman, J.M., Fyer, A.J., & Klein, D.F. (1985) Social Phobia. Review of a neglected anxiety disorder. Archives of General Psychiatry, 42(7), 729-736.

Liebowitz, M.R., Schneier, F., Campeas, R., Hollander, E., Hatterer, J., Fyer, A., Gorman, J., Papp, L., Davies, S., & Gully, R. (1992). Phenelzine vs atenolol in social phobia. A placebo-controlled comparison. Archives of General Psychiatry, 49(4), 290–300.

Liebowitz, Michael R, Gelenberg, A. J., & Munjack, D. (2005a). Venlafaxine extended release vs placebo and paroxetine in social anxiety disorder. Archives of General Psychiatry, 62(2), 190–198. doi:10.1001/archpsyc.62.2.190.

Liebowitz, Michael R, Mangano, R. M., Bradwejn, J., & Asnis, G. (2005b). A randomized controlled trial of venlafaxine extended release in generalized social anxiety disorder. The Journal of Clinical Psychiatry, 66(2), 238–247.

McCarthy, A., Lee, K., Itakura, S., Muir, D.W. (2006). Cultural display rules drive eye gaze during thinking. Journal of Cross-Cultural Psychology, 37, 717–722. doi:10.1177/0022022106292079.

McCarthy, A., Lee, K., Itakura, S., Muir, D.W. (2008). Gaze display when thinking depends on culture and context. Journal of Cross-Cultural Psychology, 39, 716–729. doi:10.1177/0022022108323807.

Mörtberg, E., Clark, D. M., Sundin, O., & Aberg Wistedt, A. (2007). Intensive group cognitive treatment and individual cognitive therapy vs. treatment as usual in social phobia: a randomized controlled trial. Acta Psychiatrica Scandinavica, 115(2), 142–154. doi:10.1111/j.1600-0447.2006.00839.x

Pallanti, S., & Quercioli, L. (2006). Resistant social anxiety disorder response to Escitalopram. Clinical Practice and Epidemiology in Mental Health: CP & EMH, 2, 35. doi:10.1186/1745-0179-2-35.

Pirkis, J., Livingston, J., Herrman, H., Schweitzer, I., Gill, L., Morley, B., Grigg, M., Tanaghow, A., Yung, A., Trauer, T., & Burgess, P. (2004). Improving collaboration between private psychiatrists, the public mental health sector and general practitioners: evaluation of the partnership project. Australian and New Zealand Journal of Psychiatry, 38(3), 125–134. doi:10.1080/j.1440-1614.2004.01314.x

Prince, R., & Tcheng-Laroche, F. (1987). Culture-bound syndromes and international disease classifications. Culture, Medicine and Psychiatry, 11(1), 3–52.

Raj, B. A., & Sheehan, D. V. (2001). Social anxiety disorder. The Medical Clinics of North America, 85(3), 711–733.

Rodrigues, H., Figueira, I., Gonçalves, R., Mendlowicz, M., Macedo, T., & Ventura, P. (2011). CBT for pharmacotherapy non-remitters--a systematic review of a next-step strategy. Journal of Affective Disorders, 129(1-3), 219–228. doi:10.1016/j.jad.2010.08.025.

Russell, J. G. (1989). Anxiety disorders in Japan: a review of the Japanese literature on shinkeishitsu and taijinkyofusho. Culture, Medicine and Psychiatry, 13(4), 391–403.

Sareen, J., Jacobi, F., Cox, B. J., Belik, S.-L., Clara, I., & Stein, M. B. (2006). Disability and poor quality of life associated with comorbid anxiety disorders and physical conditions. Archives of Internal Medicine, 166(19), 2109–2116. doi:10.1001/archinte.166.19.2109.

Schneier, F. R. (2006). Social anxiety disorder. New England Journal of Medicine, 355(10), 1029–1036. doi:10.1056/NEJMcp060145.

Schneier, F. R. (2011). Pharmacotherapy of social anxiety disorder. Expert opinion on pharmacotherapy, 12(4), 615-625. doi: 10.1517/14656566.2011.534983.

Seedat, S., & Stein, M. B. (2004). Double-blind, placebo-controlled assessment of combined clonazepam with paroxetine compared with paroxetine monotherapy for generalized social anxiety disorder. The Journal of Clinical Psychiatry, 65(2), 244–248.

Simon, N. M., Hoge, E. A., Fischmann, D., Worthington, J. J., Christian, K. M., Kinrys, G., & Pollack, M. H. (2006). An open-label trial of risperidone augmentation for refractory anxiety disorders. The Journal of Clinical Psychiatry, 67(3), 381–385.

Stangier, U, Heidenreich, T., Peitz, M., Lauterbach, W., & Clark, D. M. (2003). Cognitive therapy for social phobia: individual versus group treatment. Behaviour Research and Therapy, 41(9), 991–1007.

Stangier, Ulrich, Schramm, E., Heidenreich, T., Berger, M., & Clark, D. M. (2011). Cognitive therapy vs interpersonal psychotherapy in social anxiety disorder: a randomized controlled trial. Archives of General Psychiatry, 68(7), 692–700. doi:10.1001/archgenpsychiatry.2011.67.

Stein, D J, Ipser, J. C., & Balkom, A. J. (2004). Pharmacotherapy for social phobia. Cochrane Database of Systematic Reviews (Online), (4), CD001206. doi:10.1002/14651858.CD001206.pub2.

Stein, Dan J. (2009). Social anxiety disorder in the West and in the East. Annals of Clinical Psychiatry: Official Journal of the American Academy of Clinical Psychiatrists, 21(2), 109–117.

Stein, D.J., Baldwin, D.S., Bandelow, B., Blanco, C., Fontenelle, L.F., Lee, S., Matsunaga, H., Osser, D., Stein, M.B., & van Ameringen, M. (2010a). A 2010 evidence-based algorithm for the pharmacotherapy of social anxiety disorder. Current Psychiatry Reports, 12(5), 471–477. doi:10.1007/s11920-010-0140-8.

Stein, D.J., Ruscio, A.M., Lee, S., Petukhova, M., Alonso, J., Andrade, L.H.S.G., Benjet, C., Bromet, E., Demyttenaere, K., Florescu, S., de Girolamo, G., de Graaf, R., Gureje, O., He, Y., Hinkov, H., Hu, C., Iwata, N., Karam, E.G., Lepine, J.-P., Matschinger, H., Oakley Browne, M., Posada-Villa, J., Sagar, R., Williams, D.R., & Kessler, R.C. (2010b). Subtyping social anxiety disorder in developed and developing countries. Depression and Anxiety, 27(4), 390–403. doi:10.1002/da.20639.

Stein, Dan J, Stein, M. B., Pitts, C. D., Kumar, R., & Hunter, B. (2002). Predictors of response to pharmacotherapy in social anxiety disorder: an analysis of 3 placebo-controlled paroxetine trials. The Journal of Clinical Psychiatry, 63(2), 152–155.

Stein, M. (1996). How shy is too shy? The Lancet, 347(9009), 1131–1132. doi:10.1016/S0140-6736(96)90604-2.

Stein, M. B., Pollack, M. H., Bystritsky, A., Kelsey, J. E., & Mangano, R. M. (2005a). Efficacy of low and higher dose extended-release venlafaxine in generalized social anxiety disorder: a 6-month randomized controlled trial. Psychopharmacology, 177(3), 280–288. doi:10.1007/s00213-004-1957-9.

Stein, M.B., Roy-Byrne, P.P., Craske, M.G., Bystritsky, A., Sullivan, G., Pyne, J.M., Katon, W., & Sherbourne, C.D. (2005b). Functional impact and health utility of anxiety disorders in primary care outpatients. Medical Care, 43(12), 1164–1170.

Stein, M. B., & Stein, D. J. (2008). Social anxiety disorder. The Lancet, 371(9618), 1115–1125. doi:10.1016/S0140-6736(08)60488-2.

Sue, D.W., & Sue, D. (1977). Barriers to effective cross-cultural counseling. Journal of Counseling Psychology, 24, 420–429. doi: 10.1037//0022-0167.24.5.420.

Sugawara, N., Yasui-Furukori, N., Kaneda, A., Sato, Y., Tsuchimine, S., Fujii, A., Danjo, K., Takahashi, I., Matsuzaka, M., Kaneko, S. (2012). Factor structure of the Liebowitz Social Anxiety Scale in community-dwelling subjects in Japan. Psychiatry and Clinical Neuroscience, 66, 525–528. doi: 10.1111/j.1440-1819.2012.02381.x.

Swinson, R. P., Antony, M. M., Bleau, P., Chokka, M., Fallu, A., Katzman, M. A., Kjeristed, K., Lanius, R., Manassis, K., McIntosh, D., Plamondon, J., Rabheru, K., Van Amerigen, M., & Walker, J. R. (2006). Clinical practice guidelines: management of anxiety disorders. Canadian Journal of Psychiatry, 51(8 Suppl 2), 9S–91S.

Van Ameringen, M., Mancini, C., & Wilson, C. (1996). Buspirone augmentation of selective serotonin reuptake inhibitors (SSRIs) in social phobia. Journal of Affective Disorders, 39(2), 115–121.

Van der Linden, G. J., Stein, D. J., & van Balkom, A. J. (2000). The efficacy of the selective serotonin reuptake inhibitors for social anxiety disorder (social phobia): a meta-analysis of randomized controlled trials. International Clinical Psychopharmacology, 15 Suppl 2, S15–23.

Wang, P. S., Lane, M., Olfson, M., Pincus, H. A., Wells, K. B., & Kessler, R. C. (2005). Twelve-month use of mental health services in the United States: results from the National Comorbidity Survey Replication. Archives of General Psychiatry, 62(6), 629–640. doi:10.1001/archpsyc.62.6.629.

Wells, A. (1997). Cognitive Therapy of Anxiety Disorders: A Practice Manual and Conceptual Guide. Chichester, Sussex: Wiley.

Worthington, J. J. 3rd, Kinrys, G., Wygant, L. E., & Pollack, M. H. (2005). Aripiprazole as an augmentor of selective serotonin reuptake inhibitors in depression and anxiety disorder patients. International Clinical Psychopharmacology, 20(1), 9–11.

Yoshinaga, N., Ohshima, F., Matsuki, S., Tanaka, M., Kobayashi, T., Ibuki, H., Asano, K., Kobori, O., Shiraishi, T., Ito, E., Nakazato, M., Nakagawa, A., Iyo, M., & Shimizu, E. (2013a). A preliminary study of individual cognitive behavior therapy for social anxiety disorder in Japanese clinical settings: a single-arm, uncontrolled trial. BMC Research Notes, 6(1), 74. doi:10.1186/1756-0500-6-74.

Yoshinaga, N., Niitsu, T., Hanaoka, H., Sato, Y., Ohshima, F., Matsuki, S., Kobori, O., Nakazato, M., Nakagawa, A., Iyo, M., & Shimizu, E. (2013b). Strategy for treating selective serotonin reuptake inhibitor-resistant social anxiety disorder in the clinical setting: a randomised controlled trial protocol of cognitive behavioural therapy in combination with conventional treatment. BMJ Open, 3(2). doi:10.1136/bmjopen-2012-002242.

Young, J. E ., Beck, A. T. (1988). Cognitive Therapy Scale. Unpublished Manuscript, University of Pennsylvania, Philadelphia, PA.

On the Use of Variations in a Delayed Matching-to-Sample Procedure in a Patient with Neurocognitive Disorder

Erik Arntzen
Department of Behavioral Sciences, Faculty of Health Sciences
Oslo and Akershus University College, Norway

Hanna Steinunn Steingrimsdottir
Department of Behavioral Sciences, Faculty of Health Sciences
Oslo and Akershus University College, Norway

1   Introduction

The purpose of this paper is to give an introduction to a neurocognitive disease (NCD), dementia, and to briefly describe the use of a common assessment tool, the Mini-Mental State Examination (Folstein, Folstein, & McHugh, 1975). Then, we will describe conditional discrimination procedures, or matching-to-sample procedures, and how they have been used for research purposes within behavior analysis. For example, how fixed delayed matching-to-sample (FDMTS) and titrated delayed matching-to-sample (TDMTS) can be arranged to study variables important for analyzing short-term memory problems. Hence, we have conducted a study with a person diagnosed with dementia to illustrate how such TDMTS procedures can be arranged. We will argue that the delayed matching-to-sample (DMTS) procedures may be useful for identifying problems of short-term memory in people with dementia. Finally, we will discuss important studies within this research area and discuss further studies that will be important to conduct. In a more specific on focus of the present paper, we will argue that conditional discrimination procedures make it possible to (1) study the length of the delay of remembering in a participant and (2) map the progression of the disease.

1.1   Neurocognitive Disorder

Snarski *et al.* (2011) noted that in USA, older adults are the fastest growing age group and the prevalence of various NCD's is increasing. In a 2009 report by the Alzheimer's Association, it was estimated that approximately 35.6 million people would have an NCD diagnosis in 2010 (Prince & Jackson, 2009). Furthermore, it was estimated that by 2050, this number would increase to 115.4 million people. In the fourth edition of the Diagnostic and Statistical Manual of Mental Disorders (DSM-IV), NCD was labeled as dementia (American Psychiatric Association, 2013) and was used as an umbrella term for various types of diseases caused by different organic conditions, all of which were characterized by memory loss. Because the term dementia is well known, these terms will be used synonymously in this paper.

All types of NCDs are chronic and irreversible (Prince & Jackson, 2009), and they are most often found in adults older than age 65 years. However, younger adults may be affected by NCDs as well. As stated in the World Alzheimer Report from 2009, there is an increased awareness of NCD diagnoses in people age 65 years or younger. This is partly confirmed in the DSM-V, wherein the younger patient group receives more recognition through the modified diagnostic criteria. However, it is a fact that the likelihood of being diagnosed with dementia increases with age, and it has been noted that the prevalence of dementia diagnoses approximately "doubles with every five-year increase in age" (Prince & Jackson, 2009).

In the USA and Canada, the DSM is the most frequently used diagnostic tool, while in most of Europe, the International Classification of Diseases (ICD) is most commonly used. The Cambridge Examination for Mental Disorders of the Elderly (CAMDEX) is the most commonly used diagnostic tool in the UK. World-wide the Mini-Mental State Examination (MMSE) is the most commonly used screening test for dementia (Folstein *et al.*, 1975). The screening test is used to map the progression of the disease and also to evaluate the effect of therapeutic agents (O'Bryant *et al.*, 2008). The screening test has seven categories: (1) orientation (time and place), (2) recall, (3) registration of words, (4) attention, (5) mental arithmetic, (6) language impairment, and (7) visual-spatial skills. Each category offers a certain number of points, and the total score is 30 points. The screening test is easy to administer, which may be the reason for its frequent usage.

Albeit Folstein *et al.* (1975) suggested certain cutoff points for different degrees of dementia, and there are variations in the literature regarding the scores that form the boundaries of cognitive impairment. For example, according to Snarski *et al.* (2011), if a person scores between 24 – 30, it is concluded that there are no signs of cognitive impairment. A score of 21 – 23 indicates that the person has mild dementia symptoms, and a score of 10 – 20 indicates that the person has moderate dementia symptoms. If a person scores lower than 9, it indicates severe cognitive impairment. However, O'Bryant *et al.* (2008) suggested that when taking education into consideration, a cutoff score of 27 would be more appropriate to identify people at the early stages of the disease. It is reasonable to ask whether the test is sensitive enough as a screening test. Hence, Tombaugh and McIntyre (1992) discussed the reliability and validity of the MMSE and concluded that the test was not sensitive enough to discriminate between patients at an early stage of the disease and those without dementia. Therefore, it may be suggested that additional measurements that provide objective information about each participant's performance may be needed.

In addition, it is worth mentioning that although there are drugs that affect dementia progression by delaying the process (Geldmacher *et al.*, 2006), there is currently no cure for dementia (*e.g.*, Buchanan, Christenson, Houlihan, & Ostrom, 2011; Trahan, Kahng, Fisher, & Hausman, 2011). Therefore, Buchanan *et al.* (2011) have argued that experimental studies should be performed where the main goal is rehabilitation, to preserve the skills that the patient already has in his repertoire. The authors suggest that one of the domains that needs to be trained in each individual is remembering.

1.2 Matching-to-Sample

Conditional discrimination procedures, or matching-to sample (MTS) procedures, have been frequently used to study complex human behavior (*e.g.*, Cumming & Berryman, 1965; Sidman, 1994). In an MTS procedure, each trial starts with the presentation of a sample stimulus, and upon a response to the sample stimulus, two or more comparison stimuli are presented (see Figure 1). In this paper we have focused on identity matching. However, another type of matching is arbitrary matching which is commonly used (see for example Arntzen, 2012).The correct choice of comparison stimulus depends upon which sample stimulus was presented. The trial ends with programmed consequences for correct or incorrect choices, and an inter-trial-interval (ITI) is implemented before the start of the next trial.

There are several variables that can be manipulated when designing an experiment that uses MTS procedures (for an overview, see Arntzen, 2012). As noted by White (2013), when the studied topic is either remembering or forgetting, the delay between the offset of a sample stimulus and the onset of comparison stimuli (the temporal distance) is what "defines the behavior as remembering or its converse, forgetting" (p. 411). Therefore, the focus of this chapter will be on delayed MTS procedures (DMTS). Following that is a description of two different DMTS procedures: (1) DMTS, where there is a fixed delay between the offset of the sample stimulus and the onset of the comparison stimuli throughout the training, and (2) titrated DMTS (TDMTS), where the length of the delay changes (increases or decreases) as a function of the participants' correct or incorrect responses, respectively (see Figure 2).

1.3 Fixed DMTS Procedure

The fixed DMTS procedure has a long history as a procedure for studying remembering (Cumming & Berryman, 1965; Paule *et al.*, 1998) with both human participants (*e.g.,* Arntzen, 2006; Arntzen & Vie, 2013; Constantine & Sidman, 1975; Steingrimsdottir & Arntzen, 2011) and nonhumans (*e.g.*, Blough, 1959; Foster, Temple, Mackenzie, Demello, & Poling, 1995; Jackson & Buccafusco, 1991).

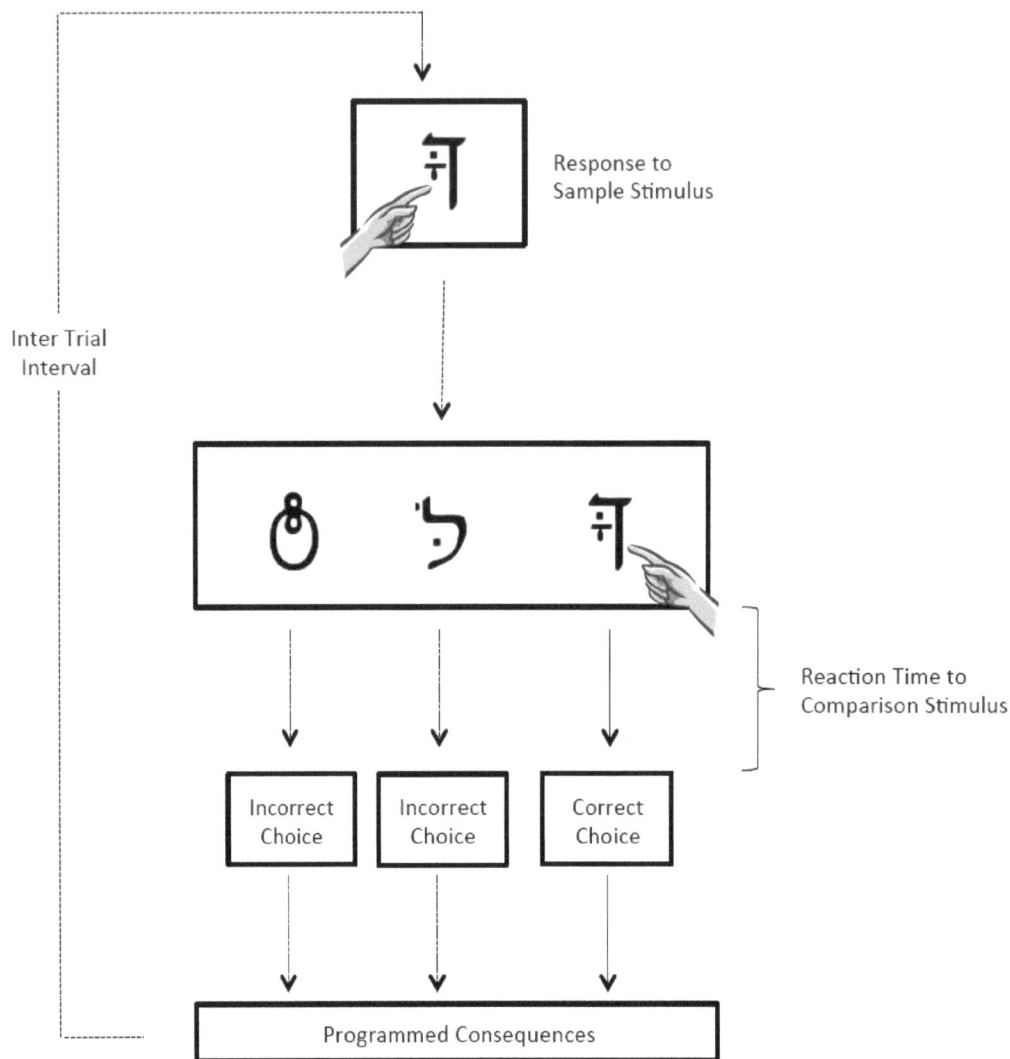

Figure 1. Example of an identity MTS training trial.

When using fixed DMTS, the length of the delay remains fixed across training trials. For example, if an experimenter uses this type of procedure to study remembering, the experimenter sets out with a certain number of training trials, such as a block of 36 trials, with a fixed 0-s delay between the offset of the sample stimulus and onset of the comparison stimuli. Thereafter, when the participant has responded correctly to 90% or more trials, the delay is increased to 2 s for the next block, then an increase to 4 s, etc. For example, Fowler, Saling, Conway, Semple, and *et al.* (1997) did a study where they used DMTS with a fixed delay to differentiate between a normal control group, a group who had dubious dementia, and a group who had early dementia of the Alzheimer type. The study had four MTS conditions: (1) simultaneous matching, (2) 0 s delay, (3) 4,000 ms delay, and (4) 12,000 ms delay. The authors concluded that the DMTS procedure might be "sensitive to cognitive decline at an earlier stage than standardized tests such as the WAIS-R and WMS-R" (p. 145). Furthermore, the authors concluded that DMTS is "sensitive to continued cognitive decline in early [dementia of Alzheimer's type] over a relatively brief period" (p. 145).

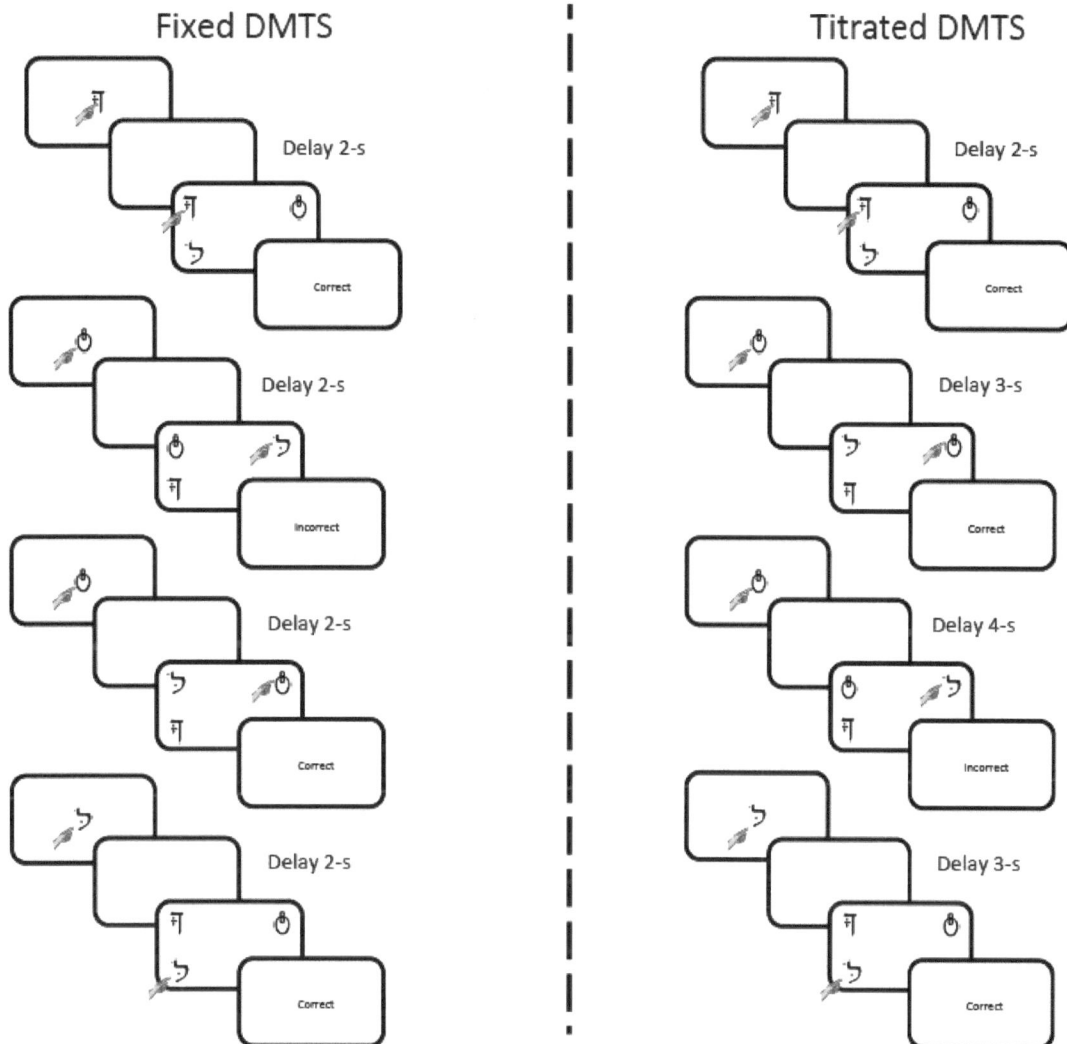

Figure 2. On the left is an example of DMTS identity with a fixed delay. On the right panel is an example of TDMTS identity with delay changing as a function of correct/incorrect responses.

Although the results from Fowler *et al.* (1997) are very interesting, it has been noted that the DMTS procedure may have an unwanted floor and ceiling effect (Han, Pierre-Louis, Scheff, & Robinson, 2000; Wenger & Kimball, 1992; Wenger & Wright, 1990). Hence, in a 2-s DMTS procedure where the participant responds correctly on all trials, it could be that the delay is not long enough to assess the longest delay the participant can remember. Hence, if the delay had been increased to 4 s, and the participant was still 100% correct on all trials in that experimental condition, it might be concluded that there were ceiling effects in the 2-s condition. Despite having increased the delay for additional 2 s, the experimental condition may still show a ceiling effect. However, by using the TDMTS procedure, these problems can be decreased.

1.4   Titrated DMTS Procedure

In the TDMTS procedure, the length of the delay is adjusted depending on the participant's responses, increasing when he or she responds in accordance with the experimenter-defined accuracy criterion and decreasing when he or she does not (Cumming & Berryman, 1965; Scheckel, 1965). TDMTS is also known as adjusting DMTS (Rosenberger, Mohr, Stoddard, & Sidman, 1968; Sidman, 2013).

TDMTS has been used to study remembering in a variety of settings. For example, Ferraro, Francis, and Perkins (1971) used the TDMTS procedure with young children of various age groups to study difference in responding as a function of increasing delay. When the children made two correct responses in a row, there was a 2-s increase in the delay. Their results showed that the youngest children in the experiment did not respond correctly when the delay was longer than 0 s, whereas the oldest children in the study responded correctly when delays were even greater than 40 s. Furthermore, in a study with nonhumans, the TDMTS procedure was used to study the effect of amnestic drug administration on rats' performance (Han et al., 2000). The authors concluded that by using TDMTS, one can "differentiate deficit patterns of amnestic drugs, and can isolate the effects of motivational side effects of drugs from working memory measures" (p. 93).

In a study by Arntzen, Steingrimsdottir, and Antonsen (2013), TDMTS was used with a patient diagnosed with dementia. The patient had first been exposed to several DMTS experimental conditions ranging from 0 – 12,000 ms. The results showed that the participant solved the DMTS task in accordance with the experimenter-defined criterion when the delay was up to 12,000 ms. However, the participant did not do so when the delay was increased to 12,000 ms. Therefore, a TDMTS procedure was used for evaluation of possible floor and ceiling effect observed in the DMTS with fixed delay. The changes in the length of delay were evaluated based on blocks of six training trials. If the participant made six out of six correct responses, the delay increased by 250 ms. If the participant made one or more errors in one block, the delay decreased by 250 ms. The results showed that over the course of approximately 1,700 training trials, the range of the titrated delay turned out to be from 7,500 ms to 12,250 ms.

In our experiment, we asked two research questions: (1) Is there a difference in matching performance when using either a 500 ms or 100 ms step size value during an identity TDMTS procedure? (2) Is it possible to find a maximum level of a delay between samples and comparison by employing an identity TDMTS procedure?

2   Method

2.1   Participant

Peter was a 62-year-old man diagnosed with dementia. His MMSE (Mini Mental State Examination; Folstein et al., 1975) was 23 at the time of the study. He lived at home but spent his days at a day care center for people with NCD. According to health care personnel and his kin, he was considered to be able to sign a consent form. Therefore, he signed the informed consent to participate in the study. The consent form provided information about the nature of the project, assured that the data would be anonymized, and explained his right to withdraw at any time from the study. Peter enjoyed participating throughout the study. Furthermore, he stated that he was happy being able to contribute to increasing understanding of NCD diseases and that it was a nice addition to the activities offered at the day care center.

2.2   Setting, Apparatus, and Stimuli

The experiment was run in a quiet room at the day-care center where Peter was during the daytime. The room was approximately 7 m^2 and had two tables and three chairs. Peter sat at one of the tables, where an HP laptop (Microsoft Windows 7 Professional 2009, Genuine Intel ® CPU T200 @ 1.83GHz, 1GB RAM) that was used to present the MTS tasks was placed. Due to a technical problem, the computer was changed (after the first three conditions, see description under Experimental Design) to an HP Computer (Microsoft Windows 7 Professional 2009, Intel® Core ™ i5-2540 M CPU @ 2.60 GHz, 4 GB RAM). A custom-made MTS program developed by Cognitive Science Partners in collaboration with the first author was used to present the stimuli on the screen and recorded the participants' responses. Since Peter had extensive experience using computers, he used a computer mouse to submit his answers. The stimuli that were used were three abstract shapes (see Figure 3).

Titrating DMTS Conditions

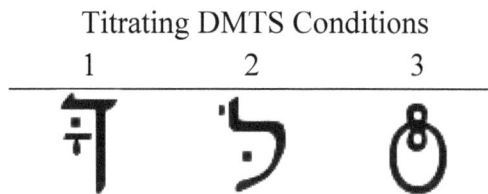

Figure 3. Stimuli used in both conditions of the study.

2.3   Procedure

2.3.1   Behavior Recorded

The computer program recorded Peter's responses. The recordings gave the experimenters information about which comparison stimulus Peter clicked on, if the chosen comparison stimulus was defined as correct or not by the experimenter, and finally the reaction time (RT) from the presentation of the comparison stimuli until a choice was made.

2.3.2   Pre-test

Peter was given a deck of nine cards, with three pictures of each stimulus that would be used during the subsequent experimental conditions. He was asked to categorize the cards.

2.3.3   Pre-training

Before starting the experimental conditions, Peter did pre-training and practiced the identity matching-to-sample behavior required during the experimental conditions. The stimuli that were used during the pre-training were color stimuli: yellow, blue, and, red. The stimuli were presented at the same locations as they would be in the subsequent experimental conditions, with the sample stimulus in the middle of the screen and the three comparison stimuli in each corner with one corner blank. A response to the sample stimulus was followed by the offset of the sample and an immediate presentation of the comparison stimuli (0 s DMTS).

2.3.4   Experimental Design

There were two experimental conditions in the experiment arranged as a withdrawal design (ABAB). In the A-condition, there was a 500 ms change in the delay depending upon the participant's responses, while in the B-condition, there was a 100 ms change in the delay. Peter was first exposed to the A-condition, followed by the B-condition. Then, the A-condition was reintroduced, followed by another exposure to the B-condition.

2.3.5   Instruction

All text, the instructions at the start of each experimental session and the programmed consequences for each trial, were originally in Norwegian. The instructions stated: "A stimulus will appear in the middle of the screen. Use the mouse to click on it. Then, three other stimuli will be presented. Choose one of them by using the mouse. If you choose the one we have defined as correct, words such as good, super etc. will appear on the screen. If you choose an incorrect stimulus, the word incorrect will appear on the screen. In the lower right corner you will see the number of correct responses. Please do your best to get everything right. Thank you and good luck!" The last instruction on the screen was: "Press here when you are ready to start."

2.3.6   Experimental Conditions

Apart from a change in the length of the titration delay, the experimental conditions (A and B) were identical across conditions. Each experimental condition started with a presentation of the sample stimulus in the middle of the screen. The 0-second DMTS condition was the same as in the pre-training. The three comparison stimuli were presented randomly, one in each corner, with one empty corner. If the participant chose the experimenter-defined correct comparison stimulus – the one that was identical to the sample – programmed consequences such as "*super*" and "*true*" were presented, whereas if the choice was incorrect, the programmed consequence "*incorrect*" was presented. The inter-trial interval (ITI) was set to 2,000 ms throughout the experiment, with a 1,500 ms display of programmed consequences. As depicted in Figure 1, one training trial begins with the presentation of the sample stimulus and ends with the ITI. The computer program was set to offer a break after every fiftieth trial, and the participant could choose whether to take the break or continue with the experiment.

The training trials were presented in blocks of six trials. For evaluation of whether there should be an increase or decrease in the length of the delay between the sample and the comparison stimuli, the computer program checked how many correct trials there were in the six-trial block. If six out of six correct trials were correct, the delay was increased. If five or fewer trials in a block were correct, the delay was decreased. In the A conditions, the length of the delay was increased or decreased by 500 ms, whereas in the B-condition, the length of the delay increased or decreased by 100 ms. Each trial was presented twice in each block, with a random order within each block.

The criterion for an asymptotic level was set as follows: The computer searched for a response pattern in which the two values were the same in three consecutive pairs of blocks, creating a clear up/down pattern of increase/decrease in the length of the delay. After minimum of 21 training blocks, the computer program started to search for this asymptotic level of responding. Upon identification of such a pattern, the computer continued to present the lowest value of the pair for the three blocks to ensure stability of the responses. If the participant correctly responded to six out of six trials in these three training blocks, the computer program terminated the session. If the participant did not respond correctly during the stability measures, the computer was programmed to go back to look for the asymptotic level again.

3 Results

The results show a quite different response pattern depending on the step size employed. As shown in Figure 4, there was a much more varied response pattern with the longer step size (500 ms) than with the shorter step size (100 ms) for the first conditions (A1 and B1). These findings were replicated in the second conditions (A2 and B2). Furthermore, the highest value before the asymptotic level was found in Condition B2 (100 ms).

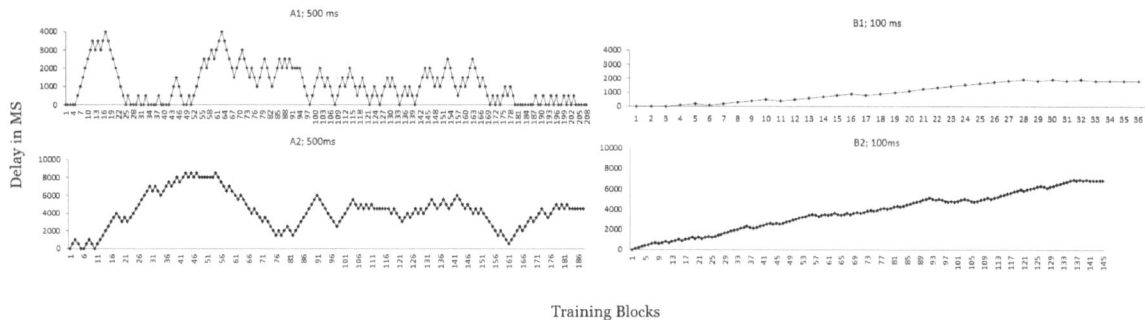

Figure 4. The four panels show the level of titrating values for the different conditions in the present experiment. The upper panels show the titration values when the step size is 500 ms, while the lower panels show the titration values when the step size is 100 ms. A1 and B1 indicate the first condition with step sizes 500 ms and 100 ms, respectively. A2 and B2 indicate the second condition with step sizes 500 ms and 100 ms, respectively.

Secondly, the results showed that stability was reached at a 0 ms delay in the first A condition (A1), at 1,800 ms in the first B condition (B1), at 4,500 ms in the second A condition (A2) and at 6,800 ms in the second B condition (B2).

Further analysis of the data revealed some systematic errors. In the first experimental condition (A1), the participant made the most errors when Stimulus 2 was the sample stimulus. The results showed that the incorrect responses were related to Stimulus 1 as the participant clicked on Stimulus 2 as the comparison stimulus instead of Stimulus 1 as the comparison stimulus (correct according to the experimenter-defined classes). However, in the second experimental condition (B1), he gave no incorrect responses when Stimulus 1 was a sample stimulus, only a few errors—7—when Stimulus 2 was the sample stimulus, and even fewer—3—when Stimulus 3 was the sample stimulus. Again, most of the errors were clicking on Stimulus 1 as the comparison stimulus when Stimulus 2 or 3 was the correct choice. In A2

(500 ms), the number of errors when the Stimulus 2 was the sample increased again to 88 incorrect responses, 16 incorrect responses to Stimulus 1 and 14 incorrect responses to Stimulus 3. The analysis of the errors showed that the participant had clicked on Stimulus 1 as the comparison stimulus most frequently when Stimulus 2 or 3 was the correct choice. In the last experimental condition (B2, 100 ms), the highest number of incorrect responses was when Stimulus 2 was presented as a sample stimulus. However, the incorrect responses were more evenly distributed between the other two incorrect comparisons (Stimulus 1 and 3).

As shown in Table 1, there was a higher RT when the participant made incorrect responses compared to correct responses. This finding holds for all conditions.

Conditions	Total RT	
	Correct	Incorrect
A1 (500 ms)	2,98	3,38
B1 (100 ms)	2,41	3,06
A2 (500 ms)	2,32	4,17
B2 (100 ms)	2,57	3,32
Average	2,57	3,48

Note. One extreme score was deleted because the participant was engaged in another behavior not relevant to the MTS task.

Table 1. The table shows the average RT from the presentation of the comparison stimuli until a response was given, for each experimental condition. All numbers are shown in milliseconds (ms). RT: reaction time.

4   Discussion

The purpose of the study was twofold: (1) to study the effect of using two different step sizes in the increased or decreased length of the delay of either 500 ms or 100 ms step sizes and (2) to find the maximum level of delay between the sample and a comparison in a person with dementia. The results from the pre-test, which used the same stimuli used later in the experiment, showed that Peter categorized the stimuli by their physical similarities. This revealed that he could do identity matching in a simultaneous matching-to-sample arrangement. Similarly, the results from the pre-training showed that he could do color matching with a 0-s delay. Taken together, these findings are important because the decrease in accuracy during the 100-ms and 500-ms conditions could not have resulted from a lack of correct matching behavior per se but rather from an issue related to stimulus control. The main findings from the present experiment were that a short step size value (100 ms) resulted in a smoother response pattern and a higher asymptotic value than a longer step size (500 ms). Finally, the RT results showed that the participant responded faster in correct choices than in incorrect choices. Thus, the participant did not respond quickly and randomly, which is in accordance with other findings (*e.g.*, Arntzen, Braaten, Lian, & Eilifsen, 2011).

The analysis of errors suggests that the matching behavior was not under optimal stimulus control. Thus, the sample did not control for the correct comparison choice across the delays. In further experiments, an extended phase with a 0 s delay should be included before starting the titration. However, it seems that the participant's responses in the current experiment were quite similar across the step size conditions.

The nature of the procedure, that is, the increases or decreases in delay as a function of the participant's correct or incorrect responses, respectively, provides an important contribution to the study of remembering in patients with dementia. By using TDMTS procedures, the length of the delay at one point can be identified, allowing for an additional measure at a later point. This information could help people working with patients or their family to understand the progress of the disease and take that into consideration when adjusting the environment to best fit the participants. Because relatively few studies have used a titrating delay with humans (see for example Lian & Arntzen, 2011; Sidman, Stoddard, Mohr, & Leicester, 1971), the present study extends the knowledge of the use of such procedures. For example, Lian and Arntzen (2011) showed that with children, the FDMTS was more efficient in establishing conditional discriminations than was the TDMTS. However, the probability of minimizing the floor and ceiling effects has been argued as one of the advantages of using TDMTS compared to FDMTS (Wenger & Kimball, 1992; Wenger & Wright, 1990). These effects are further minimized using a TDMTS procedure when titrating up to an asymptotic level (Arntzen et al., 2013).

In a study by Arntzen et al. (2013), the authors found that when using DMTS with a fixed delay between the offset of the sample stimulus and the onset of comparison stimuli, the participant could respond accurately when the delay was 10,000 ms but not when the delay was 12,000 ms. As mentioned earlier, by using the TDMTS, the floor and ceiling effects of the fixed DMTS were removed, and the results showed that the delay varied between 7,500 ms to up to 12,250 ms. It should obvious that because the asymptotic titration procedure was adapted to set the maximum delay between the sample and the comparisons for each individual, the procedure used in the present experiment was superior to FDMTS. However, as mentioned, there are other procedural variables that should be studied further to fully understand the variables that can affect TDMTS responding. For example, Kangas, Berry, & Branch (2011) found that higher titration values led to more variation in responding, whereas lower titration values resulted in more stable responding. The results from the current study are in accordance with their results. Hence, future studies may evaluate what constitutes an asymptotic level of correct responding (the number of pairs of up-and-down patterns), what are the different steps for the titration of the delay between sample and comparisons, and how many trials should be the minimum requirement before starting to look for an asymptotic level pattern of responding (criterion) for when to start searching for up-and-down patterns. Furthermore, as far as the authors know, no studies with dementia patients have used TDMTS procedures and arbitrary matching. In contrast to identity matching, arbitrary matching can give more knowledge about the deterioration of complex types of behavior, such as concept formation, the generative nature of language, etc. Responding to comparison stimuli in a DMTS procedure may be considered a form of remembering because behavior is brought under control of stimuli that, at the time of reinforcement, are no longer present in the situation (Palmer, 1991). The results support the assumption that TDMTS could be a useful procedure to study variables that influence remembering in dementia patients.

Carrying out experiments with people with dementia can be quite time-consuming. Given that dementia is a progressive disease, if an experiment extends over a longer period of time, it may lead to validity problems (Shadish, Cook, & Campbell, 2002). Therefore, it may be advantageous that this type of research is conducted within a short time period to reduce the risk of confounding variables affecting the results.

A topic related to the quite high number of sessions in each condition is the possibility of reducing the number of sessions. Some of the issues to take in consideration for further experiments are (1) the programmed consequences, (2) the criterion for increasing or decreasing the delay, and (3) how the instructions are employed. First, regarding the programmed consequences used in the present experiment, it is not quite clear what effect the text stimuli such as "super" and "incorrect" had on the participant's matching behavior. Second, we used performance within a block of six trials to evaluate an increase or decrease in the delay. It could be that blocks of 12 or 18 trials would reduce the number of errors and therefore decrease the total number of sessions. Finally, further research should include an assessment of preferences (*e.g.*, LeBlanc, Raetz, Baker, Strobel, & Feeney, 2008; Ortega, Iwata, Nogales-Gonzalez, & Frades, 2012). More specific instructions could also affect the matching behavior. However, the purpose of such studies as in the present experiment is to shape the matching behavior by contingencies arranged and not by rules or instructions. In more applied settings, the use of rules or instructions could be useful.

The present experiment was arranged as a withdrawal design, or what is commonly labeled a reversal design. It is a group of designs that are called single-case research designs or within-participant research designs. These designs ensure that each participant is in control of himself or herself. Hence, one of the main characteristics of this type of design is repeated measures within each participant, in contrast to what is usual in group designs (*e.g.*, Kazdin, 2010). The use of single-case research designs is called for in work with dementia patients because such designs are useful for adapting individual treatments and providing an understanding of functions of behavior (*e.g.*, Brooker, Snape, Johnson, Ward, & Payne, 1997). A withdrawal single case research design, as used in the present study, is quite different from what is commonly referred to as a single-case design (*e.g.*, Bakker et al., 2010); in the former, we have experimental control. It is also important to emphasize that this type of design is much more useful than group designs with regard to adapting individual treatments.

Although drawing a firm conclusion from the current experiment is a bit premature, future studies should investigate the possibility of using TDMTS procedures with dementia patients to study the possibility of training remembering behavior. At this point, it is important that the study be replicated with more participants to see whether the same results would be obtained from other participants. When more replications have been done, it will be easier to be specific on how TDMTS procedures would be suitable for the assessment of cognitive impairment in applied settings. A related issue to the need for replication is the issue of experimental control in the present experiment. Because we have arranged the conditions as ABAB, we also need replication with the conditions arranged as BABA.

The purpose of this research project was not to replace any assessment tools currently used, for example, the MMSE (see Sheean, 2012 for an overview of different assessment tools for dementia). Nevertheless, we will argue that TDMTS procedures could be an additional tool for studying important variables in short-term memory in dementia patients. Thus, we need more replications to be more specific about the how the TDMTS procedures can be used as an assessment tool in applied settings.

Limitations with the current experiment are that it does not include any parameters for evaluating the neurobiological bases of memory impairment, and one could also argue that that it does not include performances of non-demented age-matched controls. However, we will argue that the first issue, although interesting, was not a part of this research project. In addition, the second issue is related to the fact that the authors have not found any studies with elderly participants that titrate delay to an asymptotic level.

In summary, based on the previous discussion, we argue that when more knowledge is gained on the effect of other variables that affect DMTS responding, the different DMTS procedures may be useful in applied settings. For example, these procedures can be used to identify changes in or the progression of dementia, or, as already stated, they may help to identify earlier stages of dementia (Fowler, Saling, Conway, Semple, & Louis, 1995). Moreover, it appears that it is possible to use TDMTS procedures to find out details about time spans for remembering in a dementia patient in the performance of simple tasks, such as identity matching. Finally, the present experiment shows how TDMTS may be used to study important aspects of what has traditionally been characterized as short-term memory. This knowledge could in turn lead to procedures that could be used in training mnemonic techniques in people with dementia. In summary, the current experiment showed that the TDMTS procedure was more effective with a smaller (100 ms) than with a longer (500 ms) step size. The experiment was arranged as a within-participant research design and a withdrawal design and, thus, shows quite good experimental control. However, it is necessary to do more replications with a variety of people with dementia to increase the generality of the findings.

Acknowledgement

Part of this paper was presented as a poster at the Alzheimer's Association International Conference, Boston, USA, July 12–16, 2013. The authors are grateful to Kristine Gjerde for her assistance in collecting the data. There is no conflict of interest to declare for either of the authors. Corresponding author: Erik Arntzen, Oslo and Akershus University College, Department for Behavioral Science, PO Box 4 St. Olavs Plass, 0130 Oslo, Norway. E-mail: erik.arntzen@equivalence.net

References

American Psychiatric Association. (2013). Diagnostic and statistical manual of mental disorders (5th ed.). Arlington, VA: American Psychiatric Publishing.

Arntzen, E. (2006). Delayed matching to sample and stimulus equivalence: Probability of responding in accord with equivalence as a function of different delays. The Psychological Record, 56, 135–167. Retrieved from http://thepsychologicalrecord.siuc.edu/index.html.

Arntzen, E. (2012). Training and testing parameters in formation of stimulus equivalence: Methodological issues. European Journal of Behavior Analysis, 13, 123–135. Retrieved from http://www.ejoba.org/.

Arntzen, E., Braaten, L. F., Lian, T. & Eilifsen, C. (2011). Response-to-sample requirements in conditional discrimination procedures. European Journal of Behavior Analysis, 12, 505–522. Retrieved from Retrieved from http://www.ejoba.org/.

Arntzen, E., Steingrimsdottir, H. & Antonsen, A. B. (2013). Behavioral studies of dementia: Effects of different types of matching-to-sample procedures. Norwegian Journal of Behavior Analysis, 40, 17–29.

Arntzen, E. & Vie, A. (2013). On the role of distractors in delayed matching to sample. European Journal of Behavior Analysis, 14, 151–164. Retrieved from http://www.ejoba.org/.

Bakker, C., de Vugt, M. E., Vernooij-Dassen, M., van Vliet, D., Verhey, F. R. & Koopmans, R. T. (2010). Needs in early onset dementia: A qualitative case from the needyd study. American Journal of Alzheimer's Disease and Other Dementias, 25, 634-640. doi: 10.1177/1533317510385811.

Blough, D. S. (1959). Delayed matching in the pigeon. Journal of the Experimental Analysis of Behavior, 2, 151–160. doi: 10.1901/jeab.1959.2-151.

Brooker, D. J. R., Snape, M., Johnson, E., Ward, D. & Payne, M. (1997). Single case evaluation of the effects of aromatherapy and massage on disturbed behaviour in severe dementia. British Journal of Clinical Psychology, 36, 287–296. doi: 10.1111/j.2044-8260.1997.tb01415.x.

Buchanan, J. A., Christenson, A., Houlihan, D. & Ostrom, C. (2011). The role of behavior analysis in the rehabilitation of persons with dementia. Behavior Therapy, 42, 9–21. doi: 10.1016/j.beth.2010.01.003.

Constantine, B. & Sidman, M. (1975). Role of naming in delayed matching-to-sample. American Journal of Mental Deficiency, 79, 680–689. Retrieved from http://www.aaiddjournals.org/loi/ajmr.1.

Cumming, W. W. & Berryman, R. (1965). The complex discriminated operant: Studies of matching-to-sample and related problems. In D. I. Mostofsky (Ed.), Stimulus generalization (pp. 284–330). Stanford, CA: Stanford University Press.

Ferraro, D. P., Francis, E. W. & Perkins, J. J. (1971). Titrating delayed matching to sample in children. Developmental Psychology, 5, 488–493. doi: 10.1037/h0031598.

Folstein, M. E., Folstein, S. E. & McHugh, P. R. (1975). "Mini-mental state": A practical method for grading the cognitive state of patients for the clinician. Journal of Psychiatric Research, 12, 189–198. doi: 0022-3956(75)90026-6 [pii].

Foster, T. M., Temple, W., Mackenzie, C., Demello, L. R. & Poling, A. (1995). Delayed matching-to-sample performance of hens: Effects of sample duration and response requirements during the sample. Journal of the Experimental Analysis of Behavior, 64, 19–31. doi: 10.1901/jeab.1987.48-317.

Fowler, K. S., Saling, M. M., Conway, E. L., Semple, J. M. & et al. (1997). Computerized neuropsychological tests in the early detection of dementia: Prospective findings. Journal of the International Neuropsychological Society, 3, 139–146. Retrieved from http://journals.cambridge.org/action/displayJournal?jid=INS.

Fowler, K. S., Saling, M. M., Conway, E. L., Semple, J. M. & Louis, W. J. (1995). Computerized delayed matching to sample and paired associate performance in the early detection of dementia. Applied Neuropsychology, 2, 72–78. doi: 10.1207/s15324826an0202_4.

Geldmacher, D. S., Frolich, L., Doody, R. S., Erkinjuntti, T., Vellas, B., Jones, R. W., . . . Sano, M. (2006). Realistic expectations for treatment success in alzheimer's disease. J Nutr Health Aging, 10, 417-429. Retrieved from http://www.ncbi.nlm.nih.gov/pubmed/17066215.

Han, C. J., Pierre-Louis, J., Scheff, A. & Robinson, J. K. (2000). A performance-dependent adjustment of the retention interval in a delayed non-matching-to-position paradigm differentiates effects of amnestic drugs in rats. European Journal of Pharmacology, 403, 87-93. doi: 10.1016/S0014-2999(00)00480-5.

Jackson, W. J. & Buccafusco, J. J. (1991). Clonidine enhances delayed matching-to-sample performance by young and aged monkeys. Pharmacology Biochemistry and Behavior, 39, 79–84. doi: 10.1016/0091-3057(91)90400-V.

Kangas, B. D., Berry, M. S. & Branch, M. N. (2011). On the development and mechanics of delayed matching-to-sample performance. Journal of the Experimental Analysis of Behavior, 95, 221–236. doi: 10.1901/jeab.2011.95-221.

Kazdin, A. E. (2010). Singe-case research designs (2nd ed.). New York: Oxford University Press.

LeBlanc, L. A., Raetz, P. B., Baker, J. C., Strobel, M. J. & Feeney, B. J. (2008). Assessing preference in elders with dementia using multimedia and verbal pleasant events schedules. Behavioral Interventions, 23, 213-225. doi: 10.1002/bin.266.

Lian, T. & Arntzen, E. (2011). Training conditional discriminations with fixed and titrated delayed matching-to-sample in children. European Journal of Behavior Analysis, 12, 173–193. Retrieved from http://www.ejoba.org/.

O'Bryant, S. E., Humphreys, J. D., Smith, G. E., Ivnik, R. J., Graff-Radford, N. R., Petersen, R. C. & Lucas, J. A. (2008). Detecting dementia with the mini-mental state examination in highly educated individuals. Arch Neurol, 65, 963-967. doi: 10.1001/archneur.65.7.963.

Ortega, J. V., Iwata, B. A., Nogales-Gonzalez, C. & Frades, B. (2012). Assessment of preference for edible and leisure items in individuals with dementia. Journal of Applied Behavior Analysis, 45, 839-844. doi: 10.1901/jaba.2012.45-839.

Palmer, D. C. (1991). A behavioral interpretation of memory. In L. J. Hayes & P. N. Chase (Eds.), Dialogues on verbal behavior (pp. 261–279). Reno, NV: Context Press.

Paule, M. G., Bushnell, P. J., Maurissen, J. P., Wenger, G. R., Buccafusco, J. J., Chelonis, J. J. & Elliott, R. (1998). Symposium overview: The use of delayed matching-to-sample procedures in studies of short-term memory in animals and humans. Neurotoxicology and Teratology, 20, 493–502. doi: http://dx.doi.org/10.1016/S0892-0362%2898%2900013-0.

Prince, M. & Jackson, J. (2009). Alzheimer's disease international world alzheimer report 2009. Alzheimer's disease international. Alzheimer's Disease International, London, 1–96. Retrieved from http://www.alz.co.uk/.

Rosenberger, P. B., Mohr, J. P., Stoddard, L. T. & Sidman, M. (1968). Inter- and intramodality matching deficits in a dysphasic youth. Archives of Neurology, 18, 549–562. doi: 10.1001/archneur.1968.00470350107010.

Scheckel, C. L. (1965). Self-adjustment of the interval in delayed matching: Limit of delay in the rhesus monkey. Journal of Comparative and Physiological Psychology, 59, 415–418. doi: 10.1037/h0022058.

Shadish, W. R., Cook, T. D. & Campbell, D. T. (2002). Experimental and quasi-experimental designs for generalized causal inference. Boston: Houghton Mifflin Company.

Sheean, B. (2012). Assessment scales in dementia. Therapeutic Advances in Neurological Disorders, 5, 349–358. doi: 10.1177/1756285612455733.

Sidman, M. (1994). Equivalence relations and behavior: A research story. Boston, MA: Authors Cooperative.

Sidman, M. (2013). Techniques for describing and measuring behavioral changes in alzheimer's patients. European Journal of Behavior Analysis, 14, 149–149. Retrieved from http://ejoba.org.

Sidman, M., Stoddard, L. T., Mohr, J. P. & Leicester, J. (1971). Behavioral studies of aphasia: Methods of investigation and analysis. Neuropsychologia, 9, 119–140. doi: 10.1016/0028-3932(71)90038-8.

Snarski, M., Scogin, F., DiNapoli, E., Presnell, A., McAlpine, J. & Marcinak, J. (2011). The effects of behavioral activation therapy with inpatient geriatric psychiatry patients. Behavior Therapy, 42, 100-108. doi: http://dx.doi.org/10.1016/j.beth.2010.05.001.

Steingrimsdottir, H. & Arntzen, E. (2011). Using conditional discrimination procedures to study remembering in an alzheimer's patient. Behavioral Interventions, 26, 179–192. doi: 10.1002/bin.334.

Tombaugh, T. N. & McIntyre, N. J. (1992). The mini-mental state examination: A comprehensive review. Journal of American Geriatrics Society, 40, 922–935. Retrieved from http://www.ncbi.nlm.nih.gov/pubmed/1512391.

Trahan, M., Kahng, S., Fisher, A. B. & Hausman, N. L. (2011). Behavioral-analytic research on dementia in older adults. Journal of Applied Behavior Analysis, 44, 687–691. doi: 10.1901/jaba.2011.44-687.

Wenger, G. R. & Kimball, K. A. (1992). Titrating matching-to-sample performance: Effects of drugs of abuse and intertrial interval. Pharmacology, Biochemistry and Behavior, 41, 283–288. doi: 10.1016/0091-3057(92)90099-2.

Wenger, G. R. & Wright, D. W. (1990). Disruption of performance under a titrating matching-to-sample schedule of reinforcement by drugs of abuse. Journal of Pharmacology and Experimental Therapeutics, 254, 258–269. Retrieved from http://jpet.aspetjournals.org/.

White, K. G. (2013). Remembering and forgetting. In G. Madden, W. V. Dube, T. D. Hackenberg, G. P. Hanley & K. A. Lattal (Eds.), Apa handbook of behavior analysis (Vol. 1, pp. 411–437). Washington, DC: American Psychological Association.

Adult Hippocampal Neurogenesis and Mental Disorders: Building a Neurobiological Understanding toward Therapeutic Benefit

Syed Mohammed Qasim Hussaini
Department of Neurologic Surgery
Mayo Clinic College of Medicine, USA

Mi-Hyeon Jang
Department of Neurologic Surgery
Department of Biochemistry and Molecular Biology
Mayo Clinic College of Medicine, USA

1   Introduction

The neuron has a long and illustrious history in modern science. Since the first drawing by Camillo Golgi of a hippocampus stained with silver nitrate and the neuron's first recognition as a primary and structural unit in the brain by Santiago Ramon y Cajal (Lopez-Munoz *et al.*, 2006), our knowledge of the brain and its components has exponentially advanced. The process of generating newborn neurons from neural stem cells in the adult mammalian brain has received much attention in recent years. Once thought to be limited only to the pre-natal and embryonic stages of development, neurogenesis is now understood to occur well into adulthood in mammalian species. Adult neurogenesis occurs in two specialized niches of the brain: the subventricular zone (SVZ) of the lateral ventricle and the subgranular zone (SGZ) of the dentate gyrus in the hippocampus. Both comprise rich neurogenic niches that distinctly regulate progenitor cell types as they migrate, survive, mature and develop into a fully functional neuron in the circuitry (Faigle & Song, 2013; Ming & Song, 2011; C. Zhao *et al.*, 2008).

Adult neurogenesis in the hippocampus will be the central focus of this chapter because of its well-evidenced roles (C. Zhao *et al.*, 2008) in learning and memory (Dupret *et al.*, 2007; Shors *et al.*, 2001), pattern separation (Clelland *et al.*, 2009; Sahay *et al.*, 2011) and mood behavior (Santarelli *et al.*, 2003; Snyder *et al.*, 2011). These have allowed it to contribute in a unique manner to a diversity of mental disorders. We start this chapter with a general introduction on the cellular process underlying adult hippocampal neurogenesis. The microenvironment surrounding the progenitor cells is crucial to this cellular process. It is rich with regulatory signals that guide the development of the newborn neuron in both the normal and diseased condition. We discuss such regulation by signaling pathways, extracellular players, growth factors and neurotransmitters, transcription factors, inflammatory factors, cytokines and epigenetic regulators. These are connected to potential dysfunction in mental disorders. Following this we discuss physiological and pathological stimuli that can regulate neurogenesis. Stress and aging have been found to be the two major negative regulators (C. Zhao *et al.*, 2008) of adult hippocampal neurogenesis, and together with seizure have been used in a variety of disease models to study the underlying mechanisms and their treatment. Finally, we discuss the major disorders that are associated with dysfunctional neurogenesis and review the role of adult neurogenesis in disease etiology, pathogenesis and therapeutic targeting. These disorders have been logically arranged to guide the reader toward building a neurobiological understanding of the role of neurogenesis in mental disorders.

2   Adult Hippocampal Neurogenesis

In the SGZ of the dentate gyrus, a neural stem cell (NSC) upon activation can go through a number of distinct cell types before giving rise to a mature neuron that becomes integrated into the circuit and projects its axons into the hilus toward the CA3 and its dendrites into the molecular layer (Duan *et al.*, 2008; Ming & Song, 2011). Self-renewal and multipotency which define a neural stem cell (Gage, 2000) are characteristic of the Type-1 radial glia-like (RGL) cells in the SGZ (Bonaguidi *et al.*, 2011). Type-1 RGLs comprise the precursor stem cells in the SGZ that can remain quiescent, symmetrically divide to self-renew or asymmetrically divide to give rise to lineage-restricted progenitor cells of the glial or neurogenic lineage (Bonaguidi *et al.*, 2011; Encinas *et al.*, 2011; Ming & Song, 2011). In this manner, new neurons and astrocytes are generated in the SGZ. At each stage during this process, the cell types express a set of distinct markers that can be used to identify and track them (Ming & Song, 2011).

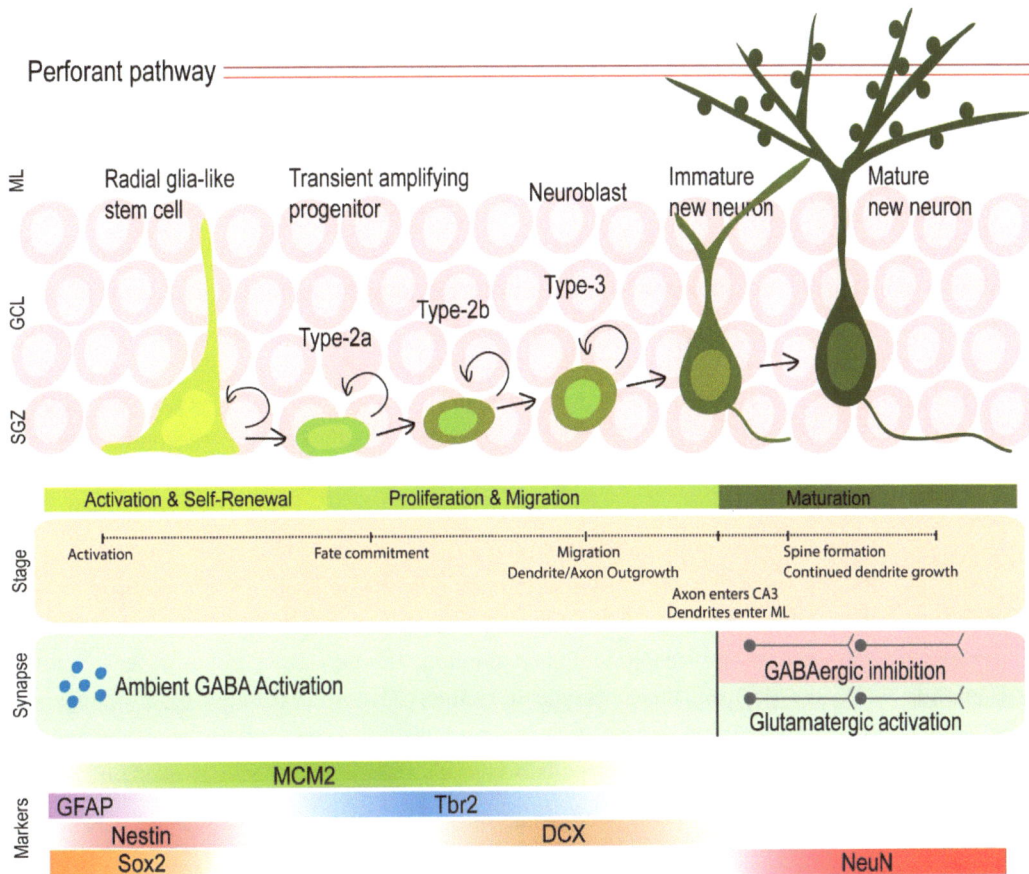

Figure 1: Figure provides a summary of the cellular process of adult hippocampal neurogenesis. A schematic diagram of adult hippocampal neurogenesis is depicted across the subgranular zone (SGZ) and granular cell layer (GCL) of the dentate gyrus, molecular layer (ML) of the hippocampus. Specific morphological changes and the cellular switch from GABAergic activation to GABAergic inhibition and glutamatergic activation following synaptic integration are shown across stage-specific time points. Finally, a schematic of various molecular markers used for identifying cell types across various stages of development are shown.

The progenitors cells belonging to the neurogenic lineage that arise from the Type-1 cells are collectively referred to as transient amplifying or the intermediate progenitor (IP) cells. These include the Type-2 cells that retain mitotic ability and can become fate committed to become the Type-3 neuroblasts (Duan *et al*., 2008; Ming & Song, 2011). The transition to the neuroblast stage can take up to 4 days (Sierra *et al*., 2010). During this critical period, a majority of cells may undergo apoptosis by microglia in the neurogenic niche (Sierra *et al*., 2010). The remaining neuroblasts migrate, undergo dendrite and axon outgrowth and by the 10th day the axon enters the CA3 region (C. Zhao *et al*., 2006). In this immature neuron, the first spines start appearing by the 16th day and undergo peak growth during the first 3-4 weeks (C. Zhao *et al*., 2006). As the mature neuron undergoes synaptic integration, dendrites continue to elaborate and spine growth can continue for a month (Ge *et al*., 2006; Ge *et al*., 2007; C. Zhao *et al*., 2006).

GABAergic and glutamatergic signaling are important in development and synaptic integration of newborn neuron in the circuit. Initially, before formation of glutamatergic input, the neurotransmitter γ-Aminobutyric acid (GABA) is depolarizing or excitatory with slow responses and consequently switches to hyperpolarizing or inhibitory with fast responses (Esposito et al., 2005). During the first week, ambient GABA in the microenvironment tonically activates the progenitor (Ge et al., 2006). During the second week, as the progenitor migrates into the GCL and dendrites appear, GABA can now depolarize through GABAergic synaptic inputs (Esposito et al., 2005). By the third week, excitatory glutamatergic input is detected and by the fourth week, the afferent glutamatergic input is abundant (Esposito et al., 2005). Following this, perisomatic GABAergic contacts can inhibit the integrated neuron (Esposito et al., 2005). Such sequential tonic and phasic GABA activity is required for synaptic integration of the immature neuron into the circuit (Ge et al., 2006). The newborn neurons are also uniquely excitable during a short, critical period following formation of glutamatergic input that mediates their survival and potentially situates them to function in learning and memory (Ge et al., 2007; Tashiro et al., 2006).

As the underlying biology of adult hippocampal neurogenesis is established, a number of studies have tried to establish the neurobiological underpinnings of this process in humans. The seminal work by Eriksson et al first directly demonstrated how the human hippocampus retained the ability to generate neurons throughout life (Eriksson et al., 1998). Similar expression patterns and age-related changes in adult hippocampal neurogenesis between rodents and humans were established for at least a number of markers including DCX across 0 to 100 years age in humans (Knoth et al., 2010). For instance, total number of DCX expressing cells in the human hippocampus decline exponentially with age and their co-expression with other markers also markedly reduces (Knoth et al., 2010). Similarly, neuroblasts in the SVZ undergo a very strong decline in number after the first year of infancy raising questions about the true extent and function of adult olfactory bulb neurogenesis in humans (Goritz & Frisen, 2012; Sanai et al., 2011; Spalding et al., 2013). A recent study utilized elevated atmospheric 14C levels in nuclear-bomb-test-derived genomic DNA of patients to retrospectively birth date hippocampal cells in humans (Spalding et al., 2013). The results show approximately one-third of the hippocampal neuronal population is subject to change, with 700 new neurons being added per day with an annual turnover rate of 1.75% within the renewing fraction (Spalding et al., 2013). A modest decline in neurogenesis was observed with age, with comparable rates of neurogenesis in middle-aged humans and mice (Spalding et al., 2013). A more quantitative assessment of adult hippocampal neurogenesis in humans has been hindered by the inability to apply several approaches from rodents in humans. As we progress through our discussion in this chapter, other relevant studies will be brought forth to discuss the role of neurogenesis in the adult hippocampus and its relationship to neurological disorders.

3   Regulation of Adult Hippocampal Neurogenesis

Adult hippocampal neurogenesis is robustly regulated in the neurogenic niche (Figure 2). There are a number of signaling pathways, extracellular pathways, intracellular mechanisms, growth factors and neurotransmitters that play key roles in regulating neurogenesis in both the normal and diseased condition (Faigle & Song, 2013). In this section, we will focus on some key signaling pathways, neurotrophins, growth factors and neurotransmitters.

PHYSIOLOGICAL & PATHOLOGICAL STIMULI	SIGNALING PATHWAYS	GROWTH FACTORS & OTHERS
Aging: Causes depletion of neural progenitors and cellular proliferation with age	Wnt Signaling sFRP3: Regulates proliferation, dendritic complexity and depression.	BDNF: required for neurogenesis, survival and LTP formation.
Exercise or environmental enrichment: Enhances neurogenesis at all ages.	DKK1: Regulates age-related changes in self-renewal, proliferation, dendritic complexity and cognition.	FGF1: required for neurogenesis. IGF-1: Inhibits BMB signaling, enhances oligodendrocyte lineage.
Stress: Reduces neurogenesis and regulates cognition. Risk factor in depression. Used in creating animal models of depression	Notch Signaling Notch1: Regulates proliferation, survival and dendritic morphology.	VEGF: required for neurogenesis, and behavior.
Seizure: Enhances proliferation but also causes aberrant migration. Used in studying epilepsy.	RBPj: Regulates quiescence, and may play a role in running and seizure activity.	NeuroD1: Mediates self-renewal, fate commitment and survival.
	Sonic Hedgehog Signaling Ptc1: Regulates neurogenesis in Down syndrome mice.	TLX: Mediates self-renewal and proliferation.

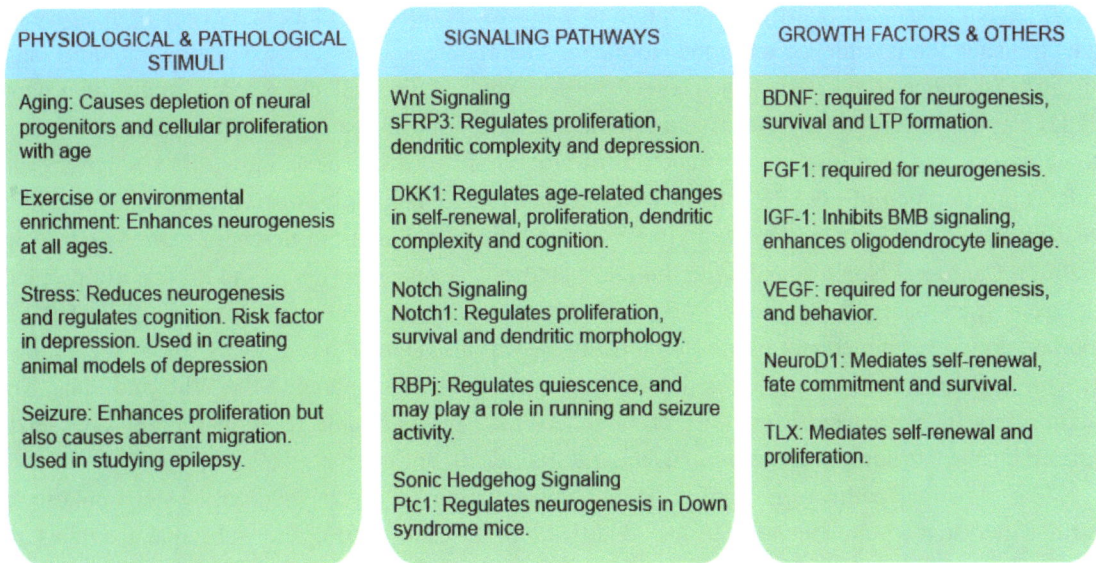

Figure 2: Adult hippocampal neurogenesis occurs in a rich neurogenic niche with factors that regulate it during both the normal and diseased condition. On its road to full development and integration into an existing neuronal circuitry, it is regulated by a variety of factors that include signaling pathways, growth factors, extracellular players and GABAergic and glutamatergic signaling. Exercise, aging and stress are potent physiological and pathological stimuli that also regulate neurogenesis. The three panels show a summary of key studies presented in sections 3 and 4.

3.1   Signaling pathways

A number of signaling pathways can regulate each step across adult hippocampal neurogenesis. These include the Wnt, Notch and Sonic hedgehog (Shh) pathways. The canonical Wnt signaling pathway, in particular, has emerged a crucial pathway in its regulation of adult neurogenesis. This pathway acts through a downstream protein called β-catenin that can translocate to the nucleus and control gene expression. Signal transduction is mediated through the Frizzled (Fzs) and LRP5/6 class of receptors that work together in binding the Wnt ligand and effecting downstream changes (MacDonald *et al.*, 2009). GSK3β is a key molecule in this pathway that can bind β-catenin and inhibit its function. It is also the therapeutic target of the mood stabilizer lithium (Contestabile *et al.*, 2013; Wexler *et al.*, 2008). Wnt pathway is robustly involved in regulating adult neurogenesis. Astrocytes in the neurogenic niche mediate proliferation of hippocampal progenitors and enhance neuronal fate commitment (H. Song *et al.*, 2002) through Wnt3-mediated activation of the Wnt pathway (Lie *et al.*, 2005). GSK3β can mediate survival and apoptosis of immature neurons (Sirerol 2011, Fuster 2013) and dendritic development (Sirerol-Piquer *et al.*, 2011), while a conditional knock-out of β-catenin can result in dendritic malformation (Gao *et al.*, 2007). Both GSK3β and β-catenin also interact with the susceptibility gene Disrupted-In-Schizophrenia 1 (DISC1) which regulates adult neurogenesis and is implicated in schizophrenia (Mao 2009). Recent evidence also shows two Wnt pathway inhibitors, sFRP3 (Jang *et al.*, 2013; Jang *et al.*, 2012) and DKK1 (Seib *et al.*, 2013) that regulate adult neurogenesis and play roles in depression and ageing. These will be discussed in the relevant sections of this chapter.

The Notch signaling pathway is another pathway regulating adult hippocampal neurogenesis. Signal transduction is achieved when the Notch transmembrane receptor is cleaved upon binding Jagged, its ligand (Pierfelice *et al.*, 2011). The cleaved portion which is also called the notch intracellular domain (NICD) can translocate to the nucleus and initiate transcription of target genes. Through the use of a Cre recombinase in the gain- and loss-of-function of Notch1 mice, it has been shown that Notch signaling regulates proliferation of GFAP+ cells *in vivo*, mediates the transition between precursor stem cells and transit-amplifying cells or neurons and alters the dendritic morphology in newborn neurons (Breunig *et al.*, 2007). Canonical Notch signaling in the DG can also distinguish between, and mark early progenitor cells from transit-amplifying progenitors, neuroblasts and neurons (Lugert *et al.*, 2010). RBPj, an important downstream mediator of the Notch pathway, was also shown to play a key role in mediating the precursor population and their proliferation (Lugert *et al.*, 2010). Compared to the Wnts and Shhs, Notch signaling may play an insufficient role in aging but may play possible roles in running and seizure-mediated changes to adult neurogenesis (Breunig & Rakic, 2010; Lugert *et al.*, 2010).

Shh signaling pathway is implicated in the regulation of central nervous system polarity and ventral patterning within the neural tube (Marti 1995, Ericson 1995), and subsequent studies have expanded its role in neuronal precursor proliferation in the cerebellum and induction of dopaminergic neurons in the midbrain (Hynes *et al.*, 1995; Wechsler-Reya & Scott, 1999). In this pathway, signal transduction is achieved when Shh binds to the transmembrane protein Patched1 (Ptc1) and inactivates it, thereby allowing the second transmembrane protein Smoothened (Smo) to active gene transcription through transcription factors belonging to the Gli family (Rohatgi *et al.*, 2007). This Patched receptor is highly expressed in the adult rat hippocampus *in vivo*, with the application of a Shh signaling inhibitor reducing progenitor proliferation *in vivo*, while a dose-dependent increase in proliferation is observed with Shh *in vitro* (Lai *et al.*, 2003). Stem cell niches in the SVZ and SGZ also respond to Shh signaling as demonstrated through an *in vivo* genetic fate-mapping strategies utilizing Gli1 to measure pathway activity (Ahn & Joyner, 2005). Further, post-natal hippocampal neurogenesis can fail in mutant mice lacking Smo function, an essential component of the Shh signaling pathway that may function through primary cilia (Han *et al.*, 2008). Mice in which the transcription factor Sox2 has been deleted during the embryonic stages or adult stages can show neurogenesis deficits, with a region-specific loss of Shh and Wnt3a in the hippocampal primordium (Favaro *et al.*, 2009). An Shh agonist could partially rescue the proliferation deficits (Favaro *et al.*, 2009). Aberrant Shh signaling through overexpression of Ptc1 has been tied to proliferation impairments in mouse model of Down syndrome using Ts65Dn mice (Trazzi *et al.*, 2011). In the mouse model of experimental autoimmune encephalomyelitis (EAE), deficits in hippocampal neurogenesis can be tied to pro-neurogenic factors and dysregulation across major pathways including Notch, Wnt and Shh involved in regulating adult hippocampal neurogenesis (Huehnchen *et al.*, 2011).

3.2   Neurotrophins, Growth Factors and Cell Adhesion Molecules

Neurotrophins and growth factors including brain derived neurotrophic factor (BDNF), fibroblast growth factor (FGF), insulin like growth factor (IGF) and vascular endothelial growth factor (VEGF) have all been shown to play crucial roles in regulating adult neurogenesis, both during the normal condition and as we will discuss later in individual sections, during the diseased condition (Faigle & Song, 2013). The role of BDNF which acts through the TrkB receptors has been studied extensively in this regard. Infusion of BDNF into the rat hippocampus increases neurogenesis (Scharfman *et al.*, 2005) and BDNF signaling is required for long-term survival of newborn neurons during neurogenesis in the mouse hippocampus

(Sairanen *et al.*, 2005). Deletion of the BDNF receptor TrkB can result in reduced growth of dendrites and spines in adult-born neurons (no effect on synapse formation), impair cell survival and neurogenesis-dependent LTP and also increase anxiety-like behavior (Bergami *et al.*, 2008). An infusion of the FGF2 into the posterior lateral ventricle of middle-aged rats can enhance hippocampal neurogenesis ipsilateral to the infusion site (Rai *et al.*, 2007). Further, in mice that lack the FGFR1 receptor for FGF2, impairments in neurogenesis, LTP and memory consolidation are observed (M. Zhao *et al.*, 2007). IGF-1 can stimulate multipotent adult rat hippocampal progenitors into oligodendrocytes through an inhibition of bone morphogenetic protein signaling (Hsieh *et al.*, 2004). The effects of an enriched environment on neurogenesis and performance on behavior tasks measuring memory may also be mediated by an increased expression of VEGF (Cao *et al.*, 2004). Administration of VEGF in rats also increased proliferation in both the SGZ and SVZ as measured by 5-Bromodeoxyuridine (BrdU) labeling *in vivo* and *in vitro* (Jin *et al.*, 2002).

Cell adhesion molecules also exert control within the neurogenic niche. The neural cell adhesion molecule (NCAM) is one such example. It belongs to the immunoglobulin (Ig) family of adhesion molecules and plays a variety of roles in the development of the nervous system and in the regulation of brain plasticity and hippocampal neurogenesis (Aonurm-Helm *et al.*, 2008). In cultured rat and mouse hippocampal progenitor cells with the ability to generate glial cells and neurons under different conditions, addition of soluble neural CAM (NCAM) reduces proliferation in a dose-dependent manner and increases differentiation to the neuronal lineage (Amoureux *et al.*, 2000). Similarly, in N-CAM deficient mice, defects may be seen in the hippocampal mossy fiber system, including impaired LTP and ectopic innervation of CA3 pyramidal neurons (Cremer *et al.*, 1998). Further, NCAM deficient mice have been associated with behavioral abnormalities such as anxiety-like behavior, deficits in spatial learning, altered exploratory behavior and increased 5-HT1A hypersensitivity (Stork *et al.*, 1999) which may be mediated through the transgenic expression of the major NCAM180 isoform (Stork *et al.*, 2000). NCAM deficient mice (NCAM$^{-/-}$) also show reduced neurogenesis along with a depression-like phenotype which is evidenced by increased freezing time in the tail suspension test and reduced preference for sucrose in the sucrose preference test (Aonurm-Helm *et al.*, 2008). Interestingly, administration of an FGL peptide, derived from the NCAM binding site for the FGF receptor, could reduce depression-like behavior in these mice and enhance survival of newborn neurons (Aonurm-Helm *et al.*, 2008). Thus, a role for NCAM has been surmised in depression and antidepressant actions, as well in other neuropsychiatric and neurodegenerative disorders (Brennaman & Maness, 2010; Sandi, 2008).

3.3   Transcription Factors

Some transcription factors have been mentioned in our discussion of the various signaling pathways above and more will be discussed as we continue our discussion below. Here we briefly summarize for the reader such important transcription factors (and others) in a logical manner across the sequential steps that occur during neurogenesis. Sox2 is one important transcription factor during embryonic and adult neurogenesis especially during the stem cell maintenance stage where its deletion can impair the Wnt signaling and Hedgehog signaling pathways (Favaro *et al.*, 2009). Maintenance of Sox2 expression may require Notch signaling (Hsieh, 2012) and may partially be mediated through the basic helix-loop-helix (bHLH) transcription factor Hes5 that colocalizes with Sox2 in controlling NSC maintenance (Hsieh, 2012; Lugert *et al.*, 2010).

Bcl11b, a Krüppel-like C2H2 zinc finger transcription factor expressed in the hippocampus, has been shown to have a dual phase-specific function during postnatal development of the dentate gyrus

(Simon *et al.*, 2012). Working via a feedback mechanism to regulate progenitor proliferation, *Bcl11b* is expressed in the postmitotic granule neurons (Simon *et al.*, 2012). In *Bcl11b* mutants, there is reduced progenitor proliferation and impaired differentiation of postmitotic neurons with failure of integration into the circuitry and thus consequent deleterious effects on learning and memory (Simon *et al.*, 2012). Another bHLH transcription factor is Ascl1, the over-expression of which can influence fate choice and generate oligodendrocytes (Jessberger *et al.*, 2008). The nuclear receptor TLX functions with the Wnt signaling pathway (Qu *et al.*, 2010) and its induced deletion selectively impairs spatial learning while also reducing NSC proliferation and neurogenesis (C. L. Zhang *et al.*, 2008). Also in regards to Wnt signaling, one of its downstream targets is the Prox1 transcription factor. Prox1 plays a stage-specific role in initial granule cell differentiation but not during the later stages (Karalay *et al.*, 2011). Finally, NeuroD1 is a crucial transcription factor essential for generation of granule neurons in the hippocampus and cerebellum and may mediate the transition between self-renewal and neuronal lineage differentiation (Kuwabara *et al.*, 2009; M. Liu *et al.*, 2000).

3.4   Neurotransmitters

The neurotransmitters comprising the microenvironment around the developing hippocampal progenitors may include GABA, glutamate, nitric oxide, dopamine and acetylcholine (Faigle & Song, 2013; Jang *et al.*, 2008). In this section, we focus on GABA and glutamate which are the major inhibitory and excitatory neurotransmitters respective. During the early stages, the developing progenitors are initially tonically activated by ambient GABA and then GABAergic synaptic input (Esposito *et al.*, 2005). This is followed by glutamatergic input and finally perisomatic GABAergic innervation (Esposito *et al.*, 2005; Ge *et al.*, 2007).

GABA can mediate a dual role during adult hippocampal neurogenesis through the GABA$_A$ receptor which allows it to be initially depolarizing (excitatory) and consequently hyperpolarizing (inhibitory) (Ge *et al.*, 2007). The balance between GABA depolarization and hyperpolarization is maintained through a chloride ion gradient across the cell membrane. This is accomplished through the ionotropic receptor channels NKCCs which increase the intracellular chloride concentration causing depolarization and the KCCs which lower the intracellular chloride concentration causing hyperpolarization (Ben-Ari, 2002). The excitatory phase of GABA is initially due to ambient GABA availability in the microenvironment which is followed by synaptic input-induced GABA activation (Ge *et al.*, 2006; Markwardt *et al.*, 2009). Ambient GABA released from the neighboring Parvalbumin (PV) interneurons can dictate RGL choice between quiescence or self-renewal (J. Song *et al.*, 2012) while conditional deletion of the γ2 subunit of GABA$_A$ can cause the RGLs to rapidly leave quiescence and asymmetrically self-renew (J. Song *et al.*, 2012). Disruption of such GABA-induced depolarization can result in significant defects in dendritic complexity and synaptic integration, and prevents formation of functional GABAergic and glutamatergic synapses in newborn cells (Ge *et al.*, 2006). Interestingly, one of the risk factors for schizophrenia, the disrupted in schizophrenia 1 (DISC1) gene, has also been shown to regulate post-natal neurogenesis by interacting with GABA signaling (Kim *et al.*, 2012). Accelerating the GABA depolarization to hyperpolarization switch can result in aberrant regulation of neurogenesis by DISC1 which is involved in the maturation and dendritic growth of newborn neurons in the circuit (Kim *et al.*, 2012).

Glutamate is the primary excitatory neurotransmitter in the brain and can exert its function in the central nervous system through a variety of ionotropic receptors which include the NMDA, kainate and AMPA receptors. Excitatory glutamate signaling follows the switch from GABA-induced excitation to inhibition, and regulates the later phases of adult hippocampal neurogenesis with the first glutamatergic afferents being detected by the fourth week in mature neurons (Esposito *et al.*, 2005). Mediating glutamatergic input to the dentate gyrus by activating or blocking the NMDA receptor can robustly regulate cell proliferation in the rat dentate gyrus (Cameron *et al.*, 1995; Nacher *et al.*, 2001). There is also a critical time period during the third week after neuronal birth when newborn neuron survival is NMDA receptor-dependent (Tashiro *et al.*, 2006). Interestingly, the subunits of the NMDA receptor, NR1 and NR2B are expressed in the GFAP-expressing type-1 precursor cells suggesting possible regulation by NMDA receptor very early in neurogenesis (Nacher *et al.*, 2007). Blocking NMDA receptor through memantine, an Alzheimer's disease medication, can enhance cell proliferation in the dentate gyrus (Maekawa *et al.*, 2009), possibly by acting on the RGL population (Namba *et al.*, 2009). Diminished medial perforant path-granule cell LTP and a reduced peak amplitude of NMDA receptor-mediated excitatory post synaptic potentials can be seen in a mouse model of Fragile X syndrome (Yun 2011). NMDA receptors in the hippocampus have also been implicated in pattern separation and the formation of context memory (Cravens *et al.*, 2006; McHugh *et al.*, 2007).

3.5   Inflammatory Response and Epigenetic Regulation

Cytokines resulting from pro-inflammatory responses mediated by the resident microglia population in the hippocampus has crucial roles in regulating the surrounding neurogenesis (Kohman 2013). Neurogenesis can be inhibited through neuroinflammation inflammation while blocking a neuroinflammatory response with an anti-inflammatory drug can restore neurogenesis after an endotoxin-induced inflammatory period (Monje *et al.*, 2003). Similarly, microglia activation can impair both basal neurogenesis or insult-induced hippocampal neurogenesis while the administration of minocycline which is an inhibitor of microglia activation can restore neurogenesis (Ekdahl *et al.*, 2003). More specifically, while both studies (Ekdahl *et al.*, 2003; Monje *et al.*, 2003) showed effects on cell survival during neurogenesis, subsequent reports have shown more varied effects of microglia activation on proliferation, differentiation and integration (Kohman & Rhodes, 2013). In a study by Belarbi *et al*, lipopolysaccharide intra-cerebroventricular infusion was administered for 28 days with consequent BrdU administration on the 29th day for 5 days (Belarbi *et al.*, 2012). Microglial activation was detected as measured by increased MHC II expression and during exploration of a novel environment, recruitment of adult-born neurons into relevant hippocampal networks functioning in spatial information was selectively impaired (Belarbi *et al.*, 2012). Fate choice and differentiation may also be affected as can be seen with the chronic administration of IL-1beta that reduces the number of new neurons but increases the number of astrocytes, an effected that may not be reduced by voluntary running (Wu *et al.*, 2012). Other signaling factors such as IL-6 have been shown to reduce proliferation, survival and neuronal differentiation (Monje *et al.*, 2003; Vallieres *et al.*, 2002). Other signaling factors such as TNF-alpha, IL-4 and IL-10 play crucial roles through the different stages of adult hippocampal neurogenesis (Kohman & Rhodes, 2013).

Epigenetic mechanisms comprise histone modifications, DNA methylation and chromatin remodeling which exert persistent biological effects requiring no change in the genomic sequence (Ma *et al.*, 2010). Such epigenetic mechanisms are able to regulate specific stages of neurogenesis and in recent years have brought into focus several important interfaces at which regulation takes place (Ma *et al.*, 2010). Several such important mechanisms have been studied in recent years. One important gene is the neuronal-activity induced Gadd45b gene (Ma *et al.*, 2009). It is an immediate early gene expressed in mature NeuN+ hippocampal neurons and spatial exploration of a novel environment can significantly induce Gadd45b expression (Ma *et al.*, 2009). Its expression can be induced by a single ECT with Gadd45b being required for DNA methylation of specific promoters and expression of genes such as BDNF and FGF (Ma *et al.*, 2009). Both shRNA-mediated reduction in Gadd45b expression or mice with Gadd45b deletion abolish ECT-induced proliferation of neural progenitors (Ma *et al.*, 2009). Mice with Gadd45b deletion also show reduced dendritic growth of newborn neurons in the adult hippocampus (Ma *et al.*, 2009).

Methyl-CpG-Binding Protein 2 (MeCP2) is another crucial epigenetic regulator that is implicated in the pathogenesis of Rett Syndrome. It is associated with neuronal maturation and maintenance in the brain (Amir *et al.*, 1999; Chahrour & Zoghbi, 2007). In the absence of astrocyte-inducing cytokines, MeCP2 expression in the neural progenitors can selectively suppress astrocytic differentiation and promote neuronal differentiation (Tsujimura *et al.*, 2009). MeCP2 also regulates glutamatergic synapse number and controls the excitatory synaptic strength (Chao *et al.*, 2007) with its deficiency leading to deficits in neuronal maturation, altered expression of presynaptic proteins and reduced spine density (Smrt *et al.*, 2007). MeCP2 may also regulate the miRNA miR-137 that modulates the proliferation and differentiation of adult neural NSCs in vivo and in vitro (Szulwach *et al.*, 2010). There is also co-regulation by the transcriptional factor Sox2 alongside MeCP2 in regulation of miR-137 activity (Szulwach *et al.*, 2010). MeCP2 will be discussed in further detail in our discussion of Rett Syndrome later in this chapter. Another crucial player is the Methyl-CpG-Binding Domain Protein 1 (MBD1). Adult MBD1-/- mice show several deficits including reduced neurogenesis and spatial learning deficits alongside which there is a significant reduction in LTP in the dentate gyrus (X. Zhao *et al.*, 2003). Other important epigenetic regulators include TET1, Bmi-1 and members of the fragile X mental retardation proteins (Faigle & Song, 2013).

4   Physiological and Pathological Stimuli Regulating Neurogenesis

4.1   Stress

Stress has been used to create preclinical animal models of depression in which to study depression. While not a prerequisite for depression, the role of stressful life events and its causal relationship with the onset of major depression has previously been shown and discussed (Kendler *et al.*, 1999; Kendler *et al.*, 1995). Stress can include foot shock, restrain stress, social isolation, social defeat and psychosocial stress through introduction of an intruder animal. In rats, chronic restraint stress over 21 days can decrease cell proliferation while repeated stress for 42 days could decrease survival rate (Pham *et al.*, 2003). Chronic restraint stress has also been shown to reduce hippocampal volume, impair hippocampus-dependent fear memory and neurogenesis as measured by Ki67, BrdU and DCX staining in the dentate gyrus (Yun *et al.*, 2010). Further, social isolation for 6 weeks in female prairie voles significantly reduced cell proliferation, survival and neuronal differentiation in the dentate gyrus and increased anxiety-like and depression-like behavior, but did not affect social recognition memory (Lieberwirth *et al.*, 2012).

The learned helplessness and the forced swimming behavior tests are two other tests that cause stress and are widely accepted in the field in studying depression and the effect of antidepressants (Cryan *et al.*, 2002). In the learned helplessness model of depression, it has been shown that animals exposed to inescapable footshock (IS) demonstrate a downregulation of neurogenesis, an effect that is rescued with the administration of the antidepressant fluoxetine (Malberg & Duman, 2003). The effect of acute psychosocial stress through introduction of an intruder animal is considered a relevant paradigm that may model human relational stress in animals, and has been shown to reduce short-term cell survival with long-lasting effects (Thomas *et al.*, 2007). Chronic psychosocial stress in rats was also shown to reduce proliferation rate and survival of hippocampal granule cells and increase stress hormone levels (Czeh *et al.*, 2002). While stress hormone levels were normalized through concomitant repetitive transcranial magnetic stimulation, the survival rate was suppressed even further with only mild effects on cell proliferation (Czeh *et al.*, 2002). In conclusion, stress is a potent negative regulator of adult hippocampal neurogenesis and due to the lack of a pathophysiologically reliable animal model, it has been used as one way of studying depression in animal models.

4.2   Aging

Adult hippocampal neurogenesis has become increasingly relevant to the effects of aging. One of the earliest studies showed there was an age-related decrease in neural progenitor proliferation in the dentate gyrus due to decreased mitotic activity of neural precursors (Kuhn *et al.*, 1996). Subsequent studies confirmed such an age-related reduction in adult hippocampal neurogenesis (Nacher *et al.*, 2003; Olariu *et al.*, 2007; Rao *et al.*, 2006). It has been debated whether the age-related decline in neurogenesis is due to the depletion of neural stem cells or a loss of their mitotic ability (Encinas & Sierra, 2012). Previous evidence supported the latter notion of increased quiescence. For instance, an analysis of the neural stem cell marker Sox2 in young, middle-aged and aged rats with other proliferative markers shows that the age-related decrease in neurogenesis can be attributed to the increased quiescence of neural stem cells (Hattiangady & Shetty, 2008). Similar observations were made in a study of aged macaque monkeys and mice (Aizawa *et al.*, 2011). Recent work, however, has attributed such an age-related decline to the continuous depletion of the resident neural stem cell population (Encinas *et al.*, 2011; Olariu *et al.*, 2007). In the "disposable stem cell" model, the neural stem cell may complete a set number of asymmetric divisions before differentiating and maturing into an astrocyte (Encinas *et al.*, 2011). Such a model takes into account the depletion of neural stem cells and the parallel increase in astrocytes with aging.

The molecular and cellular mechanisms mediating such an age-related decline in neurogenesis remain elusive. Evidence suggests important contributions from growth factors and signaling pathways. Reduced VEGF and FGF-2 signaling owing to age-related astrocytic changes can decrease neurogenesis (Bernal & Peterson, 2011) while reducing the level of corticosteroid levels in aged rats can restore hippocampal neurogenesis (Cameron & McKay, 1999). More recently, the Wnt signaling pathway inhibitor DKK1 was shown to regulate distinct stages of adult hippocampal neurogenesis through the promotion of self-renewal and survival of quiescent neural progenitors, proliferation of transit amplifying progenitors and an increase in the Type-3 neuroblast number (Seib *et al.*, 2013). Aging in the SGZ was accompanied with an increase of DKK1 levels, the subsequent loss of which improved cognitive function and restored neurogenesis (Seib *et al.*, 2013). Several other factors have been implicated in reduced neurogenesis with aging. These include cell cycle checkpoints in senescent pathways that incorporate p21, telomere shortening and DNA oxidative damage and age-related changes to the neurogenic niche (Encinas & Sierra, 2012).

Due to the functions adult neurogenesis plays in memory formation and pattern separation, an age-related decline in neurogenesis, while biologically different from the classic neuropathology involved in Alzheimer's disease, could make unique contributions to cognition. Indeed, a qualitative relationship between an age-related decline in neurogenesis and cognitive function has been suggested and confirmed (Drapeau *et al.*, 2003; Drapeau *et al.*, 2007). For instance, reduced hippocampal neurogenesis is tied to reduced spatial memory performance in aged rats and pattern separation in aged mice (Clelland *et al.*,

2009; Drapeau *et al.*, 2003). An increase in neurogenesis in aged animals has also been demonstrated through exercise therapy. For instance, following evidence that physical exercise increases cell proliferation and neurogenesis in the adult brain (van Praag *et al.*, 1999), it was shown it could also prevent an age-related decline in neurogenesis (Kronenberg 2006) and enhance learning in aged mice (van Praag *et al.*, 2005).

4.3   Seizure

Seizure is a pathological stimulus of the brain that includes excessive neuronal activity and is characteristic of the disease epilepsy. In animal studies, seizures have been modeled using drug treatment including pilocarpine, kainic acid or electrical stimulation. Taken together, such induced seizures can have distinct effects on neurogenesis and changes in expression of growth factors in the surrounding microenvironment. Seizures induced by kainic acid can increase cellular proliferation in the rat dentate gyrus (Gray & Sundstrom, 1998), and upregulate levels of neuropeptide Y (NPY) in the hippocampus (Marksteiner *et al.*, 1989) and increase basic and acidic FGF mRNA levels in the dentate gyrus and the CA1 regions (Bugra *et al.*, 1994). Similarly, pilocarpine-induced seizures can accelerate dendritic development of newborn neurons with effects that may last for upto a month (Overstreet-Wadiche *et al.*, 2006), cause aberrant migration of newborn neurons and disrupt their axon projection (Parent *et al.*, 1997) and also upregulate VEGF in the CA1 and CA3 regions of the hippocampus where VEGF may play a neuroprotective affect (Croll *et al.*, 2004).

Induced seizure activity has also demonstrated an age-related effect of hippocampal plasticity and its response to brain injury. Acute seizure (AS) activity using kainic acid can have differential effects on neurogenesis depending on age. For instance, during old age kainic acid-induced AS activity may show no enhancement of adult neurogenesis (Rao *et al.*, 2008) while during middle age it increases the number of newborn neurons and accelerates their ectopic migration (Shetty *et al.*, 2012). Interestingly, the plasticity of hippocampal neurogenesis in response to injury such as induced AS activity may progressively decrease with age (Hattiangady *et al.*, 2008). In a study of both young and aged rats, AS activity in aged rats led to significant deficits in spatial learning and increased the risk for developing chronic temporal lobe epilepsy (TLE) (Hattiangady *et al.*, 2011). Electroconvulsive seizures or stimulation (ECS) have also proven useful in studying epilepsy and neurogenesis (Hidaka *et al.*, 2008; Madsen *et al.*, 2003; Madsen *et al.*, 2000; Malberg *et al.*, 2000). ECS treatment increases adult hippocampal neurogenesis in the brain (Madsen *et al.*, 2000; Malberg *et al.*, 2000), possibly through activation of the Wnt pathway (Madsen *et al.*, 2003). Chronic ECS may also impair spontaneous alternation behavior and locomotor activity (Hidaka *et al.*, 2008). Some impairments can be rescued using antiepileptics such as phenytoin and valproate (Hidaka *et al.*, 2008). Such seizure models have been useful in studying epilepsy. Epilepsy is discussed in a further section of this chapter.

5   Anxiety Disorders

Panic disorder and post traumatic stress disorder (PTSD) are two anxiety disorders that may hold a special relationship to hippocampal function. Panic disorder is characterized by significant anxiety and behavioral changes during the course of the panic attack with a persistent fear of having similar future attacks. PTSD which is sometimes found in veterans returning from war is caused when an individual is unable to distinguish between two similar situations. In the case of veterans, auditory cues such as loud noise or visual cues that may remind them of a previous experience from war can induce extreme anxiety. The role of the hippocampus in such disorders has been narrowed down to the concept of pattern separation. The ability to distinguish between two similar experiences is termed as pattern separation. The role of the dentate gyrus in pattern separation was first founded as part of a computational theory (Marr, 1971). It has since been elaborated on through other computation models (Rolls, 2010; Rolls & Kesner, 2006).

The anatomy of the hippocampus makes it especially adept at carrying out pattern separation. In the primate brain, entorhinal cortex can pass information relayed to it such as object and spatial representations to the hippocampus (Rolls, 2010). Such information can be passed from the hippocampus through mossy fiber inputs to the CA3 region, then CA1 and subiculum before the hippocampal output can reach back to the entorhinal cortex and then to the parahippocampal gyrus and perirhinal cortex which originally relayed the signal. In such a circular network, the CA3 region plays a role in autoassociation memory and forms a recurrent collateral network that can combine inputs from different parts of brain and form associations between them (Rolls, 2010). Such a network allows for both memory formation and retrieval. When relaying a signal to the CA3, the high density of granule cells in the dentate gyrus allow it to sparsely activate unique cell populations even when faced with an experience which may be similar to a previously encountered one (Deng et al., 2013; Kheirbek et al., 2012). In this manner, the dentate gyrus can separate two events with high efficiency and provide the resulting input to the CA3 region for correct autoassociation and memory recall (Deng et al., 2013; Rolls, 2010).

Through human studies and animal models, a strong relationship has been established between the hippocampus, pattern separation and anxiety disorders. In human patients with social phobia or PTSD, a significantly reduced hippocampal volume is found using magnetic resonance imaging (MRI) (Irle et al., 2010; Kitayama et al., 2005). Other studies have shown there may be increased susceptibility to psychological trauma or depression due to a reduced hippocampal volume (Gilbertson et al., 2002; Taylor et al., 2005). In human studies, damage to the hippocampus is associated with object-place memory tasks or spatial location (Crane & Milner, 2005; Smith & Milner, 1981). Functional MRI (fMRI) has also shown pattern separation activity to occur in the CA3/dentate gyrus region (Bakker 2008). In mice, ablating young dentate granule neurons (post-integration into the circuit) can disrupt pattern separation while inhibiting the older cells can inhibit pattern completion (Nakashiba et al., 2012). Other studies in rodents have supported similar roles of the dentate gyrus in pattern separation (Gilbert et al., 2001; Leutgeb et al., 2007; McHugh et al., 2007).

In regards to pattern separation and anxiety behavior, the role of adult neurogenesis has been established and growing. In adult mice, ablating hippocampal neurogenesis impaired spatial discrimination when mice were presented with stimuli with little spatial separation (Clelland et al., 2009). Depleting adult-born neurons can disrupt contextual discrimination in mice (Tronel et al., 2012) while increasing adult hippocampal neurogenesis can enhance cognitive performance in contextual discrimination or pattern separation (Sahay et al., 2011). When such an increase was tied to voluntary running, enhanced exploratory behavior and decreased anxiety-like behavior was also observed (Sahay et al., 2011). Stimulating adult hippocampal neurogenesis may thus be a useful strategy in alleviating the symptoms in anxiety disorders such as PTSD. As will be discussed in the following sections, enhancing neurogenesis or modulating its regulation has proven useful in other brain disorders.

6   Major Depression

Major depression is among the most prevalent psychiatric disorders worldwide and is associated with high rates of morbidity, death by suicide, and significant functional disability accompanied with feelings of sadness. Hippocampus is one of the anatomical regions of the brain that has been implicated in depression, both due to the structural changes observed in major depressive disorder (MDD) patients and evidence obtained from preclinical models of depression and the action of antidepressants. In clinical studies using magnetic resonance imaging (MRI), it was observed that MDD patients in full remission show a smaller posterior hippocampal volume while the anterior hippocampus is not effected (Neumeister et al., 2005). Similar results were obtained on the association between posterior hippocampal volume and remission rates in MDD patients (MacQueen et al., 2008). In both treatment-resistant MDD patients (Maller et al., 2007) and unmedicated patients (Malykhin et al., 2010), a reduced hippocampal volume is observed in the tail section. In this latter study, medicated MDD patients showed an increased hippocampal body volume. A recent study has used regression analysis and MRI in depressed patients and healthy controls to show a relationship between depression and decrease in right hippocampal volume over a four-year period (Sawyer et al., 2012). As discussed in the physiological stimuli section, stress has been primarily been used to study depression in preclinical animal models. These stress models have been shown to typically inhibit one or more stages of adult hippocampal neurogenesis with consequent effects on anxiety and depressive behavior, and memory.

The effect of antidepressants on adult hippocampal neurogenesis is a crucial one. It has provided evidence of a strong relationship between this biological process of generating new neurons in the hippocampus, and how aberrations in it may play a causal role in depression, or at least in alleviating the associated symptoms. One of the first landmark studies in the field showed the chronic administration of antidepressants promoted adult hippocampal neurogenesis (Malberg et al., 2000). This included an increase in the proliferation of adult hippocampal progenitors in the rat hippocampus with a consequent increase in newborn neurons that matured and entered the hippocampal circuit. Electroconvulsive therapy (ECT) or electroconvulsive stimulation (ECS) is another antidepressant treatment that increases neurogenesis and can do so in a dose-dependent fashion (Madsen et al., 2000). Other studies have connected such antidepressant-induced changes in neurogenesis to changes in animal behavior. Interestingly, no significant behavioral change on locomotor activity or spontaneous alteration behavior (as measured via open field or Y-maze) was observed with single or repeated ECS treatments in rats even though both treatments increased cellular proliferation during neurogenesis. However, chronic fluoxetine treatment does influence behavior. In mice, such treatment increases the maturation of newborn neurons with increased dendritic arborization and expression of mature neuron markers, enhances neurogenesis-dependent LTP and effects performance on the Novelty Suppressed Feeding test (NSF) used in studying antidepressant action (Wang et al., 2008). In this study, the effect of fluoxetine on LTP and NSF were abolished with the ablation of neurogenesis using x-ray irradiation suggesting the requirement of neurogenesis for the antidepressant response. Previously, Santarelli et al. utilized a genetic model and X-ray irradiation of the hippocampus to establish this requirement of adult hippocampal neurogenesis in the behavioral action of antidepressants (Santarelli et al., 2003).

While a complete elucidation of the mechanism by which antidepressants may mediate such effects is lacking, recent evidence has taken us crucial steps forward in understanding molecular and cellular mechanisms at play, and their connection to human patients. Recently, two inhibitors of the Wnt signaling pathway were implicated in mediating neurogenesis and the resulting behavioral response (Jang *et al.*, 2013; Seib *et al.*, 2013). Secreted frizzled-related protein 3 (sFRP3) is a naturally secreted inhibitor of the Wnt pathway that was found to be regulated in a neuronal activity-dependent manner (Jang *et al.*, 2013). Its deletion in mice results activated the quiescent Type-1 radial NSCs, enhanced dendritic growth and spine formation (Jang *et al.*, 2013). An extension of this study revealed chronic fluoxetine treatment downregulated sFRP3 levels in the mouse hippocampus and reduced depressive-like behavior (Jang *et al.*, 2012). sFRP3 KO mice showed similar antidepressive-like behavior which wasn't increased further by fluoxetine. A human pharmacogenetic analysis revealed significant associations between single nucleotide polymorphisms in FRZB (the human sfrp3 ortholog) and the antidepressant response in clinical patients (Jang *et al.*, 2012). Another inhibitor of the Wnt pathway is Dkk1 which was previously discussed in the aging section. It regulates adult hippocampal neurogenesis and its loss in old age can reduce depressive symptoms and improve memory function (Seib *et al.*, 2013). Other studies further the relationship between antidepressants, Wnt signaling and adult hippocampal neurogenesis by showing that chronic antidepressant treatment can upregulate components of Wnt pathway in the hippocampus (Okamoto *et al.*, 2010) and that an antidepressant-like behavior could be produced through upregulating dentate gyrus expression of Wnt2 (Okamoto *et al.*, 2010) or by administering a GSK3β inhibitor (Kaidanovich-Beilin *et al.*, 2004).

The long-term effects of stress and impaired glucocorticoid signaling have also been utilized to explain the pathogenesis of depression (Anacker *et al.*, 2011; Zunszain *et al.*, 2011). The hypothalamic-pituitary-adrenal (HPA) axis comprises a set of factors and hormones across the hypothalamus, and pituitary and the adrenal glands that are responsible for regulating the body's response to external stressors (Anacker *et al.*, 2011). Cortisol is one end product of this pathway released from the adrenal cortex that exerts its effect through the glucocorticoid receptor (GR) in the brain. Both hyperactivity of the HPA axis and impaired inhibition of glucocorticoids can result in increased levels of cortisol (Anacker *et al.*, 2011). Depressed patients have been shown to have hyperactivity of the HPA axis (Pariante, 2009), and cortisol outputs can be double that of healthy controls in treatment-resistant depressed patients (Anacker *et al.*, 2011). Increased stress can effect hippocampal neurogenesis and plasticity (Zunszain *et al.*, 2011). Indeed, direct glucocorticoid treatment can reduce adult hippocampal neurogenesis in rodents (David *et al.*, 2009) with chronic administration inducing anxiety-like behavior and depression in rats (Anacker *et al.*, 2011). A growing amount of evidence has positioned the glucocorticoids as an important player in the crosstalk that happens in between the stress, neurodegenerative and inflammatory components governing the pathogenesis of depression (Anacker *et al.*, 2011; Zunszain *et al.*, 2011).

The evidence, thus far, suggests a strong relationship between adult hippocampal neurogenesis and depression. There is much evidence showing this biological process in the dentate gyrus to be a requirement for the behavioral effect of antidepressants. Recent studies have also made progress in bringing forth the potential pathways involved in mediating this antidepressant response. Other than rodent models, antidepressants also increase adult hippocampal neurogenesis in monkey (Perera *et al.*, 2007) and human MDD brains (Boldrini *et al.*, 2009). However, the role of adult hippocampal neurogenesis in a causative role in depression remains unclear. At least one clinical study showed no increase in hippocampal cell proliferation in depressed patients which remain unchanged after antidepressant medication (Reif *et al.*, 2006). Current evidence suggests adult hippocampal neurogenesis could instead be a mediator of depression allowing for therapeutic targeting of disease symptoms after the onset of depression.

7   Schizophrenia

Schizophrenia is a debilitating and complex neurodevelopmental disorder which is influenced by both genetic and environmental factors, with the role of genetics or heritability in liability to schizophrenia at 81% (Sullivan *et al.*, 2003). The disorder is characterized by aberrant throught processes, social behavior and emotional responses. There are different brain regions that have been shown to be affected in schizophrenia through a multitude of studies. One of these regions is the hippocampus and there is now ample evidence that suggests a strong relationship between aberrant neurogenesis and schizophrenia. The first study that established such a relationship looked at post-mortem tissue samples from schizophrenia patients and found significantly reduced hippocampal neural stem cell proliferation (Reif *et al.*, 2006). Previous studies had implicated hippocampal subfield abnormalities in schizophrenic patients but not looked at neurogenesis *per se*. One of these studies showed a smaller neuron size in the anatomical regions belonging to the trisynaptic pathway which includes the hippocampal subregions of subiculum, CA1, and layer II of the entorhinal cortex (Arnold *et al.*, 1995). Alterations in neuronal size and shape in other hippocampal subfields were also found in a subsequent study (Zaidel *et al.*, 1997).

Animal models of schizophrenia have, however, been the primary mode of understanding the role of adult hippocampal neurogenesis in this disorder. Current evidence suggests aberrant neurogenesis may be a risk factor in the development of schizophrenia and may prove useful in its treatment. Before we discuss the two genes that have been associated with schizophrenia and aberrant regulation of neurogenesis in both affected patients and animal models, it is worth discussing first the effect of antidepressants and antipsychotic treatment that are used in treating schizophrenia. A chronic low dose of the antipsychotic clozapine has been shown to enhance cell proliferation but not survival of newly generated neurons in the hippocampus (Halim *et al.*, 2004). The negative effect on neurogenesis of psychostimulants such as phencyclidine that induce a schizophrenia-like behavioral state in mice (J. Liu *et al.*, 2006) is prevented with the co-administration of clozapine, D-serine and glycine, suggesting NMDA receptor dysfunction in decreasing neurogenesis (Maeda *et al.*, 2007). In this regard, NMDA receptor antagonists showed a neurogenesis effect too. For instance, in the rat model of schizophrenia, ketamine has been shown to enhance neurogenesis in the SGZ of the rat hippocampus (Keilhoff *et al.*, 2004) while memantine enhanced neurogenesis in the mouse hippocampus (Maekawa *et al.*, 2009; Namba *et al.*, 2009). A role of the NMDA receptor has also directly been demonstrated in mediating migration and the correct positioning of newborn neurons via the schizophrenia risk gene, DISC1 (Namba *et al.*, 2011).

Two genes that have been strongly associated with schizophrenia are DISC1 and NPAS3. DISC1 was first identified in a large Scottish family and is considered a risk factor for major mental illness including schizophrenia, bipolar disorder and major depression (Chubb *et al.*, 2008; Millar *et al.*, 2000). Downregulating DISC1 in the mouse hippocampus increases integration of the neuron into the hippocampal circuit, but also disrupts their morphology and causes aberrant positioning of new dentate granule neurons (Duan *et al.*, 2007). Complete DISC1 knockdown also causes increased dendritic growth, enhanced excitability, and accelerated spine formation of new neurons (Duan *et al.*, 2007). Further work has shown DISC1 interacts with proteins including NDEL1 and FEZ1 (Duan *et al.*, 2007; Kang *et al.*, 2011), and may also cross talk with Wnt signaling (Mao *et al.*, 2009) and GABA signaling (Kim *et al.*, 2012) in regulating neuronal development. DISC1 can physically bind to GSK3β and regulate β-catenin stability (Mao *et al.*, 2009). DISC1 loss-of-function deficits in neurogenesis and schizophrenia- and depressive-like behavior are also normalized with GSK3β inhibition (Mao *et al.*,

2009). Previously, GABA signaling was shown to regulate newborn neuron integration with the time period between GABA-induced depolarization and hyperpolarization being crucial for dendritogenesis and synapse formation (Ge *et al.*, 2006). Interestingly, accelerating this switch from depolarization to hyperpolarization can result in the loss of DISC1-dependent regulation of early post-natal neurogenesis (Kim *et al.*, 2012).

While not as aggressively studied as DISC1, the neuronal PAS domain 3 (NPAS3), which encodes the bHLH transcription factor is another risk gene associated with schizophrenia (Kamnasaran *et al.*, 2003; Pickard *et al.*, 2009). Mice that are deficient in NPAS3 demonstrate a number of abnormalities including reduced size of anterior hippocampus, deficits in recognition memory, altered anxiety-related responses and gait defects (Brunskill *et al.*, 2005). Deficiency of both NPAS1 and NPAS3 transcription factors in mice impair behavior in social recognition and reduce amounts of reelin in the brain (Erbel-Sieler *et al.*, 2004). Newborn neurons during the maturation process in the mouse SGZ also show high immunoreactivity for NPAS3 (Sha *et al.*, 2012) and disrupting NPAS3 function can reduce cell proliferation and expression of FGFR1 in the dentate gyrus (Pieper *et al.*, 2005). Interestingly, mice that lack the FGFR1 receptor for FGF2 show impairments in neurogenesis, LTP and memory consolidation (M. Zhao *et al.*, 2007). More work is required to delineate the mechanisms and pathways through which NPAS3 may act.

8   Alzheimer's Disease

Alzheimer's disease (AD) is a common neurodegenerative disorder that is highlighted by a progressive loss of memory and mental function, and a characteristic neuropathology of β-amyloid plaque, presenilin mutations and tau phosphorylation. Because of the inherent plasticity associated with adult hippocampal neurogenesis and its role in learning and memory, it has long been considered to play a key role in AD. In mouse models of AD, amyloid β-peptide (Aβ) reduces the proliferation and survival of neuronal progenitors during adult hippocampal neurogenesis (Haughey *et al.*, 2002) while in adult mice rescuing Presenilin-1 mutation through overexpression of its wild type form can promote hippocampal neurogenesis (Wen *et al.*, 2002). Interestingly, a human study returned contradictory findings wherein an increase in hippocampal neurogenesis was actually found in brains of AD patients (Jin, Peel, *et al.*, 2004). Such a finding may be reconciled by current evidence that strongly suggests adult hippocampal neurogenesis may instead be crucial during the early stages of AD-disease progression contributing to the associated symptoms and being a prime target for therapeutic efficacy (Mu & Gage, 2011).

Recent developments in the field have shown a growing relationship between adult hippocampal neurogenesis and its role in the neuropathology associated with AD. Apolipoprotein E (ApoE) is one protein that is involved in cholesterol metabolism and its ε 4 allele (ApoE4) is associated with AD pathogenesis through its modulation of amyloid β peptide and lipid metabolism (Bu, 2009). The adult NSCs and progenitors in the hippocampus express ApoE4, and both the knock-out and knock-in of ApoE4 can decrease neurogenesis, effect cell fate commitment or impair the maturation and dendritic development of newborn neurons, possibly through GABAergic interneuron dysfunction (Li *et al.*, 2009). Another study that crossed ApoE-deficient mice to nestin-GFP reporter demonstrated an over-proliferation of progenitor cells at an early age and a consequent decrease in Type-1 nestin and GFAP-expressing NSCs at later stages; a proliferation phenotype that was rescued with an ApoE-expressing retrovirus (Yang *et al.*, 2011). Interestingly, this over-proliferation during early age and subsequent depletion of Type-1 cells also resulted in increased generation of astrocytes in the dentate gyrus (Yang *et al.*, 2011). Changes in hippocampal volume have also been associated with ApoE4 in human patients (Cohen *et al.*, 2001; Moffat *et al.*, 2000).

Another strong association has been made between Presenilin-1 (PS1) which is the catalytic core of the enzyme aspartyl protease γ-secretase which functions in cleaving membrane proteins including the amyloid precursor protein (APP) (Selkoe & Wolfe, 2007). Mutations in the *presenilin* (PS) family of genes, namely PS1 and PS2, are known to result in the accumulation of the 42-residue amyloid beta-protein and cause early-onset familial AD (FAD) (Citron *et al.*, 1997; Rogaev *et al.*, 1995; Sherrington *et al.*, 1995). In the SVZ, it has been shown that PS1 knockdown using siRNA significantly enhances cell differentiation into neurons and glia (Gadadhar *et al.*, 2011). PS1 function is also γ-secretase-dependent and it regulates neural progenitor cell proliferation through β-catenin and EGFR signaling pathways (Gadadhar *et al.*, 2011). In the hippocampus too, effects of PS1 variants tied to early-onset FAD can be seen, especially on environment enrichment (EE)-induced increase in neurogenesis. Interestingly, transgenic mice expressing these PS1 variants show an inhibition of EE-induced proliferation and neuronal lineage commitment and that the surrounding microglia may play a crucial role in mediating these changes through secretion of soluble signaling factors (Choi *et al.*, 2008). Other evidence has considered the dual effect of APP and PS1 mutations. Transgenic mice carrying mutations in both APP and PS1 exhibited amyloid deposition and microgliosis which was characteristic of AD and appeared at 6 months and 9 months respectively (C. Zhang *et al.*, 2007).

AD therapy models may also act via adult hippocampal neurogenesis. These include memantine which is an NMDA receptor antagonist that increases number of radial glia-like progenitor cells, promotes cell proliferation and production of mature granule neurons in the mouse hippocampus (Maekawa *et al.*, 2009; Namba *et al.*, 2009). Other drugs including Donepezil and Phenserine also enhance adult hippocampal neurogenesis (Kotani *et al.*, 2008; Marutle *et al.*, 2007). In APP mice, an established Alzheimer's disease animal model, administration of lithium can inhibit GSK3β and stimulate adult hippocampal neurogenesis and improve cognitive function (Fiorentini *et al.*, 2010). Interestingly, this effect was age-dependent and declined as brain Aβ deposition and pathology increased (Fiorentini *et al.*, 2010). In regards to hippocampal-dependent aging that we previously discussed, we mentioned how physical exercise can improve neurogenesis and cognitive function in aged animals (Kronenberg *et al.*, 2006; van Praag *et al.*, 2005). Similarly, in mouse models of AD, complex environmental experience can improve neurogenesis, hippocampal LTP and associated neuropathology (Hu *et al.*, 2010). In 10-12 month old transgenic mice carrying the ApoE4 allele, physical exercise can increase BDNF levels, restore TrkB receptor levels, and improve performance on hippocampal-dependent behavioral tasks (Nichol *et al.*, 2009). However, such an effect does not always hold true especially in other AD models involving PS1 mutations or variants (Choi *et al.*, 2008; Lazarov *et al.*, 2010).

9   Down syndrome

Down syndrome is the most common intellectual disability that is caused by the trisomy of chromosome 21 and results in significant deficits in language, learning and memory (Contestabile *et al.*, 2010). Hippocampal dysfunction has been associated with Down syndrome subjects (Pennington *et al.*, 2003) and previous work using mouse models of Down syndrome has suggested impaired adult neurogenesis (Ishihara *et al.*, 2010). Recently, a more direct relationship with adult hippocampal neurogenesis has been established (Bianchi *et al.*, 2010; Contestabile *et al.*, 2013; Stagni *et al.*, 2013). In the Ts65Dn Down syndrome mouse model, deficits in hippocampal-dependent memory, synaptic plasticity and adult hippocampal neurogenesis are observed (Contestabile *et al.*, 2013). Interestingly, rescuing adult hippocampal neurogenesis using the mood stabilizer lithium can fully rescue such deficits, possibly through the Wnt signaling pathway (Contestabile *et al.*, 2013). Fluoxetine administration can also rescue impairments in DG-CA3 connectivity (Stagni *et al.*, 2013) and rescue impaired neurogenesis and hippocampal-dependent memory in Ts65Dn mice (Bianchi *et al.*, 2010).

10 Rett Syndrome

Rett Syndrome (RTT) is an X-linked neurological disorder that is characterized as an ASD and has come to be associated with hippocampal dysfunction. After the first 12-18 months of normal development in an infant's life, disabilities develop that are characteristic of RTT and include deceleration of head growth, microcephaly, stereotypic hand wringing, loss of motor coordination and mental retardation (Chahrour & Zoghbi, 2007). It is caused by mutations in the Methyl CpG Binding Protein 2 (MeCP2) gene which is associated with neuronal maturation and maintenance in the brain (Amir *et al.*, 1999; Chahrour & Zoghbi, 2007). Dendritic anomalies are one of the pathological changes in the RTT brain (Chahrour & Zoghbi, 2007). Studies in cultured hippocampal slices with altered MeCP2 expression have revealed aberrant LTP or frequency of spontaneous excitatory transmission possibly due to altered glutamatergic synapse number (Chahrour & Zoghbi, 2007; Chao *et al.*, 2007; Collins *et al.*, 2004; Moretti *et al.*, 2006; Nelson *et al.*, 2006). Lower spine density in the hippocampal CA1 pyramidal neurons is present in both post-mortem RTT brains and mouse models (Belichenko *et al.*, 2009; Chapleau *et al.*, 2012; Chapleau *et al.*, 2009).

While much work is still required, a few studies have studied the relationship between MeCP2 and neurogenesis. A recent study demonstrated that MeCP2 can regulate the miRNA miR-137 (Szulwach *et al.*, 2010). miR-137 is capable of modulating the proliferation and differentiation of adult neural NSCs both in vivo and in vitro and its regulation by MeCP2 also requires cooperation by the transcription factor Sox2 (Szulwach *et al.*, 2010). Further, deletion of the MeCP2-related protein MBD1 causes reduced differentiation of neural stem cells, reduced hippocampal neurogenesis, and deficits in spatial learning and dentate gyrus LTP (X. Zhao *et al.*, 2003). In mice lacking functional MeCP2, early postnatal neurogenesis in the dentate gyrus may be normal but there is impaired maturation of neurons with consequent altered spine distribution in MeCP2-deficient mutant neurons (Smrt *et al.*, 2007). Impaired transition of immature neurons to the mature stages was evidenced by the greater number of DCX+NeuN+ neurons in 8 week old *Mecp2* KO mice (Smrt *et al.*, 2007). Another study has looked at E18 hippocampal neurons in vitro to show the effects of MeCP2 on dendritic and axonal development and how these effects may be mediated by BDNF, one of the targets of MeCP2 (Larimore *et al.*, 2009).

11 Epilepsy

Epilepsy is a chronic neurological disorder that affects approximately 50 million people worldwide, about 80% of whom live in developing countries (WHO 2012). Seizures which are defined by excessive neuronal activity are a characteristic symptom in epileptic patients. Both animal models of epilepsy and induced seizures have been utilized in the scientific community to elucidate the mechanisms at play in this disorder. The effects of induced seizures were presented in the section on pathological and physiological stimuli regulating adult neurogenesis. Kainic acid and pilocarpine have both primarily been used to study effects on adult neurogenesis. Besides enhancing it (Gray & Sundstrom, 1998; Overstreet-Wadiche et al., 2006; Shetty et al., 2012), seizures can also aberrantly regulate migration of newborn neurons (Parent et al., 1997) and have an age-dependent effect on both adult neurogenesis and cognitive performance (Hattiangady et al., 2011; Hattiangady et al., 2008). Growth factors and NPY in the hippocampus are upregulated with seizure, possibly in response to brain injury (Bugra et al., 1994; Croll et al., 2004; Marksteiner et al., 1989).

Temporal Lobe Epilepsy (TLE) is used in rodent studies as an effective model for epilepsy. In a chronic TLE model in rats that show spontaneous recurrent motor seizures (SRMS), while increased neurogenesis is initially observed with kainic acid administration at 16 days, it is significantly reduced after 5 months with chronic epilepsy (Hattiangady et al., 2004). Furthermore, the frequency and intensity of SRMS is increased in aged rats (22 months old) which when compared to young rats (5 months old) show spatial learning deficits and are at a greater risk of developing TLE (Hattiangady et al., 2008). Another study has looked at the effects of brain injury inflicted using unilateral intracerebroventricular administration of kainic acid on mood, memory and injury in rats and whether negative effects could be alleviated by grafting anterior SVZ NSCs into the hippocampus (Hattiangady & Shetty, 2012). Interestingly, the mood, memory and neurogenesis impairments in the injured mice were very effectively ameliorated with the grafting.

Increasing numbers of hippocampal GABA-producing cells has been considered a potential strategy for epilepsy (Shetty & Turner, 2000; Thompson, 2009; Turner & Shetty, 2003). More recently, an interesting therapy used in counteracting the negative effects of TLE involves the use of embryonic medial ganglionic eminence-derived NSC grafts in the adult rat hippocampus (Waldau et al., 2010). While these had no effect on improving cognitive function or neurogenesis, the grafted cells reduced the frequency of SRMS by 43% and frequency of stage V seizures by 90% which could possibly be due to the addition of new GABAergic neurons and glial-derived neurotrophic factor (GDNF) into the epileptic hippocampus (Waldau et al., 2010). Such therapies may prove useful in treating epilepsy. Further work is required to uncover the molecular mechanisms involved in the pathophysiology of epilepsy and develop feasible models of therapeutic intervention.

12   Stroke

Ischemia or the restriction of blood supply to the brain has primarily been used to model the effects of stroke and understand the role adult neurogenesis may play. A common theme that arises from these studies is an increase in neurogenesis in response to such brain injury. Transient global ischemia for 10 minutes through a bilateral common carotid artery occlusion (BCCAO) in gerbils is enough to cause a 12-fold increase in BrdU labeled cells in the SGZ which can migrate into the GCL and mature into neurons (J. Liu et al., 1998). Similarly, in other models of ischemia, such as focal cerebral ischemia, increased proliferation of cells is observed in the SVZ and SGZ of adult rats (Jin et al., 2001). In this particular study, ischemia was modeled through a middle cerebral artery occlusion (MCAO) for 90 minutes with the SGZ showing an upregulation of immature neuron markers such as DCX, but not NeuN (Jin et al., 2001). A subsequent study considered an age-related effect, and performed a similar MCAO procedure albeit for

60 minutes in 3 month and 24 month old rats (Jin, Minami, *et al.*, 2004). Results contradictory to the previous study (Jin *et al.*, 2001) were obtained in the SGZ while in the SVZ, reduced neurogenesis was observed with age which was subsequently increased with MCAO.

Behavioral impairments following ischemia and therapeutic treatments have also implicated a role for the hippocampus. In a study of transient global ischemia, subjecting gerbils to irradiation to ablate neurogenesis prior to BCCAO can cause specific behavioral deficits in water-maze task, but not affect rotor-rod or open field testing (Raber *et al.*, 2004). More recently, it was shown a 17 min BCCAO caused cell loss in the hippocampal subfields at 7, 14 or 28 days post-procedure, loss of DCX+ cells in the DG at 14 and 28 days, memory impairments and anxiety-like behavior at 7 and 14 days (Soares *et al.*, 2013). Other animal studies have shown treatment with Escin, Quetiapine, Benzamide, Melanocortin can improve cognitive impairments or hippocampal neuronal damage caused by ischemia (Kumaran *et al.*, 2008; Spaccapelo *et al.*, 2011; Yan, Bi, *et al.*, 2007; Yan, He, *et al.*, 2007; L. Zhang *et al.*, 2010). Melanocortins may produce their neuroprotective effects against global and focal ischemia through modulation of Shh and Wnt signaling pathways during melanocortin-induced neurogenesis (Spaccapelo *et al.*, 2013). Current evidence points to adult hippocampal neurogenesis playing a role in functional recovery following brain injury. Future work can further elucidate the molecular mechanisms involved.

13   Parkinson's disease

Parkinson's disease (PD) is the 2nd most common neurodegenerative disorder that is characterized by motor deficits such as bradykinesia, rigidity, tremor and postural instability (Marxreiter *et al.*, 2013). A progressive disease in nature, PD is characterized by the degeneration of the dopaminergic neurons in the central nervous system. Neurogenesis in both the SVZ and SGZ has been implicated as a possible therapeutic target in its treatment since the non-motor symptoms of the disorder include hyposmia, depression, anxiety and a lack of novelty-seeking behavior (Marxreiter *et al.*, 2013). During the pathogenesis of PD, besides the degeneration of the dopaminergic neurons in the substantia negra pars compacta region, there is formation of intracellular inclusion bodies called Lewy bodies and Lewy neurites, and consequent accumulation of a presynaptic protein called alpha-synuclein in them (Desplats *et al.*, 2012). Both overexpression of wildtype alpha-synuclein protein or human A53T mutant alpha-synuclein affect hippocampal neurogenesis (Marxreiter *et al.*, 2013). In one transgenic mouse model overexpressing human A53T mutant alpha-synuclein, the reduced dentate gyrus neurogenesis could be rescued through the administration of fluoxetine (Kohl *et al.*, 2012). In a conditional mouse model with alpha-synuclein expression under the control of neuronal promotors and a tet-regulatable system, there was hippocampal neuropathology including reduced neurogenesis and neurodegeneration, along with impaired motor performance with aging (Marxreiter *et al.*, 2013; Nuber *et al.*, 2008). The progression of the disease, but not the symptoms, could be halted by turning off alpha-synuclein expression (Nuber *et al.*, 2008). Such transgenic animal studies and other specific lesion studies have provided some supportive evidence of a possible role of the hippocampus in PD (Marxreiter *et al.*, 2013). Much work remains in establishing a more direct relationship and more importantly in harnessing the regenerative capacity of the hippocampal neurogenesis.

14 Huntington's Disease

Huntington's Disease (HD) is an autosomal dominant and inherited neurodegenerative disorder characterized by movement abnormalities and cognitive impairments (Antoniades & Watts, 2013). Caused by a mutation in the huntingtin gene (htt) on short arm of chromosome 4, other characteristics of the disease include sleep disturbances, weight problems and abnormal behavior (Antoniades & Watts, 2013). This results in increased number of CAG repeats encoding glutamines in the HTT protein (Pla *et al.*, 2013). Several mouse lines have been developed for HD including knock-in, full length or truncated transgenic mice that may differ in the size of the CAG repeats or the promoter driving the transgene (Gil-Mohapel *et al.*, 2011). The most commonly used HD animals models are the truncated transgenic R6 lines (R6/1 and R6/2) (Gil-Mohapel *et al.*, 2011). Using the R6/1 line and BrdU labeling, one study showed while cell proliferation in the hippocampus was similar in younger transgenic and wildtype control mice, there was a dramatic reduction in cell proliferation in older transgenic mice (Lazic *et al.*, 2004). Similarly, in R6/2 transgenic HD mice, the reduction in hippocampal neurogenesis may start as early as 2 weeks of age and by 11.5 weeks involve a 66% reduction in newly born cells in the dentate gyrus (Gil *et al.*, 2005). As we have previously discussed kainic acid induced seizures can upregulate neurogenesis in the dentate gyrus (Gray & Sundstrom, 1998). However, in R6/2 mice, kainic acid-induced seizures fail to upregulate dentate gyrus neurogenesis, an effect that may be attributable to impairments in the surrounding microenvironment (Phillips *et al.*, 2005). Interestingly, in R6/1 mice housed in an enriched environment, beneficial effects included increased number of BrdU+ and DCX+ cells, as well as increased migration of DCX+ cells with morphological changes such as longer neuritis (Lazic *et al.*, 2006). Besides environmental enrichment, other therapeutic strategies involving voluntary physical exercise, antidepressant treatment, cytokines and growth factors have provided further support to the role of adult hippocampal neurogenesis in HD (Gil-Mohapel *et al.*, 2011).

15 Conclusion

In this chapter, we have considered in detail the process of adult hippocampal neurogenesis and its relationship with neurological disorders. We first obtained an understanding of the cellular mechanism at play during the sequential process of adult hippocampal neurogenesis. Consequently, we have demonstrated how such a process is regulated in a stage-specific manner by signaling pathways, growth factors, neurotrophins, inflammatory cytokines, and transcription and epigenetic factors. Next, we considered three major physiological and pathological stimuli that regulate neurogenesis: stress, aging and seizures. These and other mentioned through the chapter have been extensively utilized to study adult neurogenesis both in normal and disease states. Finally, we have discussed a number of neurological disorders in relation to adult hippocampal neurogenesis. Specifically, we have reviewed its role in relation to disease etiology, pathogenesis and areas of future therapeutic targeting.

Close to two decades worth of research and technical advances has significantly advanced our understanding of adult neurogenesis. It has brought forth an appreciation of its role in learning and memory, cognition and emotional behavior. This growth spurt has also coincided with an improved understanding of neurological disorders and effective animal models have enhanced our understanding how specific stages of neurogenesis may be targeted to obtain therapeutic efficacy. Much work yet remains to be done. In this chapter, we have provided the reader a glimpse into the ongoing story in adult hippocampal neurogenesis. We have covered major focus areas of research and guided the reader to relevant review articles where necessary. In the coming decade, utilization of new technologies in quantitatively assessing neuronal activity with spatial and temporal precision in both animal models and humans in normal and disease states will provide us with an improved understanding of neurological disorders and how we may modulate neurogenesis toward therapeutic benefit.

Acknowledgements

The research in Dr. Jang laboratory was supported by NIH (R00MH090115), NARSAD (Young investigator award), Fraternal Order of Eagles Funds from Mayo Clinic Cancer Center, Accelerated Regenerative Medicine Award from Center for Regenerative Medicine at Mayo and start-up funds from Mayo foundation.

References

Ahn, S., & Joyner, A. L. (2005). In vivo analysis of quiescent adult neural stem cells responding to Sonic hedgehog. Nature, 437(7060), 894-897.

Aizawa, K., Ageyama, N., Terao, K., & Hisatsune, T. (2011). Primate-specific alterations in neural stem/progenitor cells in the aged hippocampus. Neurobiology of aging, 32(1), 140-150.

Amir, R. E., Van den Veyver, I. B., Wan, M., Tran, C. Q., Francke, U., & Zoghbi, H. Y. (1999). Rett syndrome is caused by mutations in X-linked MECP2, encoding methyl-CpG-binding protein 2. Nature genetics, 23(2), 185-188.

Amoureux, M. C., Cunningham, B. A., Edelman, G. M., & Crossin, K. L. (2000). N-CAM binding inhibits the proliferation of hippocampal progenitor cells and promotes their differentiation to a neuronal phenotype. J Neurosci, 20(10), 3631-3640.

Anacker, C., Zunszain, P. A., Carvalho, L. A., & Pariante, C. M. (2011). The glucocorticoid receptor: pivot of depression and of antidepressant treatment? Psychoneuroendocrinology, 36(3), 415-425.

Antoniades, C. A., & Watts, C. (2013). Huntington's disease and cell therapies: past, present, and future. Methods Mol Biol, 1010, 19-32.

Aonurm-Helm, A., Jurgenson, M., Zharkovsky, T., Sonn, K., Berezin, V., Bock, E., & Zharkovsky, A. (2008). Depression-like behaviour in neural cell adhesion molecule (NCAM)-deficient mice and its reversal by an NCAM-derived peptide, FGL. Eur J Neurosci, 28(8), 1618-1628.

Arnold, S. E., Franz, B. R., Gur, R. C., Gur, R. E., Shapiro, R. M., Moberg, P. J., & Trojanowski, J. Q. (1995). Smaller neuron size in schizophrenia in hippocampal subfields that mediate cortical-hippocampal interactions. The American journal of psychiatry, 152(5), 738-748.

Belarbi, K., Arellano, C., Ferguson, R., Jopson, T., & Rosi, S. (2012). Chronic neuroinflammation impacts the recruitment of adult-born neurons into behaviorally relevant hippocampal networks. Brain Behav Immun, 26(1), 18-23.

Belichenko, P. V., Wright, E. E., Belichenko, N. P., Masliah, E., Li, H. H., Mobley, W. C., & Francke, U. (2009). Widespread changes in dendritic and axonal morphology in Mecp2-mutant mouse models of Rett syndrome: evidence for disruption of neuronal networks. J Comp Neurol, 514(3), 240-258.

Ben-Ari, Y. (2002). Excitatory actions of gaba during development: the nature of the nurture. Nature reviews. Neuroscience, 3(9), 728-739.

Bergami, M., Rimondini, R., Santi, S., Blum, R., Gotz, M., & Canossa, M. (2008). Deletion of TrkB in adult progenitors alters newborn neuron integration into hippocampal circuits and increases anxiety-like behavior. Proc Natl Acad Sci U S A, 105(40), 15570-15575.

Bernal, G. M., & Peterson, D. A. (2011). Phenotypic and gene expression modification with normal brain aging in GFAP-positive astrocytes and neural stem cells. Aging Cell, 10(3), 466-482.

Bianchi, P., Ciani, E., Guidi, S., Trazzi, S., Felice, D., Grossi, G., . . . Bartesaghi, R. (2010). Early pharmacotherapy restores neurogenesis and cognitive performance in the Ts65Dn mouse model for Down syndrome. J Neurosci, 30(26), 8769-8779.

Boldrini, M., Underwood, M. D., Hen, R., Rosoklija, G. B., Dwork, A. J., John Mann, J., & Arango, V. (2009). Antidepressants increase neural progenitor cells in the human hippocampus. Neuropsychopharmacology, 34(11), 2376-2389.

Bonaguidi, M. A., Wheeler, M. A., Shapiro, J. S., Stadel, R. P., Sun, G. J., Ming, G. L., & Song, H. (2011). In vivo clonal analysis reveals self-renewing and multipotent adult neural stem cell characteristics. Cell, 145(7), 1142-1155.

Brennaman, L. H., & Maness, P. F. (2010). NCAM in neuropsychiatric and neurodegenerative disorders. Adv Exp Med Biol, 663, 299-317.

Breunig, J. J., & Rakic, P. (2010). Profiling identifies precursor suspects: notch family again! Cell Stem Cell, 6(5), 401-402.

Breunig, J. J., Silbereis, J., Vaccarino, F. M., Sestan, N., & Rakic, P. (2007). Notch regulates cell fate and dendrite morphology of newborn neurons in the postnatal dentate gyrus. Proc Natl Acad Sci U S A, 104(51), 20558-20563.

Brunskill, E. W., Ehrman, L. A., Williams, M. T., Klanke, J., Hammer, D., Schaefer, T. L., . . . Vorhees, C. V. (2005). Abnormal neurodevelopment, neurosignaling and behaviour in Npas3-deficient mice. Eur J Neurosci, 22(6), 1265-1276.

Bu, G. (2009). Apolipoprotein E and its receptors in Alzheimer's disease: pathways, pathogenesis and therapy. Nature reviews. Neuroscience, 10(5), 333-344.

Bugra, K., Pollard, H., Charton, G., Moreau, J., Ben-Ari, Y., & Khrestchatisky, M. (1994). aFGF, bFGF and flg mRNAs show distinct patterns of induction in the hippocampus following kainate-induced seizures. Eur J Neurosci, 6(1), 58-66.

Cameron, H. A., McEwen, B. S., & Gould, E. (1995). Regulation of adult neurogenesis by excitatory input and NMDA receptor activation in the dentate gyrus. J Neurosci, 15(6), 4687-4692.

Cameron, H. A., & McKay, R. D. (1999). Restoring production of hippocampal neurons in old age. Nat Neurosci, 2(10), 894-897.

Cao, L., Jiao, X., Zuzga, D. S., Liu, Y., Fong, D. M., Young, D., & During, M. J. (2004). VEGF links hippocampal activity with neurogenesis, learning and memory. Nature genetics, 36(8), 827-835.

Chahrour, M., & Zoghbi, H. Y. (2007). The story of Rett syndrome: from clinic to neurobiology. Neuron, 56(3), 422-437.

Chao, H. T., Zoghbi, H. Y., & Rosenmund, C. (2007). MeCP2 controls excitatory synaptic strength by regulating glutamatergic synapse number. Neuron, 56(1), 58-65.

Chapleau, C. A., Boggio, E. M., Calfa, G., Percy, A. K., Giustetto, M., & Pozzo-Miller, L. (2012). Hippocampal CA1 pyramidal neurons of Mecp2 mutant mice show a dendritic spine phenotype only in the presymptomatic stage. Neural plasticity, 2012, 976164.

Chapleau, C. A., Calfa, G. D., Lane, M. C., Albertson, A. J., Larimore, J. L., Kudo, S., . . . Pozzo-Miller, L. (2009). Dendritic spine pathologies in hippocampal pyramidal neurons from Rett syndrome brain and after expression of Rett-associated MECP2 mutations. Neurobiol Dis, 35(2), 219-233.

Choi, S. H., Veeraraghavalu, K., Lazarov, O., Marler, S., Ransohoff, R. M., Ramirez, J. M., & Sisodia, S. S. (2008). Non-cell-autonomous effects of presenilin 1 variants on enrichment-mediated hippocampal progenitor cell proliferation and differentiation. Neuron, 59(4), 568-580.

Chubb, J. E., Bradshaw, N. J., Soares, D. C., Porteous, D. J., & Millar, J. K. (2008). The DISC locus in psychiatric illness. Mol Psychiatry, 13(1), 36-64.

Citron, M., Westaway, D., Xia, W., Carlson, G., Diehl, T., Levesque, G., . . . Selkoe, D. J. (1997). Mutant presenilins of Alzheimer's disease increase production of 42-residue amyloid beta-protein in both transfected cells and transgenic mice. Nat Med, 3(1), 67-72.

Clelland, C. D., Choi, M., Romberg, C., Clemenson, G. D., Jr., Fragniere, A., Tyers, P., . . . Bussey, T. J. (2009). A functional role for adult hippocampal neurogenesis in spatial pattern separation. Science, 325(5937), 210-213.

Cohen, R. M., Small, C., Lalonde, F., Friz, J., & Sunderland, T. (2001). Effect of apolipoprotein E genotype on hippocampal volume loss in aging healthy women. Neurology, 57(12), 2223-2228.

Collins, A. L., Levenson, J. M., Vilaythong, A. P., Richman, R., Armstrong, D. L., Noebels, J. L., . . . Zoghbi, H. Y. (2004). Mild overexpression of MeCP2 causes a progressive neurological disorder in mice. Human molecular genetics, 13(21), 2679-2689.

Contestabile, A., Benfenati, F., & Gasparini, L. (2010). Communication breaks-Down: from neurodevelopment defects to cognitive disabilities in Down syndrome. Progress in neurobiology, 91(1), 1-22.

Contestabile, A., Greco, B., Ghezzi, D., Tucci, V., Benfenati, F., & Gasparini, L. (2013). Lithium rescues synaptic plasticity and memory in Down syndrome mice. The Journal of clinical investigation, 123(1), 348-361.

Crane, J., & Milner, B. (2005). What went where? Impaired object-location learning in patients with right hippocampal lesions. Hippocampus, 15(2), 216-231.

Cravens, C. J., Vargas-Pinto, N., Christian, K. M., & Nakazawa, K. (2006). CA3 NMDA receptors are crucial for rapid and automatic representation of context memory. Eur J Neurosci, 24(6), 1771-1780.

Cremer, H., Chazal, G., Carleton, A., Goridis, C., Vincent, J. D., & Lledo, P. M. (1998). Long-term but not short-term plasticity at mossy fiber synapses is impaired in neural cell adhesion molecule-deficient mice. Proc Natl Acad Sci U S A, 95(22), 13242-13247.

Croll, S. D., Goodman, J. H., & Scharfman, H. E. (2004). Vascular endothelial growth factor (VEGF) in seizures: a double-edged sword. Adv Exp Med Biol, 548, 57-68.

Cryan, J. F., Markou, A., & Lucki, I. (2002). Assessing antidepressant activity in rodents: recent developments and future needs. Trends in pharmacological sciences, 23(5), 238-245.

Czeh, B., Welt, T., Fischer, A. K., Erhardt, A., Schmitt, W., Muller, M. B., . . . Keck, M. E. (2002). Chronic psychosocial stress and concomitant repetitive transcranial magnetic stimulation: effects on stress hormone levels and adult hippocampal neurogenesis. Biological psychiatry, 52(11), 1057-1065.

David, D. J., Samuels, B. A., Rainer, Q., Wang, J. W., Marsteller, D., Mendez, I., . . . Hen, R. (2009). Neurogenesis-dependent and -independent effects of fluoxetine in an animal model of anxiety/depression. Neuron, 62(4), 479-493.

Deng, W., Mayford, M., & Gage, F. H. (2013). Selection of distinct populations of dentate granule cells in response to inputs as a mechanism for pattern separation in mice. eLife, 2, e00312.

Desplats, P., Spencer, B., Crews, L., Pathel, P., Morvinski-Friedmann, D., Kosberg, K., . . . Masliah, E. (2012). alpha-Synuclein induces alterations in adult neurogenesis in Parkinson disease models via p53-mediated repression of Notch1. J Biol Chem, 287(38), 31691-31702.

Drapeau, E., Mayo, W., Aurousseau, C., Le Moal, M., Piazza, P. V., & Abrous, D. N. (2003). Spatial memory performances of aged rats in the water maze predict levels of hippocampal neurogenesis. Proc Natl Acad Sci U S A, 100(24), 14385-14390.

Drapeau, E., Montaron, M. F., Aguerre, S., & Abrous, D. N. (2007). Learning-induced survival of new neurons depends on the cognitive status of aged rats. J Neurosci, 27(22), 6037-6044.

Duan, X., Chang, J. H., Ge, S., Faulkner, R. L., Kim, J. Y., Kitabatake, Y., . . . Song, H. (2007). Disrupted-In-Schizophrenia 1 regulates integration of newly generated neurons in the adult brain. Cell, 130(6), 1146-1158.

Duan, X., Kang, E., Liu, C. Y., Ming, G. L., & Song, H. (2008). Development of neural stem cell in the adult brain. Current opinion in neurobiology, 18(1), 108-115.

Dupret, D., Fabre, A., Dobrossy, M. D., Panatier, A., Rodriguez, J. J., Lamarque, S., . . . Abrous, D. N. (2007). Spatial learning depends on both the addition and removal of new hippocampal neurons. PLoS biology, 5(8), e214.

Ekdahl, C. T., Claasen, J. H., Bonde, S., Kokaia, Z., & Lindvall, O. (2003). Inflammation is detrimental for neurogenesis in adult brain. Proc Natl Acad Sci U S A, 100(23), 13632-13637.

Encinas, J. M., Michurina, T. V., Peunova, N., Park, J. H., Tordo, J., Peterson, D. A., . . . Enikolopov, G. (2011). Division-coupled astrocytic differentiation and age-related depletion of neural stem cells in the adult hippocampus. Cell Stem Cell, 8(5), 566-579.

Encinas, J. M., & Sierra, A. (2012). Neural stem cell deforestation as the main force driving the age-related decline in adult hippocampal neurogenesis. Behavioural brain research, 227(2), 433-439.

Erbel-Sieler, C., Dudley, C., Zhou, Y., Wu, X., Estill, S. J., Han, T., . . . McKnight, S. L. (2004). Behavioral and regulatory abnormalities in mice deficient in the NPAS1 and NPAS3 transcription factors. Proc Natl Acad Sci U S A, 101(37), 13648-13653.

Eriksson, P. S., Perfilieva, E., Bjork-Eriksson, T., Alborn, A. M., Nordborg, C., Peterson, D. A., & Gage, F. H. (1998). Neurogenesis in the adult human hippocampus. Nat Med, 4(11), 1313-1317.

Esposito, M. S., Piatti, V. C., Laplagne, D. A., Morgenstern, N. A., Ferrari, C. C., Pitossi, F. J., & Schinder, A. F. (2005). Neuronal differentiation in the adult hippocampus recapitulates embryonic development. J Neurosci, 25(44), 10074-10086.

Faigle, R., & Song, H. (2013). Signaling mechanisms regulating adult neural stem cells and neurogenesis. Biochimica et biophysica acta, 1830(2), 2435-2448.

Favaro, R., Valotta, M., Ferri, A. L., Latorre, E., Mariani, J., Giachino, C., . . . Nicolis, S. K. (2009). Hippocampal development and neural stem cell maintenance require Sox2-dependent regulation of Shh. Nat Neurosci, 12(10), 1248-1256.

Fiorentini, A., Rosi, M. C., Grossi, C., Luccarini, I., & Casamenti, F. (2010). Lithium improves hippocampal neurogenesis, neuropathology and cognitive functions in APP mutant mice. PLoS One, 5(12), e14382.

Gadadhar, A., Marr, R., & Lazarov, O. (2011). Presenilin-1 regulates neural progenitor cell differentiation in the adult brain. J Neurosci, 31(7), 2615-2623.

Gage, F. H. (2000). Mammalian neural stem cells. Science, 287(5457), 1433-1438.

Gao, X., Arlotta, P., Macklis, J. D., & Chen, J. (2007). Conditional knock-out of beta-catenin in postnatal-born dentate gyrus granule neurons results in dendritic malformation. J Neurosci, 27(52), 14317-14325.

Ge, S., Goh, E. L., Sailor, K. A., Kitabatake, Y., Ming, G. L., & Song, H. (2006). GABA regulates synaptic integration of newly generated neurons in the adult brain. Nature, 439(7076), 589-593.

Ge, S., Yang, C. H., Hsu, K. S., Ming, G. L., & Song, H. (2007). A critical period for enhanced synaptic plasticity in newly generated neurons of the adult brain. Neuron, 54(4), 559-566.

Gil, J. M., Mohapel, P., Araujo, I. M., Popovic, N., Li, J. Y., Brundin, P., & Petersen, A. (2005). Reduced hippocampal neurogenesis in R6/2 transgenic Huntington's disease mice. Neurobiol Dis, 20(3), 744-751.

Gil-Mohapel, J., Simpson, J. M., Ghilan, M., & Christie, B. R. (2011). Neurogenesis in Huntington's disease: can studying adult neurogenesis lead to the development of new therapeutic strategies? Brain Res, 1406, 84-105.

Gilbert, P. E., Kesner, R. P., & Lee, I. (2001). Dissociating hippocampal subregions: double dissociation between dentate gyrus and CA1. Hippocampus, 11(6), 626-636.

Gilbertson, M. W., Shenton, M. E., Ciszewski, A., Kasai, K., Lasko, N. B., Orr, S. P., & Pitman, R. K. (2002). Smaller hippocampal volume predicts pathologic vulnerability to psychological trauma. Nat Neurosci, 5(11), 1242-1247.

Goritz, C., & Frisen, J. (2012). Neural stem cells and neurogenesis in the adult. Cell Stem Cell, 10(6), 657-659.

Gray, W. P., & Sundstrom, L. E. (1998). Kainic acid increases the proliferation of granule cell progenitors in the dentate gyrus of the adult rat. Brain Res, 790(1-2), 52-59.

Halim, N. D., Weickert, C. S., McClintock, B. W., Weinberger, D. R., & Lipska, B. K. (2004). Effects of chronic haloperidol and clozapine treatment on neurogenesis in the adult rat hippocampus. Neuropsychopharmacology, 29(6), 1063-1069.

Han, Y. G., Spassky, N., Romaguera-Ros, M., Garcia-Verdugo, J. M., Aguilar, A., Schneider-Maunoury, S., & Alvarez-Buylla, A. (2008). Hedgehog signaling and primary cilia are required for the formation of adult neural stem cells. Nat Neurosci, 11(3), 277-284.

Hattiangady, B., Kuruba, R., & Shetty, A. K. (2011). Acute Seizures in Old Age Leads to a Greater Loss of CA1 Pyramidal Neurons, an Increased Propensity for Developing Chronic TLE and a Severe Cognitive Dysfunction. Aging and disease, 2(1), 1-17.

Hattiangady, B., Rao, M. S., & Shetty, A. K. (2004). Chronic temporal lobe epilepsy is associated with severely declined dentate neurogenesis in the adult hippocampus. Neurobiol Dis, 17(3), 473-490.

Hattiangady, B., Rao, M. S., & Shetty, A. K. (2008). Plasticity of hippocampal stem/progenitor cells to enhance neurogenesis in response to kainate-induced injury is lost by middle age. Aging Cell, 7(2), 207-224.

Hattiangady, B., & Shetty, A. K. (2008). Aging does not alter the number or phenotype of putative stem/progenitor cells in the neurogenic region of the hippocampus. Neurobiology of aging, 29(1), 129-147.

Hattiangady, B., & Shetty, A. K. (2012). Neural stem cell grafting counteracts hippocampal injury-mediated impairments in mood, memory, and neurogenesis. Stem cells translational medicine, 1(9), 696-708.

Haughey, N. J., Nath, A., Chan, S. L., Borchard, A. C., Rao, M. S., & Mattson, M. P. (2002). Disruption of neurogenesis by amyloid beta-peptide, and perturbed neural progenitor cell homeostasis, in models of Alzheimer's disease. Journal of neurochemistry, 83(6), 1509-1524.

Hidaka, N., Suemaru, K., Li, B., & Araki, H. (2008). Effects of repeated electroconvulsive seizures on spontaneous alternation behavior and locomotor activity in rats. Biological & pharmaceutical bulletin, 31(10), 1928-1932.

Hsieh, J. (2012). Orchestrating transcriptional control of adult neurogenesis. Genes Dev, 26(10), 1010-1021.

Hsieh, J., Aimone, J. B., Kaspar, B. K., Kuwabara, T., Nakashima, K., & Gage, F. H. (2004). IGF-I instructs multipotent adult neural progenitor cells to become oligodendrocytes. J Cell Biol, 164(1), 111-122.

Hu, Y. S., Xu, P., Pigino, G., Brady, S. T., Larson, J., & Lazarov, O. (2010). Complex environment experience rescues impaired neurogenesis, enhances synaptic plasticity, and attenuates neuropathology in familial Alzheimer's disease-linked APPswe/PS1DeltaE9 mice. FASEB journal : official publication of the Federation of American Societies for Experimental Biology, 24(6), 1667-1681.

Huehnchen, P., Prozorovski, T., Klaissle, P., Lesemann, A., Ingwersen, J., Wolf, S. A., . . . Steiner, B. (2011). Modulation of adult hippocampal neurogenesis during myelin-directed autoimmune neuroinflammation. Glia, 59(1), 132-142.

Hynes, M., Porter, J. A., Chiang, C., Chang, D., Tessier-Lavigne, M., Beachy, P. A., & Rosenthal, A. (1995). Induction of midbrain dopaminergic neurons by Sonic hedgehog. Neuron, 15(1), 35-44.

Irle, E., Ruhleder, M., Lange, C., Seidler-Brandler, U., Salzer, S., Dechent, P., . . . Leichsenring, F. (2010). Reduced amygdalar and hippocampal size in adults with generalized social phobia. Journal of psychiatry & neuroscience : JPN, 35(2), 126-131.

Ishihara, K., Amano, K., Takaki, E., Shimohata, A., Sago, H., Epstein, C. J., & Yamakawa, K. (2010). Enlarged brain ventricles and impaired neurogenesis in the Ts1Cje and Ts2Cje mouse models of Down syndrome. Cerebral cortex, 20(5), 1131-1143.

Jang, M. H., Bonaguidi, M. A., Kitabatake, Y., Sun, J., Song, J., Kang, E., . . . Song, H. (2013). Secreted frizzled-related protein 3 regulates activity-dependent adult hippocampal neurogenesis. Cell Stem Cell, 12(2), 215-223.

Jang, M. H., Kitabatake, Y., Kang, E., Jun, H., Pletnikov, M. V., Christian, K. M., . . . Ming, G. I. (2012). Secreted frizzled-related protein 3 (sFRP3) regulates antidepressant responses in mice and humans. Mol Psychiatry.

Jang, M. H., Song, H., & Ming, G. I. (2008). *Regulation of Adult Neurogenesis by Neurotransmitters. In F. H. Gage, G. Kempermann & H. Song (Eds.), Adult Neurogenesis (pp. 397-423). Cold Spring Harbor: Cold Spring Harbor Laboratory Press.*

Jessberger, S., Toni, N., Clemenson, G. D., Jr., Ray, J., & Gage, F. H. (2008). *Directed differentiation of hippocampal stem/progenitor cells in the adult brain. Nat Neurosci, 11(8), 888-893.*

Jin, K., Minami, M., Lan, J. Q., Mao, X. O., Batteur, S., Simon, R. P., & Greenberg, D. A. (2001). *Neurogenesis in dentate subgranular zone and rostral subventricular zone after focal cerebral ischemia in the rat. Proc Natl Acad Sci U S A, 98(8), 4710-4715.*

Jin, K., Minami, M., Xie, L., Sun, Y., Mao, X. O., Wang, Y., . . . Greenberg, D. A. (2004). *Ischemia-induced neurogenesis is preserved but reduced in the aged rodent brain. Aging Cell, 3(6), 373-377.*

Jin, K., Peel, A. L., Mao, X. O., Xie, L., Cottrell, B. A., Henshall, D. C., & Greenberg, D. A. (2004). *Increased hippocampal neurogenesis in Alzheimer's disease. Proc Natl Acad Sci U S A, 101(1), 343-347.*

Jin, K., Zhu, Y., Sun, Y., Mao, X. O., Xie, L., & Greenberg, D. A. (2002). *Vascular endothelial growth factor (VEGF) stimulates neurogenesis in vitro and in vivo. Proc Natl Acad Sci U S A, 99(18), 11946-11950.*

Kaidanovich-Beilin, O., Milman, A., Weizman, A., Pick, C. G., & Eldar-Finkelman, H. (2004). *Rapid antidepressive-like activity of specific glycogen synthase kinase-3 inhibitor and its effect on beta-catenin in mouse hippocampus. Biological psychiatry, 55(8), 781-784.*

Kamnasaran, D., Muir, W. J., Ferguson-Smith, M. A., & Cox, D. W. (2003). *Disruption of the neuronal PAS3 gene in a family affected with schizophrenia. Journal of medical genetics, 40(5), 325-332.*

Kang, E., Burdick, K. E., Kim, J. Y., Duan, X., Guo, J. U., Sailor, K. A., . . . Ming, G. L. (2011). *Interaction between FEZ1 and DISC1 in regulation of neuronal development and risk for schizophrenia. Neuron, 72(4), 559-571.*

Karalay, O., Doberauer, K., Vadodaria, K. C., Knobloch, M., Berti, L., Miquelajauregui, A., . . . Jessberger, S. (2011). *Prospero-related homeobox 1 gene (Prox1) is regulated by canonical Wnt signaling and has a stage-specific role in adult hippocampal neurogenesis. Proc Natl Acad Sci U S A, 108(14), 5807-5812.*

Keilhoff, G., Bernstein, H. G., Becker, A., Grecksch, G., & Wolf, G. (2004). *Increased neurogenesis in a rat ketamine model of schizophrenia. Biological psychiatry, 56(5), 317-322.*

Kendler, K. S., Karkowski, L. M., & Prescott, C. A. (1999). *Causal relationship between stressful life events and the onset of major depression. The American journal of psychiatry, 156(6), 837-841.*

Kendler, K. S., Kessler, R. C., Walters, E. E., MacLean, C., Neale, M. C., Heath, A. C., & Eaves, L. J. (1995). *Stressful life events, genetic liability, and onset of an episode of major depression in women. The American journal of psychiatry, 152(6), 833-842.*

Kheirbek, M. A., Klemenhagen, K. C., Sahay, A., & Hen, R. (2012). *Neurogenesis and generalization: a new approach to stratify and treat anxiety disorders. Nat Neurosci, 15(12), 1613-1620.*

Kim, J. Y., Liu, C. Y., Zhang, F., Duan, X., Wen, Z., Song, J., . . . Ming, G. L. (2012). *Interplay between DISC1 and GABA signaling regulates neurogenesis in mice and risk for schizophrenia. Cell, 148(5), 1051-1064.*

Kitayama, N., Vaccarino, V., Kutner, M., Weiss, P., & Bremner, J. D. (2005). *Magnetic resonance imaging (MRI) measurement of hippocampal volume in posttraumatic stress disorder: a meta-analysis. Journal of affective disorders, 88(1), 79-86.*

Knoth, R., Singec, I., Ditter, M., Pantazis, G., Capetian, P., Meyer, R. P., . . . Kempermann, G. (2010). *Murine features of neurogenesis in the human hippocampus across the lifespan from 0 to 100 years. PLoS One, 5(1), e8809.*

Kohl, Z., Winner, B., Ubhi, K., Rockenstein, E., Mante, M., Munch, M., . . . Winkler, J. (2012). *Fluoxetine rescues impaired hippocampal neurogenesis in a transgenic A53T synuclein mouse model. Eur J Neurosci, 35(1), 10-19.*

Kohman, R. A., & Rhodes, J. S. (2013). *Neurogenesis, inflammation and behavior. Brain Behav Immun, 27(1), 22-32.*

Kotani, S., Yamauchi, T., Teramoto, T., & Ogura, H. (2008). Donepezil, an acetylcholinesterase inhibitor, enhances adult hippocampal neurogenesis. Chemico-biological interactions, 175(1-3), 227-230.

Kronenberg, G., Bick-Sander, A., Bunk, E., Wolf, C., Ehninger, D., & Kempermann, G. (2006). Physical exercise prevents age-related decline in precursor cell activity in the mouse dentate gyrus. Neurobiology of aging, 27(10), 1505-1513.

Kuhn, H. G., Dickinson-Anson, H., & Gage, F. H. (1996). Neurogenesis in the dentate gyrus of the adult rat: age-related decrease of neuronal progenitor proliferation. J Neurosci, 16(6), 2027-2033.

Kumaran, D., Udayabanu, M., Nair, R. U., R, A., & Katyal, A. (2008). Benzamide protects delayed neuronal death and behavioural impairment in a mouse model of global cerebral ischemia. Behavioural brain research, 192(2), 178-184.

Kuwabara, T., Hsieh, J., Muotri, A., Yeo, G., Warashina, M., Lie, D. C., . . . Gage, F. H. (2009). Wnt-mediated activation of NeuroD1 and retro-elements during adult neurogenesis. Nat Neurosci, 12(9), 1097-1105.

Lai, K., Kaspar, B. K., Gage, F. H., & Schaffer, D. V. (2003). Sonic hedgehog regulates adult neural progenitor proliferation in vitro and in vivo. Nat Neurosci, 6(1), 21-27.

Larimore, J. L., Chapleau, C. A., Kudo, S., Theibert, A., Percy, A. K., & Pozzo-Miller, L. (2009). Bdnf overexpression in hippocampal neurons prevents dendritic atrophy caused by Rett-associated MECP2 mutations. Neurobiol Dis, 34(2), 199-211.

Lazarov, O., Mattson, M. P., Peterson, D. A., Pimplikar, S. W., & van Praag, H. (2010). When neurogenesis encounters aging and disease. Trends in neurosciences, 33(12), 569-579.

Lazic, S. E., Grote, H., Armstrong, R. J., Blakemore, C., Hannan, A. J., van Dellen, A., & Barker, R. A. (2004). Decreased hippocampal cell proliferation in R6/1 Huntington's mice. Neuroreport, 15(5), 811-813.

Lazic, S. E., Grote, H. E., Blakemore, C., Hannan, A. J., van Dellen, A., Phillips, W., & Barker, R. A. (2006). Neurogenesis in the R6/1 transgenic mouse model of Huntington's disease: effects of environmental enrichment. Eur J Neurosci, 23(7), 1829-1838.

Leutgeb, J. K., Leutgeb, S., Moser, M. B., & Moser, E. I. (2007). Pattern separation in the dentate gyrus and CA3 of the hippocampus. Science, 315(5814), 961-966.

Li, G., Bien-Ly, N., Andrews-Zwilling, Y., Xu, Q., Bernardo, A., Ring, K., . . . Huang, Y. (2009). GABAergic interneuron dysfunction impairs hippocampal neurogenesis in adult apolipoprotein E4 knockin mice. Cell Stem Cell, 5(6), 634-645.

Lie, D. C., Colamarino, S. A., Song, H. J., Desire, L., Mira, H., Consiglio, A., . . . Gage, F. H. (2005). Wnt signalling regulates adult hippocampal neurogenesis. Nature, 437(7063), 1370-1375.

Lieberwirth, C., Liu, Y., Jia, X., & Wang, Z. (2012). Social isolation impairs adult neurogenesis in the limbic system and alters behaviors in female prairie voles. Hormones and behavior, 62(4), 357-366.

Liu, J., Solway, K., Messing, R. O., & Sharp, F. R. (1998). Increased neurogenesis in the dentate gyrus after transient global ischemia in gerbils. J Neurosci, 18(19), 7768-7778.

Liu, J., Suzuki, T., Seki, T., Namba, T., Tanimura, A., & Arai, H. (2006). Effects of repeated phencyclidine administration on adult hippocampal neurogenesis in the rat. Synapse, 60(1), 56-68.

Liu, M., Pereira, F. A., Price, S. D., Chu, M. J., Shope, C., Himes, D., . . . Tsai, M. J. (2000). Essential role of BETA2/NeuroD1 in development of the vestibular and auditory systems. Genes Dev, 14(22), 2839-2854.

Lopez-Munoz, F., Boya, J., & Alamo, C. (2006). Neuron theory, the cornerstone of neuroscience, on the centenary of the Nobel Prize award to Santiago Ramon y Cajal. Brain research bulletin, 70(4-6), 391-405.

Lugert, S., Basak, O., Knuckles, P., Haussler, U., Fabel, K., Gotz, M., . . . Giachino, C. (2010). Quiescent and active hippocampal neural stem cells with distinct morphologies respond selectively to physiological and pathological stimuli and aging. Cell Stem Cell, 6(5), 445-456.

Ma, D. K., Jang, M. H., Guo, J. U., Kitabatake, Y., Chang, M. L., Pow-Anpongkul, N., . . . Song, H. (2009). *Neuronal activity-induced Gadd45b promotes epigenetic DNA demethylation and adult neurogenesis. Science, 323(5917), 1074-1077.*

Ma, D. K., Marchetto, M. C., Guo, J. U., Ming, G. L., Gage, F. H., & Song, H. (2010). *Epigenetic choreographers of neurogenesis in the adult mammalian brain. Nat Neurosci, 13(11), 1338-1344.*

MacDonald, B. T., Tamai, K., & He, X. (2009). *Wnt/beta-catenin signaling: components, mechanisms, and diseases. Developmental cell, 17(1), 9-26.*

MacQueen, G. M., Yucel, K., Taylor, V. H., Macdonald, K., & Joffe, R. (2008). *Posterior hippocampal volumes are associated with remission rates in patients with major depressive disorder. Biological psychiatry, 64(10), 880-883.*

Madsen, T. M., Newton, S. S., Eaton, M. E., Russell, D. S., & Duman, R. S. (2003). *Chronic electroconvulsive seizure up-regulates beta-catenin expression in rat hippocampus: role in adult neurogenesis. Biological psychiatry, 54(10), 1006-1014.*

Madsen, T. M., Treschow, A., Bengzon, J., Bolwig, T. G., Lindvall, O., & Tingstrom, A. (2000). *Increased neurogenesis in a model of electroconvulsive therapy. Biological psychiatry, 47(12), 1043-1049.*

Maeda, K., Sugino, H., Hirose, T., Kitagawa, H., Nagai, T., Mizoguchi, H., . . . Yamada, K. (2007). *Clozapine prevents a decrease in neurogenesis in mice repeatedly treated with phencyclidine. Journal of pharmacological sciences, 103(3), 299-308.*

Maekawa, M., Namba, T., Suzuki, E., Yuasa, S., Kohsaka, S., & Uchino, S. (2009). *NMDA receptor antagonist memantine promotes cell proliferation and production of mature granule neurons in the adult hippocampus. Neuroscience research, 63(4), 259-266.*

Malberg, J. E., & Duman, R. S. (2003). *Cell proliferation in adult hippocampus is decreased by inescapable stress: reversal by fluoxetine treatment. Neuropsychopharmacology, 28(9), 1562-1571.*

Malberg, J. E., Eisch, A. J., Nestler, E. J., & Duman, R. S. (2000). *Chronic antidepressant treatment increases neurogenesis in adult rat hippocampus. J Neurosci, 20(24), 9104-9110.*

Maller, J. J., Daskalakis, Z. J., & Fitzgerald, P. B. (2007). *Hippocampal volumetrics in depression: the importance of the posterior tail. Hippocampus, 17(11), 1023-1027.*

Malykhin, N. V., Carter, R., Seres, P., & Coupland, N. J. (2010). *Structural changes in the hippocampus in major depressive disorder: contributions of disease and treatment. Journal of psychiatry & neuroscience : JPN, 35(5), 337-343.*

Mao, Y., Ge, X., Frank, C. L., Madison, J. M., Koehler, A. N., Doud, M. K., . . . Tsai, L. H. (2009). *Disrupted in schizophrenia 1 regulates neuronal progenitor proliferation via modulation of GSK3beta/beta-catenin signaling. Cell, 136(6), 1017-1031.*

Marksteiner, J., Sperk, G., & Maas, D. (1989). *Differential increases in brain levels of neuropeptide Y and vasoactive intestinal polypeptide after kainic acid-induced seizures in the rat. Naunyn-Schmiedeberg's archives of pharmacology, 339(1-2), 173-177.*

Markwardt, S. J., Wadiche, J. I., & Overstreet-Wadiche, L. S. (2009). *Input-specific GABAergic signaling to newborn neurons in adult dentate gyrus. J Neurosci, 29(48), 15063-15072.*

Marr, D. (1971). *Simple memory: a theory for archicortex. Philosophical transactions of the Royal Society of London. Series B, Biological sciences, 262(841), 23-81.*

Marutle, A., Ohmitsu, M., Nilbratt, M., Greig, N. H., Nordberg, A., & Sugaya, K. (2007). *Modulation of human neural stem cell differentiation in Alzheimer (APP23) transgenic mice by phenserine. Proc Natl Acad Sci U S A, 104(30), 12506-12511.*

Marxreiter, F., Regensburger, M., & Winkler, J. (2013). *Adult neurogenesis in Parkinson's disease. Cell Mol Life Sci, 70(3), 459-473.*

McHugh, T. J., Jones, M. W., Quinn, J. J., Balthasar, N., Coppari, R., Elmquist, J. K., . . . Tonegawa, S. (2007). Dentate gyrus NMDA receptors mediate rapid pattern separation in the hippocampal network. Science, 317(5834), 94-99.

Millar, J. K., Wilson-Annan, J. C., Anderson, S., Christie, S., Taylor, M. S., Semple, C. A., . . . Porteous, D. J. (2000). Disruption of two novel genes by a translocation co-segregating with schizophrenia. Human molecular genetics, 9(9), 1415-1423.

Ming, G. L., & Song, H. (2011). Adult neurogenesis in the mammalian brain: significant answers and significant questions. Neuron, 70(4), 687-702.

Moffat, S. D., Szekely, C. A., Zonderman, A. B., Kabani, N. J., & Resnick, S. M. (2000). Longitudinal change in hippocampal volume as a function of apolipoprotein E genotype. Neurology, 55(1), 134-136.

Monje, M. L., Toda, H., & Palmer, T. D. (2003). Inflammatory blockade restores adult hippocampal neurogenesis. Science, 302(5651), 1760-1765.

Moretti, P., Levenson, J. M., Battaglia, F., Atkinson, R., Teague, R., Antalffy, B., . . . Zoghbi, H. Y. (2006). Learning and memory and synaptic plasticity are impaired in a mouse model of Rett syndrome. J Neurosci, 26(1), 319-327.

Mu, Y., & Gage, F. H. (2011). Adult hippocampal neurogenesis and its role in Alzheimer's disease. Molecular neurodegeneration, 6, 85.

Nacher, J., Alonso-Llosa, G., Rosell, D. R., & McEwen, B. S. (2003). NMDA receptor antagonist treatment increases the production of new neurons in the aged rat hippocampus. Neurobiology of aging, 24(2), 273-284.

Nacher, J., Rosell, D. R., Alonso-Llosa, G., & McEwen, B. S. (2001). NMDA receptor antagonist treatment induces a long-lasting increase in the number of proliferating cells, PSA-NCAM-immunoreactive granule neurons and radial glia in the adult rat dentate gyrus. Eur J Neurosci, 13(3), 512-520.

Nacher, J., Varea, E., Miguel Blasco-Ibanez, J., Gomez-Climent, M. A., Castillo-Gomez, E., Crespo, C., . . . McEwen, B. S. (2007). N-methyl-d-aspartate receptor expression during adult neurogenesis in the rat dentate gyrus. Neuroscience, 144(3), 855-864.

Nakashiba, T., Cushman, J. D., Pelkey, K. A., Renaudineau, S., Buhl, D. L., McHugh, T. J., . . . Tonegawa, S. (2012). Young dentate granule cells mediate pattern separation, whereas old granule cells facilitate pattern completion. Cell, 149(1), 188-201.

Namba, T., Maekawa, M., Yuasa, S., Kohsaka, S., & Uchino, S. (2009). The Alzheimer's disease drug memantine increases the number of radial glia-like progenitor cells in adult hippocampus. Glia, 57(10), 1082-1090.

Namba, T., Ming, G. L., Song, H., Waga, C., Enomoto, A., Kaibuchi, K., . . . Uchino, S. (2011). NMDA receptor regulates migration of newly generated neurons in the adult hippocampus via Disrupted-In-Schizophrenia 1 (DISC1). Journal of neurochemistry, 118(1), 34-44.

Nelson, E. D., Kavalali, E. T., & Monteggia, L. M. (2006). MeCP2-dependent transcriptional repression regulates excitatory neurotransmission. Current biology : CB, 16(7), 710-716.

Neumeister, A., Wood, S., Bonne, O., Nugent, A. C., Luckenbaugh, D. A., Young, T., . . . Drevets, W. C. (2005). Reduced hippocampal volume in unmedicated, remitted patients with major depression versus control subjects. Biological psychiatry, 57(8), 935-937.

Nichol, K., Deeny, S. P., Seif, J., Camaclang, K., & Cotman, C. W. (2009). Exercise improves cognition and hippocampal plasticity in APOE epsilon4 mice. Alzheimer's & dementia : the journal of the Alzheimer's Association, 5(4), 287-294.

Nuber, S., Petrasch-Parwez, E., Winner, B., Winkler, J., von Horsten, S., Schmidt, T., . . . Riess, O. (2008). Neurodegeneration and motor dysfunction in a conditional model of Parkinson's disease. J Neurosci, 28(10), 2471-2484.

Okamoto, H., Voleti, B., Banasr, M., Sarhan, M., Duric, V., Girgenti, M. J., . . . Duman, R. S. (2010). Wnt2 expression and signaling is increased by different classes of antidepressant treatments. Biological psychiatry, 68(6), 521-527.

Olariu, A., Cleaver, K. M., & Cameron, H. A. (2007). Decreased neurogenesis in aged rats results from loss of granule cell precursors without lengthening of the cell cycle. J Comp Neurol, 501(4), 659-667.

Overstreet-Wadiche, L. S., Bromberg, D. A., Bensen, A. L., & Westbrook, G. L. (2006). Seizures accelerate functional integration of adult-generated granule cells. J Neurosci, 26(15), 4095-4103.

Parent, J. M., Yu, T. W., Leibowitz, R. T., Geschwind, D. H., Sloviter, R. S., & Lowenstein, D. H. (1997). Dentate granule cell neurogenesis is increased by seizures and contributes to aberrant network reorganization in the adult rat hippocampus. J Neurosci, 17(10), 3727-3738.

Pariante, C. M. (2009). Risk factors for development of depression and psychosis. Glucocorticoid receptors and pituitary implications for treatment with antidepressant and glucocorticoids. Ann N Y Acad Sci, 1179, 144-152.

Pennington, B. F., Moon, J., Edgin, J., Stedron, J., & Nadel, L. (2003). The neuropsychology of Down syndrome: evidence for hippocampal dysfunction. Child development, 74(1), 75-93.

Perera, T. D., Coplan, J. D., Lisanby, S. H., Lipira, C. M., Arif, M., Carpio, C., . . . Dwork, A. J. (2007). Antidepressant-induced neurogenesis in the hippocampus of adult nonhuman primates. J Neurosci, 27(18), 4894-4901.

Pham, K., Nacher, J., Hof, P. R., & McEwen, B. S. (2003). Repeated restraint stress suppresses neurogenesis and induces biphasic PSA-NCAM expression in the adult rat dentate gyrus. Eur J Neurosci, 17(4), 879-886.

Phillips, W., Morton, A. J., & Barker, R. A. (2005). Abnormalities of neurogenesis in the R6/2 mouse model of Huntington's disease are attributable to the in vivo microenvironment. J Neurosci, 25(50), 11564-11576.

Pickard, B. S., Christoforou, A., Thomson, P. A., Fawkes, A., Evans, K. L., Morris, S. W., . . . Muir, W. J. (2009). Interacting haplotypes at the NPAS3 locus alter risk of schizophrenia and bipolar disorder. Mol Psychiatry, 14(9), 874-884.

Pieper, A. A., Wu, X., Han, T. W., Estill, S. J., Dang, Q., Wu, L. C., . . . McKnight, S. L. (2005). The neuronal PAS domain protein 3 transcription factor controls FGF-mediated adult hippocampal neurogenesis in mice. Proc Natl Acad Sci U S A, 102(39), 14052-14057.

Pierfelice, T., Alberi, L., & Gaiano, N. (2011). Notch in the vertebrate nervous system: an old dog with new tricks. Neuron, 69(5), 840-855.

Pla, P., Orvoen, S., Benstaali, C., Dodier, S., Gardier, A. M., David, D. J., . . . Saudou, F. (2013). Huntingtin acts non cell-autonomously on hippocampal neurogenesis and controls anxiety-related behaviors in adult mouse. PLoS One, 8(9), e73902.

Qu, Q., Sun, G., Li, W., Yang, S., Ye, P., Zhao, C., . . . Shi, Y. (2010). Orphan nuclear receptor TLX activates Wnt/beta-catenin signalling to stimulate neural stem cell proliferation and self-renewal. Nature cell biology, 12(1), 31-40; sup pp 31-39.

Raber, J., Fan, Y., Matsumori, Y., Liu, Z., Weinstein, P. R., Fike, J. R., & Liu, J. (2004). Irradiation attenuates neurogenesis and exacerbates ischemia-induced deficits. Annals of neurology, 55(3), 381-389.

Rai, K. S., Hattiangady, B., & Shetty, A. K. (2007). Enhanced production and dendritic growth of new dentate granule cells in the middle-aged hippocampus following intracerebroventricular FGF-2 infusions. Eur J Neurosci, 26(7), 1765-1779.

Rao, M. S., Hattiangady, B., & Shetty, A. K. (2006). The window and mechanisms of major age-related decline in the production of new neurons within the dentate gyrus of the hippocampus. Aging Cell, 5(6), 545-558.

Rao, M. S., Hattiangady, B., & Shetty, A. K. (2008). Status epilepticus during old age is not associated with enhanced hippocampal neurogenesis. Hippocampus, 18(9), 931-944.

Reif, A., Fritzen, S., Finger, M., Strobel, A., Lauer, M., Schmitt, A., & Lesch, K. P. (2006). Neural stem cell proliferation is decreased in schizophrenia, but not in depression. Mol Psychiatry, 11(5), 514-522.

Rogaev, E. I., Sherrington, R., Rogaeva, E. A., Levesque, G., Ikeda, M., Liang, Y., . . . et al. (1995). Familial Alzheimer's disease in kindreds with missense mutations in a gene on chromosome 1 related to the Alzheimer's disease type 3 gene. Nature, 376(6543), 775-778.

Rohatgi, R., Milenkovic, L., & Scott, M. P. (2007). Patched1 regulates hedgehog signaling at the primary cilium. Science, 317(5836), 372-376.

Rolls, E. T. (2010). A computational theory of episodic memory formation in the hippocampus. Behavioural brain research, 215(2), 180-196.

Rolls, E. T., & Kesner, R. P. (2006). A computational theory of hippocampal function, and empirical tests of the theory. Progress in neurobiology, 79(1), 1-48.

Sahay, A., Scobie, K. N., Hill, A. S., O'Carroll, C. M., Kheirbek, M. A., Burghardt, N. S., . . . Hen, R. (2011). Increasing adult hippocampal neurogenesis is sufficient to improve pattern separation. Nature, 472(7344), 466-470.

Sairanen, M., Lucas, G., Ernfors, P., Castren, M., & Castren, E. (2005). Brain-derived neurotrophic factor and antidepressant drugs have different but coordinated effects on neuronal turnover, proliferation, and survival in the adult dentate gyrus. J Neurosci, 25(5), 1089-1094.

Sanai, N., Nguyen, T., Ihrie, R. A., Mirzadeh, Z., Tsai, H. H., Wong, M., . . . Alvarez-Buylla, A. (2011). Corridors of migrating neurons in the human brain and their decline during infancy. Nature, 478(7369), 382-386.

Sandi, C. (2008). A role for NCAM in depression and antidepressant actions? (Commentary on Aonurm-Helm et al.). Eur J Neurosci, 28(8), 1617.

Santarelli, L., Saxe, M., Gross, C., Surget, A., Battaglia, F., Dulawa, S., . . . Hen, R. (2003). Requirement of hippocampal neurogenesis for the behavioral effects of antidepressants. Science, 301(5634), 805-809.

Sawyer, K., Corsentino, E., Sachs-Ericsson, N., & Steffens, D. C. (2012). Depression, hippocampal volume changes, and cognitive decline in a clinical sample of older depressed outpatients and non-depressed controls. Aging & mental health, 16(6), 753-762.

Scharfman, H., Goodman, J., Macleod, A., Phani, S., Antonelli, C., & Croll, S. (2005). Increased neurogenesis and the ectopic granule cells after intrahippocampal BDNF infusion in adult rats. Exp Neurol, 192(2), 348-356.

Seib, D. R., Corsini, N. S., Ellwanger, K., Plaas, C., Mateos, A., Pitzer, C., . . . Martin-Villalba, A. (2013). Loss of Dickkopf-1 restores neurogenesis in old age and counteracts cognitive decline. Cell Stem Cell, 12(2), 204-214.

Selkoe, D. J., & Wolfe, M. S. (2007). Presenilin: running with scissors in the membrane. Cell, 131(2), 215-221.

Sha, L., MacIntyre, L., Machell, J. A., Kelly, M. P., Porteous, D. J., Brandon, N. J., . . . Pickard, B. S. (2012). Transcriptional regulation of neurodevelopmental and metabolic pathways by NPAS3. Mol Psychiatry, 17(3), 267-279.

Sherrington, R., Rogaev, E. I., Liang, Y., Rogaeva, E. A., Levesque, G., Ikeda, M., . . . St George-Hyslop, P. H. (1995). Cloning of a gene bearing missense mutations in early-onset familial Alzheimer's disease. Nature, 375(6534), 754-760.

Shetty, A. K., Hattiangady, B., Rao, M. S., & Shuai, B. (2012). Neurogenesis response of middle-aged hippocampus to acute seizure activity. PLoS One, 7(8), e43286.

Shetty, A. K., & Turner, D. A. (2000). Fetal hippocampal grafts containing CA3 cells restore host hippocampal glutamate decarboxylase-positive interneuron numbers in a rat model of temporal lobe epilepsy. J Neurosci, 20(23), 8788-8801.

Shors, T. J., Miesegaes, G., Beylin, A., Zhao, M., Rydel, T., & Gould, E. (2001). Neurogenesis in the adult is involved in the formation of trace memories. Nature, 410(6826), 372-376.

Sierra, A., Encinas, J. M., Deudero, J. J., Chancey, J. H., Enikolopov, G., Overstreet-Wadiche, L. S., . . . Maletic-Savatic, M. (2010). Microglia shape adult hippocampal neurogenesis through apoptosis-coupled phagocytosis. Cell Stem Cell, 7(4), 483-495.

Simon, R., Brylka, H., Schwegler, H., Venkataramanappa, S., Andratschke, J., Wiegreffe, C., . . . Britsch, S. (2012). A dual function of Bcl11b/Ctip2 in hippocampal neurogenesis. EMBO J, 31(13), 2922-2936.

Sirerol-Piquer, M., Gomez-Ramos, P., Hernandez, F., Perez, M., Moran, M. A., Fuster-Matanzo, A., . . . Garcia-Verdugo, J. M. (2011). GSK3beta overexpression induces neuronal death and a depletion of the neurogenic niches in the dentate gyrus. Hippocampus, 21(8), 910-922.

Smith, M. L., & Milner, B. (1981). The role of the right hippocampus in the recall of spatial location. Neuropsychologia, 19(6), 781-793.

Smrt, R. D., Eaves-Egenes, J., Barkho, B. Z., Santistevan, N. J., Zhao, C., Aimone, J. B., . . . Zhao, X. (2007). Mecp2 deficiency leads to delayed maturation and altered gene expression in hippocampal neurons. Neurobiol Dis, 27(1), 77-89.

Snyder, J. S., Soumier, A., Brewer, M., Pickel, J., & Cameron, H. A. (2011). Adult hippocampal neurogenesis buffers stress responses and depressive behaviour. Nature, 476(7361), 458-461.

Soares, L. M., Schiavon, A. P., Milani, H., & de Oliveira, R. M. (2013). Cognitive impairment and persistent anxiety-related responses following bilateral common carotid artery occlusion in mice. Behavioural brain research, 249, 28-37.

Song, H., Stevens, C. F., & Gage, F. H. (2002). Astroglia induce neurogenesis from adult neural stem cells. Nature, 417(6884), 39-44.

Song, J., Zhong, C., Bonaguidi, M. A., Sun, G. J., Hsu, D., Gu, Y., . . . Song, H. (2012). Neuronal circuitry mechanism regulating adult quiescent neural stem-cell fate decision. Nature, 489(7414), 150-154.

Spaccapelo, L., Bitto, A., Galantucci, M., Ottani, A., Irrera, N., Minutoli, L., . . . Guarini, S. (2011). Melanocortin MC(4) receptor agonists counteract late inflammatory and apoptotic responses and improve neuronal functionality after cerebral ischemia. European journal of pharmacology, 670(2-3), 479-486.

Spaccapelo, L., Galantucci, M., Neri, L., Contri, M., Pizzala, R., D'Amico, R., . . . Guarini, S. (2013). Up-regulation of the canonical Wnt-3A and Sonic hedgehog signaling underlies melanocortin-induced neurogenesis after cerebral ischemia. European journal of pharmacology, 707(1-3), 78-86.

Spalding, K. L., Bergmann, O., Alkass, K., Bernard, S., Salehpour, M., Huttner, H. B., . . . Frisen, J. (2013). Dynamics of hippocampal neurogenesis in adult humans. Cell, 153(6), 1219-1227.

Stagni, F., Magistretti, J., Guidi, S., Ciani, E., Mangano, C., Calza, L., & Bartesaghi, R. (2013). Pharmacotherapy with fluoxetine restores functional connectivity from the dentate gyrus to field CA3 in the Ts65Dn mouse model of down syndrome. PLoS One, 8(4), e61689.

Stork, O., Welzl, H., Wolfer, D., Schuster, T., Mantei, N., Stork, S., . . . Schachner, M. (2000). Recovery of emotional behaviour in neural cell adhesion molecule (NCAM) null mutant mice through transgenic expression of NCAM180. Eur J Neurosci, 12(9), 3291-3306.

Stork, O., Welzl, H., Wotjak, C. T., Hoyer, D., Delling, M., Cremer, H., & Schachner, M. (1999). Anxiety and increased 5-HT1A receptor response in NCAM null mutant mice. J Neurobiol, 40(3), 343-355.

Sullivan, P. F., Kendler, K. S., & Neale, M. C. (2003). Schizophrenia as a complex trait: evidence from a meta-analysis of twin studies. Archives of general psychiatry, 60(12), 1187-1192.

Szulwach, K. E., Li, X., Smrt, R. D., Li, Y., Luo, Y., Lin, L., . . . Jin, P. (2010). Cross talk between microRNA and epigenetic regulation in adult neurogenesis. J Cell Biol, 189(1), 127-141.

Tashiro, A., Sandler, V. M., Toni, N., Zhao, C., & Gage, F. H. (2006). NMDA-receptor-mediated, cell-specific integration of new neurons in adult dentate gyrus. Nature, 442(7105), 929-933.

Taylor, W. D., Steffens, D. C., Payne, M. E., MacFall, J. R., Marchuk, D. A., Svenson, I. K., & Krishnan, K. R. (2005). Influence of serotonin transporter promoter region polymorphisms on hippocampal volumes in late-life depression. Archives of general psychiatry, 62(5), 537-544.

Thomas, R. M., Hotsenpiller, G., & Peterson, D. A. (2007). Acute psychosocial stress reduces cell survival in adult hippocampal neurogenesis without altering proliferation. J Neurosci, 27(11), 2734-2743.

Thompson, K. (2009). Transplantation of GABA-producing cells for seizure control in models of temporal lobe epilepsy. Neurotherapeutics : the journal of the American Society for Experimental NeuroTherapeutics, 6(2), 284-294.

Trazzi, S., Mitrugno, V. M., Valli, E., Fuchs, C., Rizzi, S., Guidi, S., . . . Ciani, E. (2011). APP-dependent up-regulation of Ptch1 underlies proliferation impairment of neural precursors in Down syndrome. Human molecular genetics, 20(8), 1560-1573.

Tronel, S., Belnoue, L., Grosjean, N., Revest, J. M., Piazza, P. V., Koehl, M., & Abrous, D. N. (2012). Adult-born neurons are necessary for extended contextual discrimination. Hippocampus, 22(2), 292-298.

Tsujimura, K., Abematsu, M., Kohyama, J., Namihira, M., & Nakashima, K. (2009). Neuronal differentiation of neural precursor cells is promoted by the methyl-CpG-binding protein MeCP2. Exp Neurol, 219(1), 104-111.

Turner, D. A., & Shetty, A. K. (2003). Clinical prospects for neural grafting therapy for hippocampal lesions and epilepsy. Neurosurgery, 52(3), 632-644; discussion 641-634.

Vallieres, L., Campbell, I. L., Gage, F. H., & Sawchenko, P. E. (2002). Reduced hippocampal neurogenesis in adult transgenic mice with chronic astrocytic production of interleukin-6. J Neurosci, 22(2), 486-492.

van Praag, H., Kempermann, G., & Gage, F. H. (1999). Running increases cell proliferation and neurogenesis in the adult mouse dentate gyrus. Nat Neurosci, 2(3), 266-270.

van Praag, H., Shubert, T., Zhao, C., & Gage, F. H. (2005). Exercise enhances learning and hippocampal neurogenesis in aged mice. J Neurosci, 25(38), 8680-8685.

Waldau, B., Hattiangady, B., Kuruba, R., & Shetty, A. K. (2010). Medial ganglionic eminence-derived neural stem cell grafts ease spontaneous seizures and restore GDNF expression in a rat model of chronic temporal lobe epilepsy. Stem Cells, 28(7), 1153-1164.

Wang, J. W., David, D. J., Monckton, J. E., Battaglia, F., & Hen, R. (2008). Chronic fluoxetine stimulates maturation and synaptic plasticity of adult-born hippocampal granule cells. J Neurosci, 28(6), 1374-1384.

Wechsler-Reya, R. J., & Scott, M. P. (1999). Control of neuronal precursor proliferation in the cerebellum by Sonic Hedgehog. Neuron, 22(1), 103-114.

Wen, P. H., Shao, X., Shao, Z., Hof, P. R., Wisniewski, T., Kelley, K., . . . Elder, G. A. (2002). Overexpression of wild type but not an FAD mutant presenilin-1 promotes neurogenesis in the hippocampus of adult mice. Neurobiol Dis, 10(1), 8-19.

Wexler, E. M., Geschwind, D. H., & Palmer, T. D. (2008). Lithium regulates adult hippocampal progenitor development through canonical Wnt pathway activation. Mol Psychiatry, 13(3), 285-292.

Wu, M. D., Hein, A. M., Moravan, M. J., Shaftel, S. S., Olschowka, J. A., & O'Banion, M. K. (2012). Adult murine hippocampal neurogenesis is inhibited by sustained IL-1beta and not rescued by voluntary running. Brain Behav Immun, 26(2), 292-300.

Yan, B., Bi, X., He, J., Zhang, Y., Thakur, S., Xu, H., . . . Li, X. M. (2007). Quetiapine attenuates spatial memory impairment and hippocampal neurodegeneration induced by bilateral common carotid artery occlusion in mice. Life sciences, 81(5), 353-361.

Yan, B., He, J., Xu, H., Zhang, Y., Bi, X., Thakur, S., . . . Li, X. M. (2007). Quetiapine attenuates the depressive and anxiolytic-like behavioural changes induced by global cerebral ischemia in mice. Behavioural brain research, 182(1), 36-41.

Yang, C. P., Gilley, J. A., Zhang, G., & Kernie, S. G. (2011). ApoE is required for maintenance of the dentate gyrus neural progenitor pool. Development, 138(20), 4351-4362.

Yun, J., Koike, H., Ibi, D., Toth, E., Mizoguchi, H., Nitta, A., . . . Yamada, K. (2010). Chronic restraint stress impairs neurogenesis and hippocampus-dependent fear memory in mice: possible involvement of a brain-specific transcription factor Npas4. Journal of neurochemistry, 114(6), 1840-1851.

Zaidel, D. W., Esiri, M. M., & Harrison, P. J. (1997). Size, shape, and orientation of neurons in the left and right hippocampus: investigation of normal asymmetries and alterations in schizophrenia. The American journal of psychiatry, 154(6), 812-818.

Zhang, C., McNeil, E., Dressler, L., & Siman, R. (2007). Long-lasting impairment in hippocampal neurogenesis associated with amyloid deposition in a knock-in mouse model of familial Alzheimer's disease. Exp Neurol, 204(1), 77-87.

Zhang, C. L., Zou, Y., He, W., Gage, F. H., & Evans, R. M. (2008). A role for adult TLX-positive neural stem cells in learning and behaviour. Nature, 451(7181), 1004-1007.

Zhang, L., Fu, F., Zhang, X., Zhu, M., Wang, T., & Fan, H. (2010). Escin attenuates cognitive deficits and hippocampal injury after transient global cerebral ischemia in mice via regulating certain inflammatory genes. Neurochemistry international, 57(2), 119-127.

Zhao, C., Deng, W., & Gage, F. H. (2008). Mechanisms and functional implications of adult neurogenesis. Cell, 132(4), 645-660.

Zhao, C., Teng, E. M., Summers, R. G., Jr., Ming, G. L., & Gage, F. H. (2006). Distinct morphological stages of dentate granule neuron maturation in the adult mouse hippocampus. J Neurosci, 26(1), 3-11.

Zhao, M., Li, D., Shimazu, K., Zhou, Y. X., Lu, B., & Deng, C. X. (2007). Fibroblast growth factor receptor-1 is required for long-term potentiation, memory consolidation, and neurogenesis. Biological psychiatry, 62(5), 381-390.

Zhao, X., Ueba, T., Christie, B. R., Barkho, B., McConnell, M. J., Nakashima, K., . . . Gage, F. H. (2003). Mice lacking methyl-CpG binding protein 1 have deficits in adult neurogenesis and hippocampal function. Proc Natl Acad Sci U S A, 100(11), 6777-6782.

Zunszain, P. A., Anacker, C., Cattaneo, A., Carvalho, L. A., & Pariante, C. M. (2011). Glucocorticoids, cytokines and brain abnormalities in depression. Prog Neuropsychopharmacol Biol Psychiatry, 35(3), 722-729.

Clinical Examination of Psychosis

Arabinda Narayan Chowdhury
Northamptonshire Healthcare NHS Foundation Trust, UK
Institute of Psychiatry, Kolkata, India

Satyadev Nagari
Crisis Home Treatment Team
Dudley and Walsall Healthcare NHS Trust, Walsall, UK

1   Introduction

Psychosis is a symptom or feature of mental illness typically characterized by radical changes in personality, impaired functioning, and a distorted or nonexistent sense of objective reality. Detection of psychotic features is an important clinical skill that not only helps for correct diagnosis but also focuses on the subsequent treatment, risk assessment and management.

The term Psychosis came from the Greek word: *ψύχωσις: ψυχή* (*psyche*), "soul" suffix *-ωσις* (-*osis*), "abnormal condition". The word *psychosis* was introduced to the psychiatric literature in 1841 by Karl Friedrich Canstatt (1807 – 1850), a German physician and medical author in his work *Handbuch der Medizinischen Klinik*. Ernst von Feuchtersleben (1806 – 1849), an Austrian poet, politician, and psychiatrist, is also credited for introducing the term in 1845, as an alternative to insanity and mania.

The term *Neurosis* was coined by the Scottish physician William Cullen in 1796 to refer to "disorders of sense of motion" due to affection of the nervous system. The term derives from the Greek word *"νεῦρον"* (neuron, "nerve") with the suffix *-osis* (diseased or abnormal condition). The phenomenological aspect of psychosis-neurosis debate spanned over hundred years with many modifications and nosological interchange (Burgy, 2008). Jaspers (1913) in his first edition of "General Psychopathology" clarified the dichotomy between psychoses and neuroses: psychosis is the result of somatic illness and neurosis results from psychological causes. Sigmund Freud (1856 – 1938), Carl Jung (1875 – 1961) and Karen Horney (1885 – 1952) elaborated further the concept and phenomenology of neurosis. They emphasized and popularized the term "psychoneuroses" at the turn of the century, and the successful treatment of apparently healthy soldiers suffering from shellshock in World War I established firmly the entity of *neuroses*, as well. DSM III (1980) and ICD 10 (WHO, 1991) however, discarded this concept of psychosis-neurosis as the basis of classification although in global literature, the terms neurosis and psychoneurosis is still appearing with its accompanying controversies (Roth, 1963; Neve, 2004; Chaturvedi & Bhugra, 2007).

Psychosis is characterized by the following main symptoms: 1. Delusions, 2. Hallucinations, 3. Disorganized speech, 4. Disorganized and/or catatonic behavior and 5. Lack of insight or inability to recognize one's illness.

2   Clinical Examination of Psychosis

The following five areas of Mental State Examination are important: (1) Thought System; (2) Perception; (3) Speech; (4) Behaviour and (5) Insight.

2.1   Examination of Thought System

Thinking refers to the ideational components of mental activity, processes used to imagine, appraise, evaluate, forecast, create and will. Individuals vary greatly in their predominant cognitive style, *i.e.,* the manner of information processing and decision-making. An obsessional style of thinking is marked by attention to detail and hypervigilence concerning the anticipated implications of a thought or event. In depression the thought process is slow and they are unable to make any decisions, often having negative thinking and may believe firmly that suicide is the only option open to them. A hysterical style of thinking is characterized by global, diffuse, emotionally laden evaluations of situation superficially. Thought process may be influenced by stress or fatigue or disease condition.

Clinical evaluation of Thought Disorder examines four components of thought process, viz., Stream, Form, Possession and Content:

A. Stream (Flow): It is the speed of the thought, the nature of which may be any of the following:

Normal	Accelerated	Retarded	Mute
Pressure of thought	Racing thoughts	Poverty of thought	Verbigeration
Incoherence	Word Salad	Stereotypy	Frequent pauses
Interrupted by cry	Interrupted by anxiety	Interrupted by Stammering	

B. Form (Continuity): It is how thought content is organized to form coherent thoughts and sentences by following the conventional semantic and syntactic rules of language. It may clinically present as:

Circumstantiality	Tangentiality	Derailment	Loosening of Association	Flight of Ideas
Thought Blocking	Paragrammatism	Neologism	Clang Association	Perseveration
Echolalia	Palilalia	Illogical Thinking	Over-inclusive thinking	Concrete thinking

Formal Thought Disorders (FTD): disturbances in speech comprehension and coherence that affect the semantic and pragmatic aspects of language in schizophrenia (Salavera *et al*., 2013).

Formal Thought Disorders: Mnemonic: NCC DIPTT

- **N** = *Neologism:* non-word phonemic combinations used as words.

- **C** = *Clang Association:* shift in frame of reference driven by phonetic similarity of words rather than tropical relationships.

- **C** = *Circumstantiality:* indirect speech, delayed in reaching the point but eventually gets from original point to desired goal, found in schizophrenia, dementia, and anxiety disorder. Circumstantial style is not necessarily pathologic. Non-patients circumstantial persons are called "long-winded".

- **D** = *Derailment:* gradual or sudden deviation in train of thought without blocking.

- **I** = *Flight of Ideas:* A special case of *Loosening of Association* (LOA) when there are rapid shifts in frame of reference and the incoherent associations occur very rapidly. Andreasen (1979) states, "flight of ideas is a derailment that occurs rapidly in the context of pressured speech". Typically this may represent increased speed of talk, increased volume and it is difficult to interrupt the patient. There are three types: with rhyming or clanging, with association by meaning, including opposites (*e.g.* white, black) and with distraction (Wing *et al*., 1974). It is not necessarily equivalent to either pressured speech (coherent but rapid speech) or racing thoughts (coherent).

- **P** = *Perseveration:* inappropriate repetition of particular word or phrases or concept during the course of speech, seen in dementia, OCD, psychosis.

- **T** = *Tangentiality:* inability to have goal-directed associations of thought. Found in psychosis and dementia. In dementia it is also called "rambling".

- **T** = *Thought Blocking:* abrupt interruption in train of thought before finishing.

The concept of FTD as diagnostic feature of schizophrenia is recently been criticized and research has shown that individuals with Autistic Spectrum Disorder also display similar language disturbances (Solomon *et al.*, 2008). *Loosening of Association* - a disturbance of thinking in which the association of ideas and thought patterns becomes so vague, fragmented, diffuse, and unfocused as to lack any logical sequences or relationship to any preceding concepts or themes. This term was introduced by Eugene Bleuler in 1911. Related terms are: Derailment, Disjointed speech, Loss of goal and Flight of ideas. LOA is a hallmark feature of schizophrenia.

- **Paragrammatism:** ungrammatical word sequences.

- **Pressured Speech:** speech produced at an abnormally high rate, rapid speech that is difficult to interrupt, usually loud and intense. Characteristic for mania.

- **Racing Thoughts:** subjective sense of one's thoughts going so fast that they're hard to keep track of, may or may not be associated with pressured speech. Seen in obsession, anxiety, substance-abusing patients undergoing detoxification.

- **Echolalia:** repetitions of a sentence just uttered by the examiner.

- **Palilalia:** repetitions of only the last uttered word or phrase said by the examiner.

- **Poverty of Speech or Thought:** reduced conversational output, very little spontaneous speech.

- **Verbigeration:** disappearance of understandable speech, replaced by strings of incoherent utterances.

- **Word Salad:** extreme version of LOA in which changes in topic are so extreme and the associations so loose that the resulting speech is completely incoherent.

- **Stereotypy:** constant repetition of a phrase (or behaviour) in many different settings, irrespective of the context.

- **Concrete thinking:** literal interpretation (superficial) rather than abstract representation of a more general concept and failure to understand metaphorical expressions. (Abstract thinking: depth thinking, ability to use concepts and to make and understand generalizations).

- **Illogical Thinking:** breakdown in reasoning, where conclusions are reached that do not follow logically (faulty inferences).

- **Over-inclusive Thinking:** tendency to include items which are only remotely relevant into the stream of thoughts, i.e., inability to preserve conceptual boundaries.

- **Drivelling:** there is a disordered intermixture of the constituent parts of one complex thought.

- **Omission:** where a thought or part of a thought is senselessly omitted.

- **Substitution:** where one thought fills the gap for another appropriate more "fitting-in" thought.

- **Fusion:** various thoughts are fused together, leading to a loss of goal direction.

- **Metonyms:** are word approximations e.g. paper skate for pen.

- **Condensation:** a single symbol or word is associated with the emotional content of several, not necessarily related, ideas, feelings, memories, or impulses, especially as expressed in dreams.

C. Possession: Alteration in the experience of one's own thought, which may be perceived by the subject as any of the following:

Thought Control	Thought Insertion	Thought Withdrawal	Thought Broadcasting	Thought Echo
Thought Blocking	Thought Diffusion	Magical Thinking	Referential Thinking	Thought Diffusion

- **Thought Control:** other people or forces controlling or directing one's thought.

- **Thought Insertion:** other person or forces are implanting thoughts in a person's mind.

- **Thought Withdrawal:** other person or forces are removing thoughts from a person's mind or thoughts have been stolen from one's mind. This is also known as Thought Alienation.

- **Thought Broadcasting:** one's own thoughts experienced as being transmitted to another person or agency.

- **Thought Echo:** hearing one's own thought being spoken aloud.

- **Thought Diffusion:** belief that as he/she is thinking, everyone else is thinking in unison with him/her (everyone else is participating in his/her thoughts)

- **Magical Thinking:** irrational belief that thoughts can change external events without intervening actions.

- **Referential Thinking:** perceptions of other people's actions or speech are directed to or are in reference to the self.

D. Content - also known as *Belief*. Two broad divisions are: (a) Non-delusional thoughts and (b) Delusional thoughts.

A. Non-delusional abnormal thoughts				
Suicidal Thought	Homicidal Thought	Worthlessness	Hopelessness	Guilt/Sin
Free-floating Anxiety	Obsession	Phobia	Overvalued Ideas	Grandiosity
Paranoia	Suspiciousness	Hypochondriasis*	Dysmorphophobia*	Eating disorders*

*Often reach to delusional proportion.

- **Suicidal thought or intent or self-harm thought** ("Do you have any thoughts of wanting to harm or kill yourself?") or *Homicidal ideation or intent* ("Do you have any thoughts of wanting to hurt anyone?") should be inquired in detail. Please note that if there is any indication of current suicidal or homicidal ideation, thought, plan or intent the person must have a thorough risk assessment and management.

- **Homicidal ideation or thoughts** spans from vague ideas of revenge to detailed plans without any act (Thienhaus & Piasecki, 1998), should always be taken seriously. Homicidal thoughts in response to command hallucination is an important issue of risk assessment in psychotic patients. Apprehension of hurting or harming others is seen as an obsessive rumination as well.

- **Worthlessness and Hopelessness:** Worthlessness is a pattern of subjective thinking where the individual thinks that he/she is without any worth, of no use, importance, or value and is good-for-nothing. *Hopelessness* causes the individual to believe that they are trapped in misery with no expectation of things ever getting better. It is a feeling that the present conditions will never improve, that there is no solution to a problem, and, for many, a feeling that dying by suicide would be better than living ("There are no solutions to my problems" or "I just want to give up"). Both are signs of depressive thinking. Beck (1988) developed a scale for hopelessness (20 item self-report inventory). Beck's "Four Ds" in depression are: Feelings of Defeated, Defective, Deserted, and Deprived.

- **Guilt/Sin:** Guilt is a normal emotion that is expressed as self-reproach and remorse for one's behavior, as if one violated a moral principle (Klass, 1987). Guilt, whether imagined or real, is an important thought content in major depressive disorder, PTSD and anxiety (pathological guilt). Guilt is an important factor in perpetuating obsessive-compulsive symptoms (Shapiro & Stewart, 2011). The feeling of guilt has a number of negative psychological impacts. It erodes self-esteem and confidence, creates self-doubt and adds negative emotions like feelings of shame, blame and worthlessness. Guilt may be of different types like Introspective guilt (bringing awareness of guilt laden act or thoughts), Perceived guilt (false sense of guilt), Retrospective guilt (discovering some past issues), Religious guilt (concept of sin and punishment by God) and Pathological guilt (out of proportion to the real or imagined event or act).

- **Free-floating Anxiety:** sense of dread and/or impending doom or preoccupation with health related or situational factor in anxiety disorder.

- **Obsession:** repetitive preoccupation with a thought, acknowledged by the patient to be irrational and associated with anxiety. Main four types: Ruminations (single or series of thoughts around a theme); Imagery (distressing images often of erotic nature involving relatives); Ideas (distressing) and Memories (distressing). The most common Obsessions are: thinking or feeling objects are dirty or contaminated/ worrying about health and hygiene/ fear about safety and security, *e.g.*, doors left unlocked or appliances left switched on/ pre-occupation with order and symmetry/ religious or anti-religious thoughts/ disturbing thoughts about aggression or sex/ the urge to hoard useless things/ superstitions; excessive attention to something considered lucky or unlucky. Obsessional phobias are obsessional thoughts with a fearful content (fear of contracted HIV infection). Though Compulsion (repetitive acts (rituals) based on obsession) is not an item of thought content but a motor behavior and in clinical situation most of the compulsive acts are associated with obsessive thoughts of some kind. So it would be better to delineate during assessment that whether the subject has only obsessional thoughts or it is accompanied by compulsive acts as well.

- **Phobia:** persistent and irrational fear of delineated aspects of nonhuman object or environment. Common three types: Simple phobia (fear of animals, heights, bridges etc); Social phobia (fear of social situations where he/she may do wrong thing, being looked at or asked to speak) and Agoraphobia (fear of open spaces or crowds).

- **Other patterns of thinking:** Following five types may be seen as a pattern of thinking, strongly held, not always illogical and culturally inappropriate, usually occur singly or unassociated with other psychopathology - carefully distinguish whether such thoughts have reached delusional intensity.

    o *Overvalued ideas:* unreasonable, sustained false beliefs or ideas maintained less firmly than a delusion (*i.e.*, the person is able to acknowledge the possibility that the belief may not be true). The belief is not one that is ordinarily accepted by other members of the person's culture or subculture. Clinical difficulties often arise to separate it from delusion.

    o *Grandiosity:* Beliefs that one's ideas, capacities or actions are generally superior to those of others.

    o *Mystical experience:* feels that the mystery of the universe has been suddenly revealed to him, may be associated with superior power and regarded as very valuable and auspicious.

    o *Suspiciousness:* a cautious attitude based on possible malevolent intuitions of others. Simple suspiciousness is not paranoia, not if it is based on past experience or expectations learned from the experience of others.

    o *Paranoia:* level of suspiciousness altering thinking and behavior in nonadaptive ways. It is a mistrust that is either highly exaggerated or not warranted at all.

- **Idea** is a mental impression or conception that potentially or actually exists in the mind as a product of mental activity. Usual five types are:

    o *Autochthonous idea* - a persistent idea originating within the mind but seeming to have come from an outside source and often therefore felt to be of malevolent origin.

    o *Dominant idea* - one that controls or colors every action and thought.

    o *Fixed idea* - a persistent morbid impression or belief that cannot be changed by reason.

    o *Overvalued idea* - a false or exaggerated belief sustained beyond reason or logic but with less rigidity than a delusion, also often being less patently unbelievable.

    o *Idea of reference* - the incorrect idea that words and actions of others refer to oneself or the projection of the causes of one's own imaginary difficulties upon someone else.

- **Overvalued idea:** first described by German neurologist Carl Wernicke (1848–1905), who refers to a solitary, abnormal belief that is neither delusional nor obsessional in nature, but which is preoccupying to the extent of dominating the sufferer's life (McKenna, 1984). The relationship between delusions and overvalued ideas is complex and uncertain, and thus has clinical as well as conceptual implications. Richard & Richard (2010) provided the following distinction between delusion and overvalued ideas:

    o Deluded individuals are less likely to identify what might modify their belief, less preoccupied, and less concerned about others' reactions than those with overvalued ideas.

    o Delusions are less plausible and their onset less likely to appear reasonable.

    o   Delusions are more likely to have abrupt onset and overvalued ideas a gradual onset.

    o   Conviction and insight are similar in both the groups.

    o   Belief conviction and insight may be an inadequate basis for separating delusions from overvalued ideas. Abrupt onset, implausible content, and relative indifference to the opinions of others may be better distinguishing features.

- **Hypochondriasis:** is excessive fear and anxiety of having a serious disease. These fears are not relieved when a medical examination finds no evidence of disease. They are often able to acknowledge that their fears are unrealistic, but this intellectual realization is not enough to reduce their anxiety. Most people occasionally fear they have an illness, but people with hypochondriasis are constantly preoccupied with their fear. This fear is severe and persistent and interferes with work as well as relationships and frequently leads to multiple health consultations.

- **Dysmorphophobia:** the affected person is excessively concerned about and preoccupied by a perceived defect in his or her physical features (body image). Now it is known as Body Dysmorphic Disorder (BDD). In cases where a minor defect truly exists, the individual with BDD exhibits an inordinate amount of anguish. BDD is often encountered in dermatologic and cosmetic surgery settings.

- **Eating disorders:** Eating disorders are characterized by an abnormal attitude and beliefs towards food that causes someone to change their eating habits and behavior. They may focus excessively on their weight and shape, leading them to make unhealthy choices about food with damaging results to their health. Eating disorders include a range of conditions that can affect someone physically, psychologically and socially. The most common eating disorders are Anorexia nervosa; Bulimia; Binge eating and Compulsive overeating.

B. Delusional thoughts: Delusions are false and firm beliefs not endorsed by social group, relatively impervious to invalidation.	
Delusion	According to Type: • *Simple* - Contain few elements • *Complex* - Contain extensive elaborations of people, motives and situations

	According to Onset:
	a) *Primary (autochthonous):* Instant, without identifiable preceding events – like an unexpected flash of insight, like a bolt from the blue. Jaspers (1913) described four types:
	    i. *Delusional intuition* - where delusions arrive "out of the blue", without external cause.
	    ii. *Delusional perception* - Interpreting a normal perception with a delusional meaning
	    iii. *Delusional atmosphere or mood* - A strange sense that something uncanny or odd is going on that threatens the patient, but in unspecified ways.
	    iv. *Delusional memory* - Patient recalls a remembered event or idea that is clearly delusional- here delusion is retrojected in time, often called retrospective delusion
	
	b) *Secondary:* Arises out of an underlying mood or from another psychotic phenomenon or from a defect in cognition or perception.

	According to Fixity: • *Complete* - Held firmly without any doubt. • *Partial* - Have doubts about the delusional beliefs.
	According to Span: • *Systematized* – restricted to well-delineated areas, usually with a clear sensorium and absence of hallucination • *Non-systematized* - Extend into many areas of life, new people and situations are constantly incorporated with concurrent mental confusion, hallucination and affective lability.
	According to number of content: • *Monothematic* – that concerns only one particular topic • *Poly or multi-thematic* - where the person has a range of delusions
	According to nature of content: • *Non-bizarre* - referred to real life situations which could be true, but are not or greatly exaggerated • *Bizarre* - when the delusional theme is totally impossible or absurd

Delusional Ideas / Themes	*Mood Congruent/ Incongruent*: whether match with the prevailing mood state?				
	Paranoid	Grandiose	Somatic	Religious	Guilt/Sin
	Nihilistic (Cotard's syndrome)	Jealousy/ Infidelity	Hypochondrical	Technological	Poverty
	Erotic (de Clerembault's syndrome)	Delusion of pregnancy	Delusion of rape	Bizarre	
Delusions of misidentification	Of replacement (Capgras's syndrome)/ Of disguise (Fregoli's phenomenon)/ Intermetamorphosis/ Subjective doubles/ Mirrored self-misidentification/ Reduplicative paramnesia/ Delusional companion/ Clonal pluralization of self.				
Communicated Delusions	Folie a deux		Folie a trois	Folie a famille	Shared or Mass delusion

- **Be sure about identifying delusion:** Clinically, a delusion is a false belief that is held with absolute passion and conviction that are impervious to reasoning and is out of proportion to the subject's educational, cultural and social background. Delusions beliefs may be absolutely impossible, simply improbable, or possible but incorrect or without any evidence. Delusions are multidimensional constructs comprising mainly of five dimensions (Combs *et al.*, 2006) as follows: *Conviction* (how strongly a belief is held); *Preoccupation* (how often the person focuses or thinks about their belief); *Pervasiveness* (how widespread and influential the belief is); *Negative emotionality* (whether the belief is linked to negative emotional states like anger, depression or anxiety) and *Action-inaction* (whether the belief is linked to behaviours). In addition, for a belief to qualify as a true delusion, it must have the following features (Kendler *et al.*, 1983):

  o **Influence or Extension:** That idea appears to exert an undue influence on his/ her life (even to an inexplicable extent).

  o **Pressure:** The degree to which the patient is preoccupied and concerned with the expressed delusional beliefs.

o **Bizarreness:** The degree to which the delusional belief departs from culturally determined consensual reality.

o **Disorganization:** The degree to which the delusional beliefs are internally consistent, logical and systematized.

o **Secretiveness:** Despite his/her total conviction, there is often a quality of secretiveness or suspicion when the patient is questioned about it.

o **Reactivity:** Any attempt to contradict the belief is likely to arouse an inappropriately strong emotional reaction, often with irritability and hostility.

o **Odd:** The belief is mostly unlikely, and out of keeping with the patient's social, cultural and religious background.

o **Deviant Behaviour:** The delusion, if acted out, often leads to behaviors which are abnormal and/or out of character of the person.

o **Unusual:** Individuals who know the patient will observe that his/her belief and behavior are uncharacteristic and alien.

o **Not Shared by Family or Community:** Sometimes a belief of delusional proportion may be held by a cultural or ethnic group as a part of their world-views.

2.2   Different types of Delusions

2.2.1   Paranoid Delusions

Most common single delusion, affecting about 60% of patients.

- **Persecutory delusion:** most common type, involve the theme of being followed, harassed, cheated, poisoned or drugged, conspired against, attacked or harmed (by poisoning or plotting to murder) or spied on by extraordinary gadgets like radio-imaging or computer-assisted micro-wave monitoring or photography etc or obstructed in the pursuit of goals by a person or group of persons.

- **Querulous or Litigious paranoia:** manifested in querulant behavior. A querulant (meaning "complaining") is a person who obsessively feels wronged, particularly about minor causes of action and they usually repeatedly petition authorities or pursue legal actions based on manifestly unfounded or too trivial grounds. Currently this term is rarely used.

- **Delusions of Reference:** casual events have a special, usually dangerous, significance in reference to him/her (other persons are talking about him/ people on television or radio are talking about him or headlines or stories in newspapers are written especially for them), either overtly or covertly.

- **Delusions of Control or Influence or passivity:** some outside force or agency is controlling thoughts and feelings. Common symptoms are *thought broadcasting*- private thoughts are being transmitted to others; *thought insertion* – someone is planting thoughts into patient's head; and *thought withdrawal* – FBI or police is robbing his/her own thoughts, obviously with a malicious intent.

- **Delusion of mind being read**: other people can know one's thoughts. This is different from thought broadcasting in that the person does not believe that his or her thoughts are heard aloud.

- **Delusions of Jealousy or infidelity:** A belief that one's spouse is unfaithful, despite no supporting evidence. Commoner in men with alcohol problems and is associated with a risk of violence.

2.2.2 Somatic Delusions

Usually three main types:

- **Delusion of Infestation or Delusional parasitosis (Ekbom's syndrome):** Patient believes that insects or worms or tiny animals are infesting the skin or body. Usually the imaginary parasites are reported as being "bugs" or insects crawling on or under the skin; the experience of this sensation is called formication. Karl Axel Ekbon (1907 – 1977) a Swedish neurologist published seminal account on this in 1937 – 1938. The term "delusions of parasitosis" was introduced in 1946 by Wilson & Miller.

- **Delusions of dysmorphophobia:** Patient believes that he/she is having ugly look or defective/abnormal size of body parts. Associated with obsessive and compulsive behaviours related to perceived defects.

- **Delusion of foul body odors (Halitosis):** Patient believes he/she is having foul body odor, also known as *Olfactory reference syndrome.*

2.2.3 Grandiose Delusions

Belief that one has special powers and is accomplishing or will accomplish extraordinary things for good of the community. Grandiose delusions are characterized by profound beliefs that one is famous, having special powers or ability (*e.g.*, communicating with deceased relatives or extraterrestrial objects or persons), omnipotent, often with a supernatural, science-fictional or religious bent. Usually an elaborate loosely formed plan or programme of activity is attached with this delusion. Most common in manic psychosis.

2.2.4 Religious Delusions

Any delusion with a religious or spiritual content. Belief that one has special power of God or God-like and has sacred duties towards mankind or chosen by God. Beliefs that would be considered normal for an individual's religious or cultural background are not delusions.

2.2.5 Technological Delusions

Patient believes that he/she is somehow connected to computers or other extraordinary (electrical or magnetic) gadgets, allowing him/her to exert immense power (one pt said by this power he may "create chaos in the cosmos").

2.2.6 Other delusions:

- **Erotic or amorous delusion (de Clerembault's syndrome):** Patient believes another person, usually of a higher social status and standing, is secretly in love with the patient and communicates this in oblique ways. This was described by Gaëtan Gatian de Clérambault (1872 – 1934), a French psychiatrist, in his publication of *Les Psychoses Passionelles* in 1921.

- **Nihilistic delusion (Cotard's syndrome):** Patient thinks that internal organs have disappeared or rotted away or the family, possessions or even the whole world has been destroyed or disappeared or things (or everything, including the self) do not exist; a sense that everything is unreal. This syndrome was first described by Jules Cotard (1840 – 1889), a French neurologist.

- **Delusion of guilt or sin (delusion of self-accusation):** Patient thinks they are guilty of any minor or imagined behaviour or event that may be related or unrelated with him/her.

- **Delusion of Poverty:** a false belief that one is impoverished or will be deprived of material possessions. Depressed patients are prone to *delusions of poverty* and *delusions of nihilism*. Negative thoughts like "the future is hopeless, the present is desolate and the patient is destitute and abandoned to a bleak fate" are common. Depressed patients may also suffer from inordinate *guilt*, the most extreme punishments being meted out to them for unremarkable, ancient transgressions.

- **Hypochondriacal delusion:** These are false beliefs about illness. Despite effective medical evidence to the contrary the patient believes that he/she is suffering from serious diseases.

2.2.7 Delusional misidentification syndrome

It is an umbrella term, introduced by Christodoulou (1986) for a group of delusional beliefs that occur in the context of psychiatric or neurological disorders. The core delusional belief is relating to the changed or altered identity of a person, object or place. As these delusions typically only concern one particular topic they are also called monothematic delusions.

- **Capgras delusion:** the belief that a close relative or spouse has been replaced by an identical-looking impostor. First reported in 1923 by Capgras and Reboul-Lachaux. Joseph Capgras (1873 – 1950) was a French psychiatrist and J Reboul-Lachaux was his intern. They named it as "Illusions of double".

- **Reverse Capgras:** The patient believes others think he is an imposter.

- **Fregoli delusion:** the belief that different people are in fact a single person who changes appearance or is in disguise. This was named after the famous Italian stage actor Leopold Fregoli (1867 – 1936) who had extraordinary ability in impersonations and his quickness in exchanging roles. P. Courbon and G. Fail first reported the condition in a 1927 (Ellis *et al.*, 1994).

- **Reverse Fregoli:** The patient believes that he looks like a famous person.

- **Intermetamorphosis:** the belief that people in one's environment swap identities with each other whilst maintaining the same appearance, so that A becomes B, B becomes C and so on. P Courbon and J Tusques reported this in 1932 (Ellis *et al.*, 1994).

- **Subjective doubles** (Christodoulou, 1978): the delusional belief that the person has a double or doppelganger with the same appearance, but usually with different character traits and leading a life of its own. Sometimes the patient has the idea that there is more than one double.

- **Mirrored self misidentification:** The belief that one's reflection is of another person's. A related rare phenomenon is "negative autoscopy", characterized by the failure to perceive one's mirror image while looking into a mirror, often found in dementia, traumatic brain injury or neuro-logical illness (Dening & Berrios, 1994).

- **Reduplicative paramnesia :** Characterized by the belief that a familiar person, place, object or body part is duplicated, existing in two or more places simultaneously, *e.g.* the patient thinks his real home has been moved and that he is living in identical looking home (Taylor & Vaidya, 2009). This term was used first by Czech neurologist Arnold Pick in 1903.

- **Delusional companions:** Characterized by the belief that certain non-living objects (like toys) possess consciousness and can think independently and feel emotion. This belief is transient and normal in childhood but abnormal in adult.

- **Clonal pluralization of self:** Characterized by the belief that he/she exists in plural numbers – there are many physically and psychologically identical copies of a given original (Voros *et al.*, 2003).

2.2.8   Communicated delusions
Communicated delusions seen in couples (folie a deux) or in families (folie a famille) – usually there is one dominant member who induced the delusion in the passive partner or other members.

- **Folie a deux ("madness for two") or Folie impose**: also called induced psychosis, is a delu-sional disorder shared by two or more people (folie a plusieurs) who are closely related emotion-ally. One suffers from "real" psychosis while the symptoms of psychosis are induced in the other or others, due to close attachment to the one with psychosis. Separation usually results in symp-tomatic improvement in the one who is not psychotic.

- **Folie simultanee:** a delusional system emerges simultaneously and independently in two closely related persons, and the separation of the two would not be beneficial in the resolution of psy-chopathology.

- **Folie communiqué**: occurs when a normal person suffers a contagion of his ideas after resisting them for a long time. Once he acquires these beliefs he maintains them despite separation.

- **Folie induite:** a person, who is already psychotic, adds the delusions of a closely associated per-son to his own.

- **Shared or Mass delusion:** Spontaneous, en masse development of an irrational belief leading to identical physical or mental symptoms among a group of individuals (usually as reaction to a re-cent event). Also known as collective hysteria, epidemic hysteria, mass psychogenic illness. It is the operative force in psychiatric epidemics (koro, penis loss, fainting/ dancing epidemics).

2.2.9   Pseudocyesis or "false pregnancy" or "phantom pregnancy"
It is a state when a non-pregnant woman has a false belief that she is pregnant and presents marked bodily signs of pregnancy (*i.e.,* amenorrhea, breast changes, nausea, abdominal enlargement, reported fetal movements, weight gain, etc.). It usually occurs in hysterical women with infantile personalities and ab-normal sexual histories, also when a woman is either desperate for a child, or is overwhelmed by fears that she may be pregnant or in relation to infertility in women with normal sexual behaviour. Pseudocye-sis can be delusional, when the false belief of pregnancy is firm and unshakable. Pseudocyesis and delu-

sional pregnancy can be differentiated by absence or presence of somatic manifestations of the gravid state.

2.2.10 Delusion of pregnancy

It is a special form of hypochondriacal/ somatic delusion. It is nosologically non-specific, occurring in schizophrenia and schizo-affective disorder, delusional disorders, affective disorders, epilepsy, dementia, and other organic brain syndromes, as well as in medical conditions like urinary tract infection, drug-induced lactation, and polydypsia and hyponatremia syndrome (Simon *et al.*, 2009).

2.2.11 Delusion of Rape

It represent a complex mixture of delusional belief and somatic delusion (of genital penetration), usually complained that occurred during sleep by schizophrenic female patients. Almost similar to that is the complaint of injections (muscular or intravenous) of blood or other chemical by malevolent force or person, during sleep.

2.2.12 Bizarre and Non-Bizarre Delusion

Categorization of delusion on the basis of content as Bizarre and Non-bizarre is important from the diagnostic point of view. DSM IV considered the presence of bizarre delusion as one of the criteria in the diagnosis of schizophrenia so long as dysfunction/suffering and length-of-illness criteria are satisfied. The concept of bizarreness is defined in DSMs through the following notions (Cermolacce *et al.*, 2010) as: a. physical (or perhaps logical) impossibility, b. generally not shared in cultural context, and c. overall implausibility or incomprehensibility with emphasis on grounding in ordinary experience, although some authors have raised the issue of reliability (Mojtabi & Nichilson, 1995) and validity (Nakaya *et al.*, 2002) of bizarre delusion as diagnostic criteria (Flaum *et al.*, 1991) for schizophrenia. In DSM V this diagnostic requirement is omitted (as also the Schneiderian first rank auditory hallucination- two or more voices conversing) in Criterion A and is replaced by core positive symptoms (*e.g.* delusion, hallucination and disorganized speech) – at least one of which should be present (APA, 2013). Non-bizarre delusion was considered as diagnostic for Delusional Disorder in DSM IV-TR but eliminated as diagnostic criteria in DSM 5. Non-bizarre delusions, in contrast to bizarre delusions, are those delusions that reflect real life situations (which, though false belief, is at least possible or could be true) and may include feelings of being followed, poisoned, infected, deceived or conspired against, or loved at a distance.

2.2.13 Therianthropy

Belief in metamorphosis of humans into animals. It is also known as "Shapeshifting" that refers to alteration of physical appearance, from human to animal. Lycanthropy (transformation into a wolf) is the most well known form, followed by Cynanthropy (transformation into a dog) and Ailuranthropy (transformation into a cat or feline). This has a strong relation with cultural folk myths and is now a rare psychiatric disorder.

2.3 Examination of Perception

- **Perception:** Mental process by which all kinds of data, intellectual, emotional, sensory and environmental, are meaningfully organized. (*Imagery* - A sensory experience over which the subject has voluntary control and experiences as taking place within the mind. *Apperception* – awareness of the meaning and significance of a particular sensory stimulus as modified by one's own experiences, knowledge, thoughts and emotions.)

- **Clinical Evaluation of perceptual disturbances:** Following issues should be clarified-

  o *Which sensory modality is involved* - One (simple hallucination) or multiple (complex hallucination)?

  o *Nature of perception* –Intensity, clarity and frequency. Time of the day - in waking state or while drowsy? On medication?

  o *Content of perception* – Personal comments? Commands? Accusatory? Threatening? (narrative should be cited), Fear producing voice or images?

  o *Location of their sources of origin* – Inside the head, outer space, from any object or place?

  o *Degree of volitional control over them* - Can they be initiated voluntarily or stopped at will by the patient?

  o *Level of conviction (Insight) about their reality* - Is the experience factual or product of patient's imagination?

  o *Attitude* – pleasant, disturbing or neutral

  o *Nature and degree of influence on the behaviour*- patient's reaction: Unbothered? Trying to avoid? Obey commands? Reply or converse with the voices? Attempt to escape? Feeling stressed or fearful?

2.3.1   Disorder of Perceptions – Perceptual Distortions

There is a *real* perceptual object but perceived in a distorted way. The common distortions are:

- *Changes in intensity* - perception may be altered - either heightened or diminished, *e.g.* Hyperacusis: sounds of normal intensity are perceived as abnormally loud. Seen in migraine, hangover from alcohol excess, depressive disorders. Visual hyperaesthesia: Colours look more intense or vivid. Seen in hypomanics, epileptic aura, effect of LSD, and situation of intense emotion like religious fervour.

- *Changes in quality*- mainly visual perception are affected, brought about by toxic substances *e.g.* colouring of yellow, green, or red, seen in mescaline or digitalis poisoning.

- *Changes in spatial form* (Dysmegalopsia) - an inability to judge the size or measure of an object accurately: Micropsia (objects are perceived to be smaller than they actually are), macropsia (objects within an affected section of the visual field appear larger than normal), porropsia (visual distortion in which stationary objects appear to be moving away from the observer), metamorphosia (a distorted vision in which a grid of straight lines appears wavy and parts of the grid may appear blank). Seen in temporal and parietal lobe lesions, retinal disease, disorders of accommodation and convergence.

- *Distortion of experience of time* - There are two varieties of time: physical and personal. It is the latter that is affected by psychiatric disorders, *e.g.* in severe depression patient may feel time passes slowly and even stands still. By contrast the manic patient feels that time speeds by.

- *Splitting of perception* - Changes in the emotional quality and associations of real percepts. It is a psychoanalytic concept (child during the early years splits his/her perception of mother as good or bad mother and in time, that becomes the mental relationship that is re-enacted in life relationships.)

2.3.2   Disorder of Perceptions – Perceptual Deceptions

2.3.2.1   Illusions

Illusions are misinterpretations of real sensory stimuli. An illusion may be:

- *Optical illusion*: characterized by visually perceived images that is deceptive or misleading.

- *Auditory illusion:* an illusion of hearing. The listener hears either sounds which are not present in the stimulus, or "impossible" sounds.

- *Tactile illusion (e.g. phantom limb)*: can occur with other senses including that of taste and smell.

- *Completion illusion*: They depend on inattention for their occurrence *e.g.* misreading words or missing misprints.

- *Affect illusions*: They arise in the context of a particular mood state *e.g.* a bereaved person may momentarily believe that they see the deceased person.

- *Fantastic illusion*: Are perceived as extraordinary modifications of the environment. Frank Fish gave an example of one of his patient who, during examination, saw Fish's head changed into a rabbit's head.

- *Muller–Lyer illusions*: refer to perceptions that do not agree with the physical stimulus.

- *Autokinetic illusion*: a visual perception in which there is an apparent movement of a stationary single point of light or small object at the background of dark field when observed continuously.

- *Eidetic image:* a vivid and detailed reproduction of a previous perception as in a "photographic memory".

- *Pareidolias*: playful, voluntary illusions from ambiguous or evanescent images, *e.g.*, flames or clouds (without any conscious effort).

- *Trailing*: a visual illusion, is the perception that an object moving steadily in space is followed by temporary, distinct after-images. Occur in fatigue, marijuana and mescaline intoxication.

2.3.2.2   Hallucination

A *hallucination* is a false perception that occurs in the waking state in the absence of a sensory stimulus. It is not merely a sensory distortion or misinterpretation but also carries a subjective sense of conviction.

A true hallucination appears to the subject to be substantial and occurs in external objective space. In contrast, a mental imagery is insubstantial and experienced within internal subjective space.

Hallucinatory experience may involve all the main sensory modalities, viz. olfactory, gustatory, visual, auditory and tactile. In addition it may involve somatic (bodily) sensations, sexual sensations, vibrations, sensation of heat and cold, kinaesthetic and proprioceptic sensations and the experience of time. Depending on the modalities involved, hallucinations can be grouped as: Elementary hallucinations are simple phenomena that confine themselves to a single sensory modality. Organized hallucinations are more complex in nature, ranging from simple geometrical patterns (or tunes, in the auditory modality) to full-colour, three-dimensional images (or symphonies), within a single sensory modality. Complex hallucination is used to denote hallucinated symphonies, three-dimensional images, occurring in more than one sensory modality. Often referred to as compound or multimodal hallucinations.

- **Hallucinosis:** a pathologic mental state in which awareness consists primarily or exclusively of hallucinations, not associated with clouding of consciousness (*e.g.*, alcoholic hallucinosis, organic hallucinosis in dementia). Sensory deprivation may produce visual and auditory hallucinosis in many subjects. Hallucinosis and Delirium (*e.g.*, following cataract surgery) probably act by the same mechanism, especially in association with dementia. Diencephalic and cortical disease may be associated with hallucinations (usually visual). Tumors of the olfactory or basal temporal regions may cause olfactory hallucinosis, for example, as an aura.

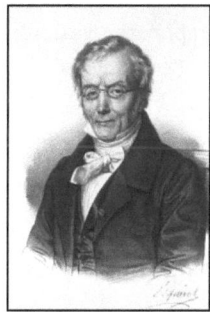

Johann Kaspar Lavater
(1741 – 1801)

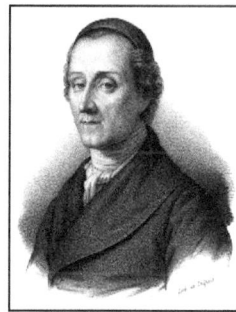

Esquirol
(1772 – 1840)

Figure 1. The word "hallucinatory" has its roots in the Latin *hallucinari* or *allucinari*, which means to *wander in mind.* Lavater, a Swiss poet and physiognomist, introduced "hallucination" in the English language in 1572 to refer to "ghosts and spirits walking the night". The word was first used in its current sense in 1837 by Jean-Etienne Dominique Esquirol, a French psychiatrist. In the middle ages, hallucinations were thought to be manifestations of demons or angels. A religious person who experienced such phenomena was seen as a saint, whereas a commoner was believed to be possessed by the devil. In certain cultures, hallucinations are still perceived as the work of Satan or as a result of magic (Wahass & Kent, 1997).

Types of Hallucinations

- **Auditory hallucination**: false perception of sound without outside stimulus, usually voices but also other noises and music. Most common form involves hearing one or more talking voices. It is the most common hallucination in psychiatric disorders. It is also known as Paracusia. **Com-**

mand hallucinations are hallucinations in the form of "hearing commands"- that instruct the patient to act in specific ways. The contents here can range from neutral comments or simple directives like "do this" or "do that", "don't go out" etc to asking to inflict harm to self or others. It is usually associated with schizophrenia. People experiencing command hallucinations may or may not comply with the hallucinated commands, sometimes ignore or resist the command and sometimes there is a compulsion to carry out the commands. Compliance is more common for non-violent commands (Lee *et al.*, 2004). Research has shown many potential determinants of compliance like beliefs about the command (Beck-Sander *et al.*, 1997); a voice known to the patient, emotional involvement during the hallucination and perceiving the voice as real (Erkwoh *et al.*, 2002); and command hallucination with hallucination related delusion (Junginger, 1995). Generally, patients who experience command hallucination are at risk for dangerous behavior (Rogers *et al.*, 1990). Dangerousness of command hallucinations and subsequent violent acts (to self or to others) are of forensic importance and if present, needs detailed clinical evaluation for risk assessment and management (Hersh & Borum, 1998).

- **Auditory Hallucinations in Schizophrenia:** Usually 5 types: (i) audible thoughts described as hallucinated voices that speak aloud what the patient is thinking (*echo de la pensee*); (ii) voices that give a running commentary on the patient's actions; (iii) hearing two or more voices arguing with each other, often about the patient who is referred to in the third person; (iv) command hallucination – order patients to do things; and (v) various meaningless sounds, *e.g.*, buzzes, hums or rumbles

  o **Second person hallucinations:** a voice appears to address the patient in the second person, *e.g.*, the voice may be talking directly to the patient- "You are going to die" – or the voice may direct the patient to do some action- "kill him". These types of auditory hallucinations are not diagnostic in the same way as third person auditory hallucinations, but the content of the hallucination, and the patient's reaction to it, may help the diagnosis.

  o **Third person hallucinations:** patients hear voices talking about them, referring to them in third person, for example "he is a bad person".

  o **Voices or Phoneme:** Phoneme is a term from linguistics, which denotes the set of speech sounds in any given language. German neuropathologist Carl Wernicke (1848 – 1905) used this term to designate hallucinated voices in 1900. It is also known as Verbal Auditory Hallucination (VAH) that is primarily verbal in nature and different from other auditory hallucinations (*e.g.*, musical hallucination or nonverbal auditory hallucinations (Sommer *et al.*, 2003). Phonemes are the commonest form of hallucinations in patients with manic-depressive illness and schizophrenia. Voices may have the following characters:

  i.   May consist of one or more voices

  ii. Frequency: Intermittent or constant, may be related with any specific situation, location or activity.

  iii. Type of Voice: May be heard in a regular tone of voice, whisper or a shout, may be intelligible or unintelligible, may be clear or vague and may speak in a foreign language. It may be **Inchoate (***e.g.*, humming, rushing water, inaudible murmurs) or **Fragmentary** (*e.g.*, words or phrases such as "fag", "get him," or "beastly") or **Complex -** Typically a schizophrenic patient identifies complex hallucinations in inner or outer space, as a voice or voices speaking to or about him/ her.

iv. Source: May be perceived as coming from within the head or other body parts like abdomen (internal auditory hallucination) or from outside the head (external auditory hallucination) or may be swapping the location. They may be perceived as originating from alleged implants (*e.g.* transmitter or camera in the brain) or electronic devices like TV or radio or from nearby locations (from outside the window), or even from a distant place or from space.

v. Nature: Voices may be benign (they may give valuable advice or make pleasant comments) or malignant (insulting and threatening). When they consist of spoken orders or incentives, they are referred to as **command hallucinations.** They may also give **a running commentary** on the individual's thoughts or behaviour.

- **Visual hallucination:** false perception involving sight consisting of both formed images (people, animal, insect) and unformed or elemental images (flashes of light or colour). In general, visual hallucination suggests organic brain disorder, alcohol-related illness and tends to occur in a setting of confusion or obtundation. In delirium, insects or other small objects may be seen moving on the bed. Lilliputian hallucinations, of little people on the bed, may occur in delirium and other organic brain syndromes. Complex audiovisual hallucinations may occur in temporal lobe epilepsy. Sometimes, however, a schizophrenic patient may report visual hallucinations (*e.g.,* trips in flying saucers) aligned with his/ her prevailing delusions. The visual hallucinations of hysteria or dissociative disorder have a pseudo-hallucinatory quality and sometimes represent a past traumatic event. Closed eye hallucinations, which occur in darkness, seen after psychedelic drug (LSD, mescaline) use.

- **Olfactory hallucination (Phantosmia):** false perception of smell, most common in medical disorder (*e.g.,* smell of burning rubber, steak and onions or smells rotting flesh, vomit, smoke; may occur in epilepsy and damage to the olfactory system. Schizophrenic patients may perceive the odor of gas being pumped into their bedrooms by persecutors.) *Parosmia* - smell is actually present, but perceived differently from its usual smell.

- **Gustatory:** false perception of taste such as unpleasant taste, caused by an uncinate fits of complex partial seizure. Schizophrenic patient may think they taste poisonous substances in their food. *Phantageusia* is a sudden, vague taste without the presence of the substance normally causing the sensation. Olfactory and Gustatory hallucinations most often associated with organic brain diseases, particularly with the uncinate fits of complex partial seizures.

- **Haptic or Tactile:** false perception of touch or surface sensation as from an amputed limb (phantom limb) or crawling sensation on or under the skin (**formication** in alcohol withdrawal syndrome, cocaine intoxication). May be associated with delusion of **parasitosis**. Some tactile hallucinations like having intercourse with God or some other particular alleged person (**sexual hallucinations** – erection, orgasm, and penetration) is highly suggestive of schizophrenia.

- **Somatic:** Perception of things occurring in or to the body, most often of visceral origin. Somatic hallucinations occur in Schizophrenia, where genital, visceral, intracerebral or kinesthetic sensations are often referred to being the influence of persecutors or machines. A depressed patient may have the sense of having no stomach, with food dropping from the throat into a void, a schizophrenic patient complaints that persecutors made his mouth cavity smaller by tricks.

- **Somaesthetic hallucination:** Hallucination of bodily sensations are often classified as *external bodily hallucinations* like tactile or haptic hallucinations (sensation of touch); thermic (an abnormal perception of heat and cold) and hygric (a perception of fluid) hallucination, kinaesthetic (hallucinations felt in muscles and joints) and *internal visceral sensation* that arise from the internal organs and perceived as pain, heaviness, stretching or distension and palpitation (Kathirvel & Mortimer, 2013). Visceral hallucination is found in schizophrenia, often in a bizarre way or may present as delusional infestation (one patient believes that a leech is wandering into her abdomen); present as "epigastric aura" in complex partial seizure; as a feeling of "butterflies in the throat" in limbic epilepsy; in multiple sclerosis, in thalamic pain syndrome and secondary to antiparkinsonian medications.

- **Autoscopic hallucination (phantom mirror image):** Hallucinations of one's own physical self - experience of seeing one's own body projected into external space, usually in front of oneself for short periods. This may stimulate the delusion that one has a double. In **internal autoscopy** the subject sees his or her own internal organs. In **negative autoscopy** the patient looks at the mirror and sees no image at all. Seen in acute and subacute delirious state, epilepsy, focal lesions affecting parietal-occipital regions. Reported in near-death and out-of-body experiences of hospitalized subjects.

- **Functional hallucinations:** Hallucinations that occur in connection with a specific external perception (in the same sensory modality), *e.g.*, sound of running water triggers a hallucinatory voice or wallpaper pattern triggers visual hallucination of dreadful faces or traffic noise triggers command hallucination. Very often found in schizophrenia, delirium, toxic states, seizure disorder and focal brain vascular disease.

- **Reflex hallucinations:** A stimulus in one sensory field leads to a hallucination in another, *e.g.* a schizophrenia patient would feel a sharp chest pain every time a certain family member called his name. It is a form of synesthesia.

- **Extracampine hallucinations:** Hallucination that occurs outside the patient's sensory field, *e.g.*, a young schizophrenia patient hearing verbal command of Bill Clinton in USA from India.

- **Musical hallucination:** A form of auditory hallucination in which music is heard, often the same piece of music. In most cases the music is familiar to the person. It is most common in older people, especially women, with hearing loss. It is suggested that sensory deprivation from the deafness is the cause. It may also result from specific lesions in the dorsal pons, brain tumour or abscess and epileptic activity. It is also reported from patients with depression, OCD, schizophrenia and alcoholism.

- **Synesthesia:** Stimulation of one sensory modality evokes perceptual distortions in another, as if sensory modalities seem fused, *e.g.*, sound seen or colours felt. Found in marijuana and mescaline intoxication, also a normal experience in many people.

- **Migrainous hallucinations:** reported by 50% patients with migraine – visual hallucinations of geometric patterns, sometimes with micropsia and macropsia. Also known as the *Alice in Wonderland syndrome*.

- **Ictal hallucinations:** occurring as a part of seizure activity, typically brief and stereotyped, in a state of altered consciousness or a twilight sleep.

- **Hypnagogic:** false sensory perception occurring while falling asleep, generally considered non-pathological. Severe sleep deprivation can cause hypnagogic hallucination.

- **Hypnopompic:** false sensory perception occurring while awakening from sleep, generally considered nonpathological. May occur in healthy people and are characteristic symptoms of narcolepsy.

- **Mood congruent:** hallucinatory content is consistent with either a depressed or manic mood.

- **Mood incongruent:** hallucinatory content is not consistent with either a depressed or manic mood.

- **Pseudohallucinations:** perceptions experienced as coming from within the mind (vivid images that are heard or seen from within – Jasper, 1911). Usually the patient says that the voices are "inside the head" and many clinicians preferred the term *nonpsychotic hallucination* over pseudohallucination (van der Zwaard & Polak, 2001). Obsessional ruminations or intra-psychic self-reproach in severe depressive guilt are sometimes expressed as "voices". Borderline Personality disorder cases often complained of nonpsychotic hallucination (Yee *et al..*, 2005).

- **Experiential hallucinations:** The term coined by Canadian neurosurgeon Wilder Graves Penfield (1891-1976) and defined as "hallucinations made up of elements from the individual's past experiences. They may seem to him so strange that he calls them dreams, but when they can be carefully analyzed it is evident that the hallucination is a shorter or longer sequence of past experience. *The subject re-lives a period of the past although he is still aware of the present.*"

- **Panoramic hallucination:** Also known as scenic or holocampine hallucination that denotes a compound hallucination in which the entire sensory input is replaced by hallucinatory percepts, thus giving rise to a totally different perceptual reality. It is similar to experiential hallucination and is usually found in temporal lobe psycho-sensory epilepsy, catatonic schizophrenia, delirium, PTSD flashbacks, brainstem lesions and hallucinogen use.

- **Flashback:** an intense visual re-experience of highly charged past events, which are often replays of hallucinations. These images are usually triggered by a trivial reminder of the past experiences (*e.g.* a smell or sound) and usually brief and intensely upsetting. Typically seen in LSD and mescaline use, in PTSD.

- **Delusional perception:** A true perception, to which a patient attributes a false meaning, *e.g.*, a perfectly normal event such as the traffic lights turning red may be interpreted by the patient as meaning that the aliens are about to land. It is one of Schneider's first rank symptoms. Though it is highly indicative of Schizophrenia, it can also occur in other psychoses, including mania with grandiose colour.

- **Charles Bonnet syndrome:** Patients who are visually impaired often develop pseudohallucinations (visual hallucinations) with preserved cognitive status. A similar phenomenon is the musical hallucination in individual with acquired deafness.

- **Schneider's First Rank Symptoms in schizophrenia (FRS):**

- o Delusional perception (a normal perception is suddenly interpreted in a delusional manner)

- o Thought insertion, withdrawal or broadcast

- o Somatic passivity (Delusional belief that one is a passive recipient of bodily sensations from an external agency)

- o Passivity of impulse, affect and volition (made impulse, affect and volition)

- o Thought echo (audible thoughts)

- o Third-person auditory hallucinations discussing or arguing about the patient

- o Auditory hallucination of running commentary of patient's actions

[**ABCD**: **A**uditory hallucinations, **B**roadcasting of thought, **C**ontrolled thought (delusions of control), **D**elusional perception.]

The reliability of using first-rank symptoms for the diagnosis of schizophrenia has since been questioned, although the terms might still be used descriptively by mental health professionals who do not use them as diagnostic aids. FRS is not exclusive to schizophrenia, it also occurs in patients with manic-depressive illness, delirium or intoxication, dementia, seizure disorder, and stroke. Individuals with Dissociative Identity Disorder (DID) may experience first-rank symptoms more commonly than even patients with schizophrenia though patients with DID lack negative symptoms of schizophrenia and normally do not mistake hallucinations for reality.

- **Frequency of Hallucinations** (Yager & Gitlin, 2004):

  - o 10 – 27% of general population have visual hallucination

  - o 50% grieving spouses have auditory or visual hallucinations

  - o 90% of patients with hallucinations also have delusions

  - o 35% of patients with delusions also have hallucinations

  - o 60 – 90% patients of schizophrenia have auditory hallucinations

  - o 20% manic patients have auditory hallucinations

  - o 10% of depressed patients experience auditory hallucination

- **Deliberate or Fake Hallucinations** (Resnick & Knoll, 2005)

  - o **Malingered Psychotic Symptoms:** Detecting malingered mental illness is considered an advanced psychiatric skill. Malingerers may have inadequate or incomplete knowledge of the mental illness they are faking. Indeed, malingerers are like actors who can portray a role only as they understand it. They often overact their part or mistakenly believe that the more bizarre their behavior, the more convincing they will be. Conversely, "successful" malingerers are more likely to endorse fewer symptoms and avoid endorsing overly bizarre or unusual symptoms. Several clinical factors suggest malingering. Malingerers are more likely to eagerly "thrust forward" their illness, whereas patients with genuine schizophrenia are often reluctant to discuss their symptoms. There must be a hidden agenda or goal behind the symptom presentation, *e.g.*, either to avoid some stressful situation like arrest, criminal prosecution or imminent joining a job or military or to seek controlled substances, compensation or disability benefits. Some important points in clinical examination are:

o   **Hallucinations:** If a patient alleges atypical hallucinations, ask about them in detail. Hallucinations are usually (88%) associated with delusions (Lewinsohn, 1970). Genuine hallucinations are typically intermittent rather than continuous.

o   **Auditory hallucinations** are usually clear, not vague (7%) or inaudible. Both male and female voices are commonly heard (75%), and voices are usually perceived as originating outside the head (88%) (Goodwin *et al.*, 1971). In Schizophrenia, the major themes are persecutory or instructive (Small *et al.*, 1966). Comparing with the norm is another clinical way to identify fake hallucination (Rogers *et al.*, 1984; Rogers, 1987): 88% of real auditory hallucinations are from outside the head (usually outside the body or sometimes from a body part); 75% of real psychotics hear both male and female voices; 76% hear the hallucination in both ears and 98% of hallucinations are spoken in the person's native language. Most auditory hallucinations are brief (<20 seconds) and real psychotics can identify sex, race, age, and emotional state of the voice; the tone, volume, and rate of the voice and most auditory hallucinations ask for an interaction or a response from the person.

o   **Command auditory hallucinations** are easy to fabricate. Persons experiencing genuine command hallucinations do not always obey the voices, especially if doing so would be dangerous and usually present with non-command hallucinations (85%) and delusions (75%) as well (Thompson *et al.*, 1992). Solitary command hallucination without other psychotic symptoms raises the index of suspicion of malingering.

o   **Visual hallucinations** are experienced by an estimated 24% to 30% of psychotic individuals but are reported much more often by malingerers (46%) than by persons with genuine psychosis (4%) (Cornell & Hawk, 1989). Genuine visual hallucinations are usually of normal sized people and are seen in color. On rare occasions, genuine visual hallucinations of small people (Lilliputian hallucinations) may be associated with alcohol use, organic disease, or toxic psychosis (such as anticholinergic toxicity) but are rarely seen by persons with schizophrenia. Psychotic visual hallucinations do not typically change if the eyes are closed or open, whereas drug-induced hallucinations are more readily seen with eyes closed or in the dark. Unformed hallucinations—such as flashes of light, shadows, or moving objects—are typically associated with neurologic disease and substance use. Suspect malingering if the patient reports dramatic or atypical visual hallucinations.

2.3.2.3   Distortions of body image

Body image is a multifaceted cognitive construct involving perceptions, thoughts and feelings about one's physical being. It is the self-perception of appearance reflecting perceptual experience and subjective evaluation. The phrase *body image* was first coined by the Austrian psychiatrist and psychoanalyst Paul Ferdinand Schilder (1886 – 1940) in his book *The Image and Appearance of the Human Body* (1935). Body image distortions are an inaccurate perception of one's body shape, size or weight. Body dysmorphic disorder (BDD) is the extreme preoccupation and concern with body image, viz. a perceived defect in the physical appearance. In ICD 10 it bears the code F45.2 and placed under Somatoform disorder (F 45). In DSM IV, it was "delusional disorder, somatic type" but in DSMV it is included under the chapter on Obsessive –Compulsive and Related disorder. Several studies found abnormalities in different dimensions of body image in schizophrenia, viz. cognitive (thoughts, beliefs – body concept); affective (body satisfaction – body cathaxis) and perceptual (body size estimation – body schema) (Chapman *et al.*, 1978; Priebe & Rohricht, 2001).

- **Cenesthesias:** Cenesthesias are abnormal body sensations and are not uncommon in schizophrenia. This term was coined by Johann Christain Reil (1759 – 1813), a German physician and psychiatrist who also coined the term "Psychiatry" 100 years ago. Patients with schizophrenia frequently report abnormal body sensations like sensations of pain, numbness, stiffness and feeling strange, abnormal heaviness, lightness, extension, diminution, shrinking, and enlargement of limbs etc. (Rajender *et al.*, 2009) and body experience like underestimation of lower extremities, desomatization, boundary loss and diminution (Rohricht & Priebe, 2002) and underestimation of body size (Kim *et al.*, 2012). Varieties of disorders of body awareness- body schema disorder has been reported in the literature, mainly in the context of organic brain pathology but some may be found in schizophrenic disorder (Barr, 1998) like: phantom limb (perception of presence of amputed limb); macrosomatognosia (where either a part of the body, or the body as a whole, is experienced as disproportionally large and microsomatognosia (where the body, in part or in whole, is experienced as disproportionally small). Usually the last two types are associated with epileptic seizures, migraine, delirium, delirium tremens, alcohol withdrawal, mesencephalic lesions, and intoxication with hallucinogens such as LSD and mescaline.

2.4   Disorganized Speech

Patients with psychosis in addition to their dysfunctional thinking process also display disorganized speech. Following is a clinical guide to assess speech abnormalities.

1	**Volume** average amplitude at which speech is generated	audible		excessively loud		abnormally soft	
2	**Pitch** the highness or lowness of a sound based on the frequency of the sound waves	normal		low		high	
3	**Tone**: variation of spoken pitch	Normal fluctuation/ Prosody		monotonous			
4	**Reaction time** time to answer question	normal		delayed			
5	**Rate**	normal	very slow	rapid		pressure of speech	
6	**Flow** progression of speech	spontaneous	hesitant	slurring		stammering / stuttering	
		speaks only on question		muttering		mute	
7	**Relevance**	Relevant		Irrelevant			
8	**Coherence**	Coherent		Incoherent			
9	**Goal direction**	goal directed		circumstantial		tangential	
10	**Productivity**	normal		abundant		scanty	
11	**Deviation**	rhyming		punning		stereotypy	
		perseveration		clang association		talking past the point	
12	**Word/ Letter Substitution**	phonemic paraphasia		semantic paraphasia		neologism	
13	**Speech Defects**	dysphasia	dysarthria	dysphonia		mutism	

The functional aspects of voice, speech, and language are interrelated. **Voice** or vocalization is the sound produced by the individual. Disorders of the voice involve problems with pitch, loudness, and quality - usually occurs in neurological pathology or malignancy of larynx, may occur in hysterical or manic presentation. **Speech** is the vocalized form of communication, based upon the syntactic combination of lexical and names and with set grammatical rules and structure. Speech or communication disorder disrupted the normal speech pattern, usually found in both psychiatric and neurological disorders. **Language** is the expressive part of communication through either abstract concept or specific linguistic system in which knowledge, belief, and behavior can be experienced, explained, and shared. This sharing is guided by systematic, conventionally used signs, sounds, gestures, or marks that convey understood meanings within a group or community. Language disorders may be receptive (impaired language comprehension) or expressive (impaired language production) or both and are usually of organic origin.

Clinical guide to Disorders of Speech and Language (Taylor & Vaidya, 2008):

Speech Articulation	Speech Production	Speech Organization
Dysarthia	Pressured speech	Circumstantial speech
Manneristic speech: using foreign accents, robotic or stilted speech, odd rhythms or unexpected stress on some words	Paucity of speech (associated with loss of emotional expression and avolition in schizophrenia)	Flight of ideas/tangential speech/looseness of associations
Stammering and stuttering	Aphonia / Dysphonia /Mutism	Taking past to the point
Prosody (Modulation)	Thought blocking and speech arrest	Clang associations
	Stereotypic speech: words and phrases are delivered repetitively and automatically without any control- verbigeration/ palilalia/ logoconia	Rambling speech
	Perseveration	Formal Thought Disorder

- **Prosody:** It is the rhythm, stress and intonation of speech. It reflects different aspect of the speaker and his speech, *e.g.*, emotional state, nature and form of utterance (statement, question or command) and the presence of emphasis, contrast or focus.

- **Dysprosody:** loss of normal speech melody (called prosody)

- **Rate:** speed at which one speaks, *i.e.*, number of words spoken per minute (Wong, 2009). Slow speech is < 110wpm; conversational speech ranged between 120 – 150 wpm, Radio or TV broadcaster- 150 – 160 wpm and Auctioneers – 250 – 400 wpm.

- **Slow speech:** may be a feature of retardation. Usually associated with a lack of spontaneous and reduced speed of reply.

- **Fast Speech:** often results from "normal" anxiety, but may indicate mania or schizophrenia.

- **Pressure of speech:** rapid speech that is increased in amount and difficult to interrupt.

- **Push of speech:** rapid speech that is increased in amount but can be interrupted.

- **Volubility (logorrhoea):** copious, coherent and logical speech.

- **Poverty of Speech:** restriction in the amount of speech, replies may be monosyllabic.

- **Nonspontaneous Speech:** verbal responses given only when asked or spoken to directly, no self initiation of speech.

- **Poverty of content of speech:** speech is adequate in amount but covers little information because of vagueness, emptiness or stereotyped phrases.

- **Bradylalia:** abnormally slow speech.

- **Aprosodia:** inability to articulate or comprehend emotional voice tone. They miss the "affective or feeling" content of speech. Usually occurs in right frontal lobe damage (flat and monotone voice).

- **Aphonia:** speaks, but fails to produce any volume of sound or merely whispers. Found in disorders of larynx and vocal cord. If, despite this, the patient is able to cough normally, the origin is probably hysterical.

- **Dysphonia:** abnormal fluctuation in speech sound levels or difficulty or pain in speaking.

- **Dysarthria:** volume of sound and content is normal, but the articulation and enunciation of individual words and phrases is distorted. Found in disorders of control of muscles producing speech – upper or lower motor neuron lesions.

- **Dysphasia:** failure to put properly constructed words or phrases for expression. Lesion is in the dominant cerebral hemisphere. Dysphasic state also includes disturbances of writing (dysgraphia) and failure to comprehend the spoken word (receptive dysphasia) or the written word (dyslexia).

- **Stammering:** frequent repetition or prolongation of a sound or syllabi leading to markedly interrupted speech fluency, usually associated with tick disorder.

- **Stuttering:** difficulties in uttering speech sounds at the beginning of words, may be primary (from childhood) or secondary (after stroke, traumatic brain injury or extrapyramidal disease).

- **Muttering:** a low continuous indistinct sound; often accompanied by movement of the lips without the production of articulate speech.

- **Slurring speech:** or difficulty articulating words, commonly associated with drunkenness. Other causes are drug intoxication, hypoglycemic attacks, brain pathology like stroke or TIA and physical disorders of the face or oral region that interfere with speech. Slurred speech is not the same as poorly articulated speech or overly rapid speech.

- **Paraphasia:** Abnormal speech in which one word is substituted for another- two types: Semantic paraphasia- problem in the selection of right word thus substituted a word (words) for the correct one. Phonemic paraphasia – does errors by adding or omitting phonemes or missequencing the order of the phonemes in a word (treen for train).

- **Circumloculatory speech:** patient refers to an object, event, or person by descriptive terms (*e.g.*, its function or physical characteristics) rather than by its name, usually associated with paraphasias (word-finding difficulties).

- **Allusory speech:** vague, imprecise and hard to comprehend speech because too few details are provided.

- **Rhyming***:* using of words that sounds alike, as used in poetry.

- **Punning:** A play on words, sometimes on different senses of the same word and sometimes on the similar sense or sound of different words.

- **Clang association**: A thought disorder wherein words are chosen or repeated based on similar sounds, instead of semantic meaning.

- **Talking past to the point**: patient understands the question but deliberately give incorrect answers.

- **Cryptolalia:** A private language, which is spoken aloud.

- **Telegraphic speech:** conjunctions and articles are missed out in a sentence but meaning is retained and few words are used.

- **Rambling speech:** non-goal-directed, distractible speech. Meaningful connections are lost between phrases and sentences, but the syntax and meanings of the components may remain intact, found in delirium and intoxication.

- **Mutism:** The inability or unwillingness to speak. Akinetic mutism - A state in which a person is unspeaking (mute) and unmoving (akinetic). A person with akinetic mutism has sleep-waking cycles but, when apparently awake, with eyes open, lies mute, immobile and unresponsive. Akinetic mutism is often due to damage to the frontal lobes of the brain. *Selective mutism* is a childhood disorder in which a child does not speak in some social situations although he or she is able to talk normally at other times, usually associated with social anxiety.

2.5   Disorganized or Catatonic Behaviour

Grossly disorganized behavior may manifest in a variety of ways. People with schizophrenia usually display odd behaviours and have difficulty in formulating and producing goal-directed behavior and activity. Some examples are: Wandering about/ talking to themselves/ childlike silliness / unpredictable anger and untriggered agitation, *e.g.* swearing or shouting/ disheveled and malnourished / difficulties with daily activities of living such as preparing meal or maintaining hygiene / unusual dressing like wearing multiple overcoats and gloves on a hot day/ odd movements or mannerisms/ lack of inhibition and impulse control and inappropriate sexual behavior, *e.g.* masturbation in public place and Catatonic features – completely unaware of the environment, patient reacts to the environment by either remaining and maintaining a rigid or immobile body posture and resist efforts to be moved or engaging in excessive motor activity.

- **Catatonia:** Catatonia is a state of motor immobility and behavioural abnormality, commonly manifested by stupor and was first described by Karl Ludwig Kahlbaum (1828 – 1899), a German psychiatrist in 1874 in his monograph "Die Katatonie oder das Spannungsirresein" (Catatonia or Tension Insanity). Catatonia is a neuropsychiatric syndrome that can occur due to medical or psychiatric disorder. Rajagopal (2007) provided a very comprehensive review of Catatonia. The three main clinical types are: Catatonic Stupor, Catatonic Excitement and Malignant Catatonia. The main symptoms of catatonia (adopted from Rajagopal, 2007) are as follows:

Clinical feature	Description
Stupor	It is a motionless motor immobility with nonreactivity to external stimuli, often accompanied by mutism and rigidity.
Posturing	Patient maintains same posture for long periods.
Waxy flexibility (cerea flexibilities)	Patient maintains highly uncomfortable postures for long periods of time.
Negativism	Patient resists the attempt to move parts of their body and the resistance offered is equal to the strength applied.
Automatic obedience	Patient demonstrates exaggerated cooperation, automatically obeying every instruction of the clinician.
Ambitendency	Patient alternates between resistance to and cooperation with the clinician's instruction (*e.g.*, when asked shake hands, the patient repeatedly extends and withdraws hands)
Forced grasping	The patient forcibly and repeatedly grasps the clinician's hand when offered.
Obstruction	The patient stops suddenly in the course of a movement and is generally unable to offer any reason. This appears to be the motor counterpart of thought block.
Echopraxia	The patient imitates the action of the interviewer.
Aversion	The patient turns away from the examiner when addressed.
Mannerisms	Repetitive goal directed movements (*e.g.* saluting).
Stereotypies	Repetitive, non-goal directed regular movements (*e.g.* rocking)
Motor perseveration	The patient persists with a particular movement that has lost its initial relevance.
Excitement	Patient displays excessive, purposeless motor activity that is not influenced by external stimuli.
Speech abnormalities	Three main speech abnormalities: *Echolalia*: repetition of the examiner's words; *Logorrhoea*: incessant, incoherent and monotonous speech; *Verbigeration*: a form of verbal perseversion in which the patient repeats certain syllables (*logoclonia*), words (*palilalia*) or phrases or sentences.
Malignant Catatonia	Is an acute onset of excitement with fever, autonomic instability, delirium and may be fatal.

2.5.1   Symptom Triad: Positive- Negative-Cognitive symptoms

Clinically the signs and symptoms of schizophrenia generally divided into three categories: Positive, Negative and Cognitive symptoms as follows:

Positive Symptoms: Those are *added* to the personality, *i.e.*, symptoms that are "extra" due to additional brain activity, reflect loss of touch with reality.	*Negative Symptoms:* Reflects under-functioning or "loss" of personality- loss of emotional range and interpersonal function.	*Cognitive Symptoms:* Cognitive dysfunction involving multiple areas of brain functioning.
i. Delusions: Bizarre delusions are considered characteristic of Schizophrenia. Delusions of persecution are most common.	**i. Affective flattening:** Diminished range of emotional expression, flat or blunted affect, poor eye contract, reduced body language.	**i. Difficulty maintaining attention:** Difficulty in getting and remaining focused on any task or even a thought; not being able to pay attention to instructions or directions.

ii. Hallucinations: These may occur in all the sensory modalities, but auditory hallucinations are most common.	**ii. Alogia :** Decreased fluency and productivity of speech - poverty of speech, such as brief, empty replies.	**ii. Memory problems:** Difficulties with normal "working memory", which involves the capacity to use information immediately after it has been presented and/or learned.
iii. Thought Disorder: Difficult speaking and organizing thoughts, "Formal Thought Disorder" is considered typical for schizophrenia.	**iii. Avolition** : Lack of motivation, inability to initiate and persist in goal-directed activities, show little interest in participating in work or social activities.	**iii. Low Executive functioning:** Problem with understanding information and acting upon that to make decisions.
iv. Disorganized Behaviour: Difficulties in goal directed behavior or odd and inappropriate behavior.	**iv. Anhedonia:** Inability to experience pleasure in things that they once found enjoyable.	**iv. Difficulty planning and structuring activities:** Caused by reduced executive control.
v. Catatonic Motor Behaviour: any type: extreme degree of complete unawareness (catatonic stupor) or maintaining a rigid posture and resisting efforts to be moved (catatonic negativism) or the assumption of inappropriate or bizarre postures (catatonic posturing), or purposeless and unstimulated excessive motor activity (catatonic excitement).	**v. Asociality:** Lack of desire to form relationships.	**v. Lack of insight:** Caused by loss of reality testing, having a specific cognitive blind spot that prevents them from understanding that they are ill and need treatment.

2.6 Insight

Definition: Subject's degree of awareness and understanding about being ill. The term "insight" has many meanings, but for psychiatric interview it implies five dimensions (Amador & David, 1998): (i) awareness of mental illness, (ii) awareness of specific signs and symptoms of the disorder; (iii) attribution of symptoms to the disorder; (iv) understanding the social consequence of the disorder; and (v) awareness of the need of medical treatment.

Insight may be measured in terms of the patient's understanding of his or her health condition as being primarily either psychological or medical condition. Insight has deep influence on assessment as well as on treatment compliance. Complete lack of insight is often seen in psychotic disorders or dementia and is an important consideration in treatment planning and in assessing the capacity to consent to treatment. Poor insight is common in schizophrenia. Approximately one half of all patients exhibit severe, pervasive, and persistent problems with insight. Poor insight has a strong correlation with noncompliance and thus effectiveness of treatment (Amador & Gorman, 1998). Poor insight may also be found in personality disorder or low intelligence.

Insight is not an all or none phenomenon and there are degrees of insight. Insight is subjective, and the reason for assessing this is to examine whether the patient and the psychiatrist share the same ideas about what is wrong and what to do about it (treatment). Psychiatric Illnesses in which the patient has an altered sense of reality can affect insight. The patients understanding of their condition and their perceived need for treatment can vary from day to day, hour to hour. Remember, insight fluctuates and can be present in variable measure.

Grade I	Complete denial of illness
Grade II	Slight awareness of being sick but denying it at the same time.
Grade III	Awareness of being sick but blaming it on external factors
Grade IV	Awareness that illness is due to something unknown to/ in the patient.
Grade V	Intellectual Insight: admission that the patient is ill and the symptoms or failure in social adjustments are due to the patient's own particular irrational feelings or disturbances without applying this knowledge to future experiences.
Grade VI	True Emotional Insight: emotional awareness of the motives and feelings within the patient and the important persons in his/her life, which can lead to basic changes in behavior.

References

Amador, X.F. & David, A.S . (1998). Insight and Psychosis. ISBN 0198525680. New York: Oxford University Press.

Amador, X. F. & Gorman, J.M. (1998). Psychopathologic domains and insight in schizophrenia. Psychiatric Clinics of North America, 21, 27-42.

Andreasen, N.C. (1979). Thought, language and communication disorders. Archives of General Psychiatry, 36, 1315-1321.

APA (1994). Diagnostic and Statistical Manual of Mental Disorders. American Psychiatric Association, ISBN: 0-89042-062-9. Washington DC: American Psychiatric Publishing.

APA (2013). Highlights of changes from DSM IV-TR to DSM5. Availabe at: www.psych.org/File%20Library/Practice/DSM/DSM-5/Changes-from-DSM...

Barr, W.B. (1998). Neurobehavioral disorders of awareness and their relevance to schizophrenia. In, Amador, X.F. & David, A.S. (Eds) Insight and Psychosis. New York: Oxford University Press, (pp. 107-141).

Beck, A.T. (1988). Beck Hopelessness Scale. San Antonio, TX: Pearson Education, Inc.

Beck-Sander, A., Birchwood, M., Chadwick, P. (1997). Acting on command hallucinations: A cognitive approach. British Journal of Clinical Psychology, 36(Pt 1), 139-148.

Burgy, M. (2008). The concept of psychosis: Historical and phenomenological aspects. Schizophrenia Bulletin, 34, 1200-1210.

Cermolacce, M., Sass, L., Parnas, J. (2010). What is bizarre in bizarre delusion? A critical review. Schizophrenia Bulletin, 36, 667-679.

Chapman, L.J., Chapman, J.P., Rau-lin, M.L. (1978). Body-image aberration in schizophrenia. Journal of Abnormal Psychology, 87,399–407.

Chaturvedi, S.K. & Bhugra, D. (2007). The concept of neurosis in a cross-cultural perspective. Current Opinion in Psychiatry, 20, 47-51.

Christodoulou, G.N. (1978). Syndrome of subjective doubles. American Journal of Psychiatry, 135,249.

Christodoulou, G.N. (1986). Delusional Misidentification Syndromes. Basel: Karger.

Combs, D.R., Adams, S.D., Michael, C.O., Penn, D.L., Basso, M.R., Gouvier, W.D. (2006). The conviction of delusional beliefs scale: Reliability and validity. Schizophrenia Research, 86, 80-88.

Cornell, D.G. & Hawk, G.L. (1989). Clinical presentation of malingerers diagnosed by experienced forensic psychologists. Law and Human Behavior, 13,375–383.

Dening, T.R. & Berrios, G.E. (1994). Autoscopic phenomena. British Journal of Psychiatry, 165, 808-817.

Ellis, H.D., Whitley, J., Luaute ,J.P. (1994). Delusional misidentification: The three original papers on the Capgras, Frégoli and intermetamorphosis delusions. History of Psychiatry, 5, 117-146.

Erkwoh, R., Willmes, K., Eming-Erdmanna, A., Kunert, H.J. (2002). Command hallucinations: Who obeys and who resists when? Psychopathology, 35, 272-279.

Flaum, M., Arndt, S., Andreasen, N.C. (1991). The reliability of "bizarre" delusions. Comprehensive Psychiatry, 32,59–65.

Goodwin, D.W., Anderson, P., Rosenthal, R. (1971). Clinical significance of hallucinations in psychiatric disorders: a study of 116 hallucinatory patients. Achieves of General Psychiatry, 24,76–80.

Hersh, K. & Borum, R. (1998). Command hallucinations, compliance and risk assessment. Journal of the American Academy of Psychiatry and the Law, 26, 353-359.

Jaspers, K. (1913). Allgemeine Psychopathologie. Berlin, Germany: Springer.

Junginger, J. (1995). Command hallucinations and the prediction of dangerousness. Psychiatric Services, 46, 911-914.

Kathirvel, N. & Mortimer, A. (2013). Causes, diagnosis and treatment of visceral hallucinations. Progress in Neurology and Psychiatry, 17(1), 6-10.

Kendler, K.S., Glazer, W.M., Morgenstern, H. (1983). Dimensions of delusional experience. American Journal of Psychiatry, 140, 466-469.

Kim, S.J., Moon, S.W., Kim, D. (2012). Body image distortions among inpatients with schizophrenia. Korean Journal of Biological Psychiatry, 19,211-218.

Klass, E.T. (1987). Situational approach to the assessment of guilt: development and validation of a self-report measure. Journal of Psychopathological Behavior, 9, 35-48.

Lee, T.M., Chong, S.A., Chan, Y.H., Sathyadevan, G. (2004). Command hallucinations among Asian patients with schizophrenia. Canadian Journal of Psychiatry, 49(12), 838-842.

Lewinsohn, P.M. (1970). An empirical test of several popular notions about hallucinations in schizophrenic patients. In, Origin and mechanisms of hallucinations (Ed. W. Keup). New York: Plenum Press, (pp. 401–403).

McKenna, P.J. (1984). Disorders with overvalued ideas. British Journal of Psychiatry, 145, 579-585.

Mojtabai, R. & Nicholson, R.A. (1995). Interrater reliability of ratings of delusions and bizarre delusions. American Journal of Psychiatry, 152, 1804–1806.

Nakaya, M., Kusumoto, K., Okada, T., Ohmori, K. (2002). Bizarre delusions and DSM-IV schizophrenia. Psychiatry and Clinical Neurosciences, 56,391–395.

Neve ,M. (2004). Neurosis. Lancet, 363 (9415),1170.

Priebe, S. & Rohricht, F. (2001). Specific body image pathology in acute schizophrenia. Psychiatry Research, 101, 289-301.

Rajagopal, S. (2007). Catatonia. Advances in Psychiatric Treatment, 13,51-59.

Rajender, G., Kanwal, K., Rathore, D.M., Chaudhary, .D (2009). Study of cenesthesias and body image aberration in schizophrenia. Indian Journal of Psychiatry, 51,195-198.

Resnick .P.J. & Knoll, J. (2005). Feigned schizophrenia symptoms usually won't deceive the clinician who watches for clues and is skilled in recognizing the real thing. The Journal of Family Practice, 4(11), available at: http://www.jfponline.com/Pages.asp?AID=2821

Richard, M. & Richard, L. (2010). A comparison of delusions and overvalued ideas. Journal of Nervous and Mental Disease, 198, 35-38.

Rogers, R. (1987). Assessment of malingering within a forensic context. In, Law and psychiatry: international perspectives (Ed. D.W. Weisstub), New York: Plenum Press, (pp. 209–237).

Rogers, R., Gillis, J.R., Turner, R.E., Frise-Smith, T. (1990). The clinical presentation of command hallucinations in forensic population. American Journal of Psychiatry, 147, 1304-1307.

Rogers, R., Thatcher, A., Cavanaugh, J. (1984). Use of SADS diagnostic interview in evaluating legal insanity. Journal of Clinical Psychology, 40, 1537–1541

Rohricht, F. & Priebe, S. (2002). Do cenesthesias and body image aberration characterize a subgroup in schizophrenia? Acta Psychiatrica Scandinavica, 105,276-282.

Roth, M. (1963). Neurosis, psychosis and the concept of disease in psychiatry. Acta Psychiatrica Scandinavika, 39,128-145.

Salavera,C., Puyuelo, M., Antonanzas, J.L., Teruel,P. (2013). Semantics, pragmatics, and formal thought disorders in people with schizophrenia. Neuropsychiatric Disease and Treatment, 9, 177-183.

Schilder, P. (1935). The Image and Appearance of the Human Body: Studies in the Constructive Energies of the Psyche. London: K. Paul, Trench, Trubner & co. ltd

Shapiro, L.J. & Stewart, S.E. (2011). Pathological guilt: A persistent yet overlooked treatment factor in obsessive-compulsive disorder. Annals of Clinical Psychiatry, 23, 63-70.

Simon, M., Vörös, V., Herold, R., Fekete, S., Tenyi, T. (2009). Delusions of pregnancy with post-partum onset: an integrated individualized view. European Journal of Psychiatry, 23 (4), available at: http://scielo.isciii.es/scielo.php?pid=S0213-61632009000400004&script=sci_arttext

Small, I.F., Small, J.G., Andersen, J.M. (1966). Clinical characteristics of hallucinations of schizophrenia. Disease of the Nervous System, 27,349–53.

Solomon, M., Ozonoff, S., Carter, C., Caplan, R. (2008). Formal thought disorder and the autism spectrum: relationship with symptoms, executive control, and anxiety. Journal of Autism and Developmental Disorder, 38 (8), 1474–84

Sommer, I.E.C., Aleman, A., Kahn, R.S. (2003). Left with the voices or hearing right? Lateralization of auditory verbal hallucinations in schizophrenia. Journal of Psychiatry and Neuroscience, 28, 17-18.

Taylor, M.A. & Vaidya, N.A. (2008). Descriptive Psychopathology. New York: Cambridge University Press, (pp. 279; 230-243).

Thienhaus, O.J. & Piasecki, M. (1998). Emergency psychiatry: Assessment of psychiatric patients' risk of violence toward others. Psychiatric Services, 49, 1129–1147.

Thompson, J.S., Stuart, G.L., Holden, C.E. (1992). Command hallucinations and legal insanity. Forensic Report, 5, 29–43.

van der Zwaaed, R. & Polak, M. (2001).). Pseudohallucinations: A pseudoconcept? A review of the validity of the concept, related to associate symptomatology. Comprehensive Psychiatry 42(1), 42–50.

Voros, V., Tenyi, M., Trixler, M. (2003). Clonal Pluralization of the self: A new form of delusional misidentification syndrome. Psychopathology, 36, 46-48.

Wahass, S. & Kent, G. (1997). Coping with auditory hallucinations: A cross-cultural comparison between Western (British) and non-Western (Saudi Arabian) patients. Journal of Nervous and Mental Disease, 185, 664-668.

Wilson, J.W. & Miller, H.E. (1946). Delusion of parasitosis. Archives of Dermatology and Syphilology, Chicago, 54, 39-56.

Wing, J., Cooper, J., Sartorius, N. (1974). Measurement and Classification of Psychiatric Symptoms. Cambridge: Cambridge University Press.

Wong, L. (2009). Essential study skill. Stamford, USA: Cengage Learning (pp. 348).

World Health Organisation (1991). ICD-10 Classification of mental and behavioural disorders. New York: Churchill Livingstone.

Yager, J. & Gitlin, M.J. (2000). Clinical manifestations of psychiatric disorders. In, Comprehensive Textbook of Psychiatry,(Eds. B.J.Sadock & V.A.Sadock), vol.1, 7th Ed. Philadelphia: Lippincott Williams & Wilkins, (pp. 964-1002).

Yee, L., Korner, A.J., McSwiggan, S., Meares, R.A., Stevenson, J. (2005). Persistent hallucinosis in borderline personality disorder. Comprehensive Psychiatry, 46, 147-154.

Photo of Lavater: http://en.wikipedia.org/wiki/Johann_Kaspar_Lavater

Photo of Esquirol: https://en.wikipedia.org/wiki/Jean-%C3%89tienne_Dominique_Esquirol

www.ingramcontent.com/pod-product-compliance
Lightning Source LLC
Chambersburg PA
CBHW050846220326
41598CB00006B/441